PSYCHIATRIC/MENTAL HEALTH NURSING: AN IRISH PERSPECTIVE

PSYCHIATRIC/MENTAL HEALTH NURSING: AN IRISH PERSPECTIVE

*Jean Morrissey, Brian Keogh
& Louise Doyle (Eds)*

Gill & Macmillan

Gill & Macmillan
Hume Avenue
Park West
Dublin 12
with associated companies throughout the world
www.gillmacmillan.ie

© Morrissey, Keogh & Doyle 2008

978 07171 4459 4

Index compiled by Cover to Cover
Print origination in Ireland by Carole Lynch

The paper used in this book is made from the wood pulp of managed forests.
For every tree felled, at least one tree is planted, thereby renewing natural resources.

A CIP catalogue record for this book is available from the British Library.

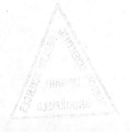

Contents

Acknowledgments

Jean Morrissey would like to dedicate this book to the memory of Katherine Waters, who always had time to listen and encourage. She is remembered with fond memories.

Brian Keogh would like to dedicate this book to the memory of Michael Keogh. Gratitude is also extended to Paul Kelly for his assistance and support in completing this project.

Louise Doyle would like to remember her grandmother Rita Quigley, also a psychiatric nurse, who was and continues to be a strong presence.

We would like to thank all the contributors who have given so generously their time and effort in writing their chapters. As editors, we have enjoyed learning with and from each other. Finally, we particularly wish to acknowledge the learning and experience we have gained from all the clients, students and colleagues we have worked with over the years.

Editors and Contributors

EDITORS

Jean Morrissey, Brian Keogh and **Louise Doyle** are lecturers in mental health nursing at the School of Nursing and Midwifery, University of Dublin, Trinity College.

CONTRIBUTORS

Padraig Byrne is a Clinical Nurse Manager II at Waterford Regional Hospital.

Professor Seamus Cowman is Head of Department at the School of Nursing, Royal College of Surgeons in Ireland.

Christine Deasy is a lecturer in the Nursing and Midwifery Department, University of Limerick.

Catherine Delaney is a research nurse at St Patrick's Hospital, Dublin.

Suzanne Denieffe is a lecturer at the Department of Nursing, Waterford Institute of Technology.

Margaret Denny is a lecturer at the Department of Nursing, Waterford Institute of Technology.

Mary Farrelly is a professional development officer with the National Council for the Professional Development of Nursing and Midwifery, Ireland.

Dr Agnes Higgins is Head of the Psychiatric/Mental Health Nursing Forum, University of Dublin, Trinity College.

Dr Mary Keys is a lecturer in law at the Law Faculty, National University of Ireland, Galway.

Gordon Lynch is an Advanced Nurse Practitioner in Child and Adolescent Mental Health.

Gerry Maguire is a lecturer at the School of Nursing and Midwifery, University of Dublin Trinity College.

Jim Maguire is a lecturer at the Department of Nursing Studies and Health Sciences, Athlone Institute of Technology.

Dr John McCardle is a Clinical Nurse Manager III at the Donegal Mental Health Services in Letterkenny.

John McDonald is a lecturer in midwifery, health and applied science at the School of Nursing, Dundalk Institute of Technology.

Liam Mac Gabhann is a lecturer in practice at the School of Nursing, Dublin City University, and practises at St Vincent's Hospital, Fairview, Dublin.

Mark Monahan is a lecturer at the School of Nursing and Midwifery, University of Dublin, Trinity College.

Gerry Moore is a lecturer at the School of Nursing, Dublin City University.

Declan Patton is a lecturer at the School of Nursing, Midwifery and Health Systems, University College Dublin.

Dr Denis Ryan is a senior lecturer at the Department of Nursing and Midwifery, University of Limerick.

Frances Ryan is a lecturer at the School of Nursing and Midwifery, Trinity College Dublin.

Dr Ann Sheridan is a lecturer in the school of Nursing, Midwifery and Health Systems in University College Dublin.

Professor Chris Stevenson is Acting Head of School/Professor of Mental Health Nursing/Director of Research, School of Nursing, Dublin City University.

Agnes Tully is a lecturer in the Department of Nursing Studies at the National University of Ireland, Galway.

Mark Tyrrell is a lecturer at the School of Nursing and Midwifery, National University of Ireland, Cork.

Mike Watts is National Programme Co-ordinator for GROW in Ireland, a mutual help organisation in the area of mental health.

Dr John S. G. Wells is Head of the Department of Nursing, Waterford Institute of Technology.

Foreword

A psychiatric/mental health nursing text, written with the Irish context in mind, is both original and important, and it is my great honour and privilege to welcome readers to this book. Some readers will be students, embarking on a career in psychiatric/mental health nursing. Others will be more mature practitioners, seeking to update knowledge of their chosen field. A smaller group will doubtless be those with the onerous responsibility of teaching and supervising students. This book should inform and inspire you all. One is never too old to learn and there is much that is new in this book; much to whet the appetite for knowledge, among students, expert practitioners and lecturers alike. By the time you have finished reading, I am confident that you will be as informed and stimulated as was I. Reading is, of course, only the first step. The vital next step is to put this knowledge to work, within your practice. Making use of knowledge is rarely easy, but this book should help inspire confidence.

The concept of 'psychiatric/mental health nursing' is quite a mouthful, and one that is not easily digested. This book attempts to break it down into bite-sized chunks, without losing any of the flavour of the complex practice of nursing, in its more complete sense. You may well have doubts as to what exactly *is* psychiatric/mental health nursing. However, these doubts should be resolved by reading about its practice, illustrated so well by the many authors who address a wide range of settings across the human lifespan.

Traditionally, psychiatric nursing has been seen as managing or otherwise helping people cope with a 'mental illness'. Mental health nursing appears to be more about helping people grow and develop in such a way that their 'illness', or life difficulties, become just another part of their existence. How do nurses help people lead such a purposeful, satisfying life? How do they help them grow through their difficulties? There may well be no definitive answers as yet, but this book will help you to begin to answer such questions for yourself.

Changes in the way we talk about our work are important because they illustrate that, at some point, it was recognised that the practice of nursing was changing, or needed to change. From this simple acknowledgement has flowed a whole vocabulary of change. *Patients* became *clients*, who in turn became *service users*. Perhaps, in the fullness of time, we shall be comfortable calling people who receive psychiatric/mental health care, *people* — plain and simple! Nurses, once defined narrowly as custodians, began to be recognised as carers, then as therapeutic agents. In time we may recognise that genuine caring is inherently therapeutic. Perhaps we shall also recognise that people's madness needs to be contained, as a step towards helping them resolve this bitter affliction of the human spirit.

Another important change has been the move away from *psychiatric* care associated with hospitals and containment, in favour of *mental health* care in the community; where personal development, social integration and recovery have become the main focus. We need to remember, however, that ideas like 'recovery', if not the whole emphasis on health rather than illness, have long been promoted by non-government organisations (NGOs) and other mental health activists. Such developments are all part of an increasing sense of consumerism, which emphasises co-operation, collaboration and creative ways of helping people deal with their various mental health problems. This change of emphasis is of vital importance. People who receive psychiatric and mental health care are no different from those receiving other human services. They can judge whether or not the care meets their needs. They can assess to what extent they feel any benefit from the service on offer. They can also contribute to or begin to take over aspects of their own care. We cannot begin to think about rehabilitation, far less recovery, without acknowledging the part the person, their family and friends will play in translating such paper dreams into a full, living reality. Before we get side-tracked by inflated concepts like 'evidence-based-practice', we might consider if there is a simpler way of judging if something 'works'. The American psychologist George Kelly was once asked, 'How do you know what makes people tick?' His answer was simple and profound: 'If you want to know what someone thinks — ask him!' We risk spending too much time quantifying and analysing, measuring and monitoring, when a simple, direct question might give us the information we need to judge the value of our care.

Like many other Western countries, Ireland is a society in transition. Various economic, social and cultural changes, especially over the past twenty years, have had a dramatic and far-reaching effect on Irish society. In turn these effects have been felt in the ever-changing mental health services. Nursing itself has moved very quickly, from hospital school training to a full graduate education. Nursing research has also developed rapidly and new knowledge is emerging that will change the shape of nursing practice in the years ahead. Ultimately, the most vital changes are occurring on the ground — at the *care-face* — where nurses are developing and extending their practice, in part to keep up with the changes occurring in the society around them, but also as part of their mission to strengthen the therapeutic value of nursing within the healthcare team.

This book is unashamedly focused on informing readers about practice and is central to the mission to strengthen the professional standing of psychiatric and mental health nursing in Ireland. I congratulate the editors for their foresight in organising this book and I congratulate all the authors on their obvious knowledge and commitment to their chosen field of practice.

I hope that all readers — whether novice or expert — will use the wide body of knowledge contained within this book wisely, to enhance practice and to advance the professional standing of psychiatric/mental health nursing, at home and abroad.

Phil Barker PhD RN FRCN

Introduction

The landscape of psychiatric/mental health nursing in Ireland has changed considerably over the last two decades. Changes in nursing education, research and practice, professional and ethical guidelines, legislation and the provision and delivery of mental health services have had a major impact on the practice of psychiatric/mental health nursing in Ireland today. In addition, economic, social and cultural changes, along with the demands of lifelong learning, will also impact upon the approaches to care and therapeutic interventions that nurses will have to embrace over the next decade. We believe that the challenges in the practice of psychiatric/mental health nursing in an Irish context are one of the things that make this book an interesting and unique one. Our aim in producing this book was to make it as comprehensive as possible. Inevitably, constraints of space meant that we had to omit many areas we might have liked to include, so we decided to include the areas we believe take into account the core concepts underpinning the theory and practice of psychiatric/mental health nursing and the contemporary context of its practice.

Throughout this book particular emphasis is placed on providing the foundation of knowledge and skills required by nurses to participate in the provision of safe, comprehensive and high-quality nursing care along with the promotion of mental health for clients with different mental health problems in a variety of settings. Therefore each author was asked to focus on the particular issues in his or her area of expertise and the challenges they present in clinical practice. Social, ethical and legal influences specifically relating to the provision and delivery of mental healthcare in Ireland are also examined. The importance of applying theory to practice is paramount and this theme is illustrated by clinical case examples. Different authors have used different vocabulary to describe what they do — *psychiatric nursing* and *mental health nursing* — and whom they work with or care for — *patients, clients, service users* — which may be guided by different cultures of practice and training that have many similarities and some differences.

The book is divided into four sections. Each chapter is written by someone who is an experienced practitioner or specialist in the area of practice that they have written about. Section One, 'Foundations of Psychiatric/Mental Health Nursing', begins with a historical overview of the development of psychiatric nursing as a profession in Ireland. The following chapter addresses core concepts related to psychiatric/mental health nursing, including the social construction of mental health and mental illness. Chapter 3 examines the application of the Mental Health Act 2001 and the role of the mental health nurse. The next chapter focuses on ethical challenges in mental health nursing and how they relate specifically to contemporary mental health nursing practice; Chapter 5 covers care planning; and Chapter 6 discusses the practice of mental health nursing within the understanding of mental health promotion. The final chapter in this section examines the components of community mental health nursing and rehabilitation.

The first chapter in Section Two, 'Therapeutic Modalities in Psychiatric/Mental Health Nursing', examines the use of basic skills and more sophisticated approaches in therapeutic communication in mental health nursing. This is followed by an overview of the different psychotherapeutic approaches commonly used in mental healthcare. Chapter 10 focuses on the therapeutic modalities concerning the principles and approaches of psychosocial interventions; and this is followed by an overview of the common medications used in the treatment of different mental illnesses and the role of the nurse in medication administration and ECT.

The penultimate section, 'Clinical Application to Practice', looks at specific mental illnesses that can occur across the life span, their aetiology, presenting features, the range of treatments available and the appropriate assessment and nursing care principles for a client experiencing the illness.

The first chapter in the final section, 'Contemporary Issues and Challenges in Psychiatric/Mental Health Nursing' describes the personal experience of mental breakdown and recovery. This is followed by an examination of sexuality in the context of people who are experiencing mental distress, followed by an overview of the principles and practice of clinical supervision in mental health nursing. The remaining chapters focus on mental health nursing in an ethnically diverse society and the principles underpinning liaison nursing as a sub-speciality of psychiatric nursing and its areas of practice.

Finally, as editors we hope the reflective questions at the end of each chapter will act as a springboard to prompt further discussion of the respective issues both in the classroom and clinical setting.

Jean Morrissey, Brian Keogh and Louise Doyle

SECTION 1

Foundations of Psychiatric/ Mental Health Nursing

1

Psychiatric Nursing Practice: A Historical Overview

Ann Sheridan

To a large extent the history of nursing is one that presents the views of those individuals recognised as important or great. However, this generally fails to address the accounts of the 'ordinary' participants in that history. This chapter attempts to redress this balance by bringing to light evidence about psychiatric nursing in Ireland from the perspective of Irish psychiatric nurses. The study on which this chapter is based was concerned with the accounts of 'ordinary nurses' practising in Irish psychiatric services, and gaining an understanding of their role and how it has changed over the past fifty years. This chapter reviews the development of psychiatric nursing in Ireland, and training programmes leading to nursing registration, together with the practice of psychiatric nursing within Irish asylums, hospitals and subsequently community-based services.

ORIGINS OF IRISH PSYCHIATRIC NURSING — NINETEENTH-CENTURY ASYLUMS

In Ireland the development of psychiatric nursing was closely aligned with the building of asylums as the primary means of providing care for the insane. While this pattern of development is similar to that of psychiatric nursing in other European countries, particularly the United Kingdom, there are a number of features that make its development in Ireland distinctive. Central to this distinctiveness is Ireland's history of political governance. Ireland's particular political, social, economic and religious dimensions that prevailed throughout the nineteenth century and until the last third of the twentieth century converged to create a set of circumstances in psychiatric care that made it different from that of other countries in Western Europe and the United States. This difference was emphasised in the aftermath of the founding of the Irish Free State with the explicit governmental policies of rejecting foreign influences and focusing specifically on attempting to establish a nation that could be identified as distinctly 'Gaelic and Catholic'. The policies of the new Irish Government resulted in a degree of isolation, with the result that changes and developments in the wider international context failed to have an impact in Ireland, and this was evident with regard to changes in practices associated with the care of the mentally ill.

As with many other countries, the asylum system in Ireland was established during the nineteenth century and by the first decade of the twentieth century had become the primary means of providing care for the insane. From the opening of the first public asylum in 1815, Ireland moved from a situation in which there was virtually no public provision for care of the mentally ill to one in which accommodation was being provided for approximately 17,000 patients in public asylums throughout the island of Ireland (Finnane 1981). The first public asylum built was the Richmond Lunatic Asylum in Dublin. Prior to this, the insane had been housed with the poor in workhouses, in houses of industry or incarcerated with prisoners in gaols. By 1835 ten asylums had been constructed throughout Ireland including Armagh, Limerick, Derry, Belfast, Carlow and Portlaoise, Waterford, Clonmel and Ballinasloe. These ten asylums represent the first stage of the foundation of an asylum system in Ireland, which at this stage tended to be small with provision for about 150 patients (Finnane 1981; Reynolds 1992).

The second phase of asylum development was initiated in 1852. The primary factor contributing to this second phase was the seemingly ever-increasing numbers of mentally ill people in Ireland who required accommodation in asylums. More important, however, was the large number of these who were considered to be 'incurable'. The second phase of development saw the construction of a further twelve asylums throughout the island of Ireland. In contrast to earlier asylums, these new asylums were larger, providing accommodation for up to 500 inmates in an attempt to relieve the by now chronic problem of overcrowding (Finnane 1981).

The establishment of such a monolithic system brought with it the demand for a workforce to ensure its optimal functioning. Care of the mentally ill in these early asylums was provided primarily by keepers or attendants — terms generally used to refer to males; and nurses — a term reserved for female carers. While relatively little has been written about the overall role and function of attendants and nurses in early Irish asylums, their function appears to have been related principally to ensuring the smooth functioning of the institution. No special training or preparation was provided and their role was more akin to domestic servants. They were expected to get the patients out of bed, wash and dress them, provide clean bedding if required and ensure patients were ready for breakfast. They were also to provide constant observation of patients and had a role in the control of violent patients (Malcolm 1989; Reynolds 1992).

Associated with the continued development and consolidation of the asylum system as the primary means of providing for the mentally ill was the desire to establish an associated group of workers in asylums for the insane similar to those that existed in hospitals caring for the physically sick. Thus the attendants and nurses, whose initial primary function in the asylum system had been the custody of the mentally ill and maintenance of the institution, were recognised as requiring training if they were to be effective in their emerging role of 'doctor's assistant' (Nolan 1991, 1993).

INTRODUCTION OF TRAINING FOR ATTENDANTS

The Medico-Psychological Association (MPA), founded in 1841 as the Society of Medical Officers for the Insane of Great Britain and Ireland, provided a medium through which knowledge and ideas about insanity could be shared. In 1889 a special committee of the MPA was formed to examine the possibilities of establishing a formal system of training for asylum nurses. This committee identified the need for systematic training of asylum attendants, the granting of certificates following examination of proficiency in nursing and the keeping of an efficient register of such nurses and attendants (Henry 1989). The committee believed that once established, training should be of 'the highest possible standard but not so exacting as to deter attendants from formally entering it; be of two years duration with practical instruction provided by matron/head attendant' (Henry 1989: 455). The recommendations of the sub-committee were adopted by the MPA in 1891 and the first examinations leading to the award of the Certificate of Proficiency in Nursing and Attending on the Insane were held in 1892. The first account of attendants and nurses in Irish asylums being prepared for the examination of the MPA was in 1894 at the Richmond Asylum in Dublin. In 1895, 27 registrations are recorded for staff from Irish asylums in the Register of Certificate of Proficiency in Nursing and Attending on the Insane of the MPA: 21 males and six females representing two Irish asylums, the Richmond Asylum in Dublin (13 males); and the Limerick Asylum, with eight males and six females (Sheridan 1999, 2004, 2006). In 1896 the number of Irish attendants/nurses successful in the examination of the MPA had risen to 98, representing 11 Irish asylums, one of which was a private asylum. This year also saw the beginning of a trend in which the number of females presenting for examination from Ireland outnumbered males, a trend that has continued to present times. Within the first three years of the commencement of training in Ireland, 195 nurses had been awarded the Certificate of Proficiency in Nursing and Attending on the Insane (Sheridan 1999, 2006).

The final phase of development of the asylum system in Ireland occurred at the beginning of the twentieth century with the building of extensions to a number of district asylums and the building of auxiliary asylums; again, these were primarily designed to deal with the problems of overcrowding within the district asylums.

NURSING REGISTRATION

As developments in medical knowledge and science advanced, the skills and competencies required by both physicians and nurses became increasingly complex. Thus it became even more desirable to train nursing personnel to enable them to function more effectively within a changing healthcare environment. While advancement in medical science was largely associated with identifying causes of physical disease and developing associated treatments such as antibiotics, the disease model also had an impact in institutions concerned with the care of the mentally ill. Associated with these developments was the drive among a number of occupational groups for recognition of their special skills and knowledge, which would ultimately lead, they hoped, to being identified as professional. Among the occupational groups seeking recognition was nursing.

In the United Kingdom, the Nurses' Registration Act received Royal Assent in 1919. While Ireland was still effectively under British rule, this Act provided for the separate and distinct registration of nurses in Ireland by authorising a General Nursing Council (GNC) for Ireland. The Irish GNC established a supplementary Register for Mental Nursing in 1921, the year independence was achieved. Between 1921 and 1922 the names of five nurses who were admitted on the basis of their MPA qualification are recorded in the register. However, in 1923, two years after independence, the names of 703 nurses are recorded; and a further 80 names are recorded in 1924 (Sheridan 2006). Courses in Mental Nursing continued to be offered by the now Royal Medico-Psychological Association (RMPA) until 1951, and in practice two parallel systems existed for 28 years. While nurses from Ireland continued to undertake the RMPA certificate until 1947, from 1935 onwards the number of Irish registrations recorded in the RMPA register began to decline, while those registering with the GNC Ireland began to increase. This was due primarily to the holding of the first examinations of GNC (Ireland) for Mental Nurses in 1935. At the end of 1949 a total of 2,617 entries were recorded for Mental Nurses in the GNC Ireland register (Sheridan 1999). This was intended to replace the RMPA registration, with no reciprocal recognition being intended after this date.

The GNC established in 1919, while Ireland was still under British rule, continued to be responsible for the regulation of education and registration of nurses in the new independent state until 1950. In this year a new Nurses Act was introduced, which dissolved existing statutory bodies including the General Nursing Council and Central Midwives Board and replaced them with a single body known as An Bord Altranais (Irish Nursing Board). This new body was established in June 1951.

While the first half of the twentieth century saw no fundamental change in the system of care for the mentally ill in Ireland, the nomenclature associated with insanity and the insane began to change: gradually asylums became hospitals, insanity was renamed mental illness and lunatics were now called patients (Hensey 1988). In 1945 the Mental Treatment Act repealed all previous legislation other than that related to the care of criminal lunatics and wards of court, and firmly established the jurisdiction of the medical profession as the sole legitimising profession in determining the existence of mental illness and the detention of patients in mental hospitals.

CHANGING PATTERNS OF CARE

During the 1940s and 1950s the care of the mentally ill and the existing systems of provision began to attract more attention internationally. In spite of the emergence of new treatment approaches for the mentally ill during the war years, namely psychodynamic and group therapy, the existing care and treatment of this group remained primarily institutionally based (Sheridan 2000, 2004, 2005). More and more these institutions, now re-named hospitals, were being identified as inappropriate and indeed damaging places; and were frequently associated with harsh regimes resulting in a range of damaging effects collectively termed 'institutionalisation' (Barton 1959).

However, the recognition of the importance of the environment in which care was delivered was not a new concept. The 'moral' management of patients promoted by Tuke at York and Pinel in Paris in the eighteenth century had recognised the value of providing an environment in which patients benefited by being exposed to friendly association, discussion of their difficulties and productive and purposeful activity (Digby 1984). In particular the works of Maxwell Jones (1953), Russell Barton (1959) and Erving Goffman (1961) focused attention on the negative effects of institutions and their prevailing systems of rules, regulations and paternalistic attitudes, while promoting recognition of the care environment as a potentially therapeutic entity. This process of liberalising the care environment, coupled with an emphasis on providing interventions aimed at developing the patient's personality, became a primary focus for debate surrounding developments in psychiatry and the role of the psychiatric nurse.

In 1956, the World Health Organisation (WHO) addressed the issue of psychiatric nursing, producing a seminal international report on the topic which was to prove instrumental in directing changes in psychiatric nursing globally over the next two decades. The intention of this report was to drive change in the existing patterns of psychiatric nursing practice away from the predominantly custodial approach towards one that was therapeutic and interpersonal. In delimiting the future role of the psychiatric nurse, the WHO's expert committee drew heavily on the dual theoretical concepts of interpersonal relations and therapeutic community.

IDENTIFYING THE PRACTICE OF IRISH PSYCHIATRIC NURSING

This section is based on the first comprehensive study of psychiatric nursing practice in Ireland between 1950 and 2000 undertaken by the author. The findings provide an account of what nurses did with and for patients, what it was like to work and live in an institutional setting and what nurse training was like during these periods. This study provides a unique insight into both the practice of psychiatric nursing and how practice has changed over the intervening decades.

1950s and 1960s
Looking at records of the care and treatment provided to patients in psychiatric hospitals is one way of discovering what it was that nurses did with and for patients. Initially asylum records consisted of a system of 'casebooks', with separate books for male and female patients. The records contained in these books

provide a summarised and retrospective version of the patient's stay in hospital from admission through to either discharge or death. Because of their composite nature, casebooks contain only selective elements of the patient's care and treatment. However, what is evident is that accounts of what took place during the period of a year were informed by those who were intimately associated with patients over prolonged periods of time; in reality nurses were the only group intimately associated and present with patients in the asylum during these extended periods. These records show that nurses had a significant role in monitoring, observing and reporting on patient activities such as attendance at work, patients' behaviour, physical illness, and particular incidents such as accidents, and aggressive and violent episodes. However, there were no accounts of what nurses did beyond this.

Casebooks remained in use until the introduction of individualised patient records in mid-1957, in which a separate sheet for 'nursing notes' was included. Initially, the majority of entries made by nurses focused on patients' existing physical or medical conditions. Furthermore, when nursing entries were made, it was often on an ad hoc basis: in some instances notes were documented daily, sometimes weekly and sometimes only occasionally throughout the patient's stay in hospital. Thus, as in previous decades, a significant proportion of the patient's stay in hospital went undocumented, as did the care and treatment they received. As these records are the primary source records of nursing activity during this period they provide only scant evidence of nurses' contribution to the care of the mentally ill.

However, nurses' records during the 1960s were more likely to be completed, and by virtue of this fact alone, there is increasing evidence of the contribution of nurses to the care of the mentally ill in Irish psychiatric hospitals. There is also a notable shift in the nature of the records made. While physical care and treatment still dominated these written accounts, nurses' records during the 1960s began to include more detailed accounts of the mental state of the patient, their prescribed treatments and activities engaged in, as well as the nursing activities undertaken by nurses. From examination of records made by nurses during the 1960s and supplemented with data from interviews with retired nurses who had practised during this period, a clearer picture of what psychiatric nurses did with and for patients begins to emerge. This data identified that the role of the psychiatric nurse involved a range of activities relating to observing and reporting about patients' behaviour and daily activities — these activities were predominantly associated with work, the patient's physical and mental condition and the treatments received by the patient. The nurse's role also involved assisting and supporting the work of doctors, providing physical care to patients, and engaging in social and leisure activities with patients. Finally, nurses engaged in supervising and teaching student nurses and managing the ward.

However, what needs to be emphasised and appreciated is that nurses were intimately engaged with patients within the mental hospitals over prolonged periods of time. During these years, patients stayed in hospital for extended periods and, in a significant number of cases, some patients spent the majority of their adult lives within psychiatric hospitals. Nurses worked long hours and were frequently accommodated in rooms adjacent to the wards, so that they were within easy reach should a crisis arise and extra assistance was required. Thus the relationships between patients and nurses were sustained with frequent and regular contact both within the confines of the ward and throughout the wider hospital environment.

Daily Work

Daily work for both patients and nurses consisted mainly of domestic-type activities, with females generally engaged in 'indoor' activities including cleaning, cooking, and other domestic chores. Males, on the other hand, generally engaged in 'outdoor' activities, dominated by farm work and grounds maintenance, and tailoring, shoemaking, and working in the hospital kitchens. Interestingly, the kitchen appears to be the only area where both male and female patients and nurses worked alongside each other. These activities have been described as 'institutional maintenance' activities in that patients were considered a primary workforce in the institution and the activities of both patients and nurses were directed towards sustaining the institution rather than towards individualised therapeutic interventions (Sheridan 2005).

Physical Care and Assisting the Doctor

Providing physical care to patients and assisting the work of doctors represented an interrelated aspect of nurses' work. Physical care included a wide range of activities from bathing patients, toileting, dressing, and managing their oral hygiene and hair care, to dressing wounds, administering prescribed treatments and monitoring routine observations such as temperature and pulse. The role of the nurse in assisting doctors included setting up for a procedure and assisting with treatments and investigations such as insulin therapy, electroconvulsive therapy, and taking blood. However, as the majority of specialised treatments such as insulin or narcosis therapy were undertaken in special wards, not all nurses were involved in these activities. Furthermore, as these treatments were physical in nature it was often the practice to employ general trained nurses in these specialist wards, including the infirmary, as they were deemed to have the appropriate skills required.

Social and Leisure

Engaging in social and leisure activities with patients constituted a significant element of the work of psychiatric nurses. As with domestic-type activities, nurses were charged with arranging, organising and participating in social and leisure activities for patients. These activities ranged from those undertaken in individual wards to special events in the wider hospital such as dances, theatre and sporting events. These activities were as important for the nurses as they were for patients in that they provided welcome relief from a life dictated by daily rituals and routines. They also provided one of the few legitimate opportunities for nurses and patients to fraternise with members of the opposite sex within the institution. However, these events were strictly managed and monitored by senior institutional personnel to prevent any transgressions by either patients or nurses. Attending religious services, while different in nature and purpose to social activities, also provided a further opportunity for both patients and nurses to be relieved of the daily burden of activities and to mix legitimately with the opposite sex. A number of other activities in the institution, including hospital bands, sports teams and acting as assistants to clergy during religious services, provided male nurses with additional opportunities to be relieved of 'normal duties'.

Training

Until relatively recently, being prepared to occupy the role of psychiatric nurse relied on an apprenticeship model in which nurses learned about nursing and mental illness in the wards and units where they worked. While a formal system of block study and the appointment of nurse tutors had been introduced in some hospitals during the 1950s, both were ad hoc and haphazard in nature. Likewise, the recruitment of student nurses was not confined to a particular time of year: new recruits arrived throughout the year. On arrival they were given a uniform and dispatched to 'the wards' without any formal period of induction or preparation. The primary emphasis was on learning the ward routines as quickly as possible to ensure the continued smooth functioning of the ward and the wider institution.

Student nurses often worked closely with 'trusted patients'. These patients guided students and 'showed them the ropes'. Trusted patients frequently held keys of stock rooms, controlling ward supplies of patient clothing, soap, detergents and food supplies. Ward work was based on a hierarchical division of tasks, with different grades of nurses undertaking different tasks. Students and junior registered nurses tended to undertake the majority of domestic and basic care activities with and for patients, while more senior registered nurses and ward sisters/charge nurses attended to ward administration and management activities and 'dealt with the doctors'.

Living and Working Conditions of Nurses

All the nurses interviewed had 'lived in' at the hospital during their training and the majority did not move out of hospital accommodation until they got married. The hospitals also provided some housing for married staff. From descriptions of hospital accommodation, the majority began by sharing large dormitories with other nurses: these were situated within the hospital buildings and generally in close proximity to the wards. They consisted of twenty or so beds curtained off from each other. Each nurse had a locker and shared bathroom and toilet facilities. There were no facilities for nurses to cook their own meals, and these had to be taken in the nurses' dining room(s). During the early years of the 1960s nurses' homes were built, with separate homes for male and female nurses. In these homes nurses now had their personal bedroom with a washbasin, storage for clothing and a dressing table. Bathroom and toilet facilities continued to be shared, but kitchen facilities were provided. Nurses' accommodation rules were strict and a 'home sister' policed the system. Nurses were called at 6.30am and had to be on duty by 7.00am; lights had to be out by 11.00pm. Late passes (permission to stay out beyond 9.30 to either 11.00pm or midnight) were given at the discretion of matron. Nurses on late passes were checked into the home at the appointed times. Failure to return at the appointed time resulted in the nurse being 'in front' of matron the next morning and usually being deprived of future late passes for a period of time or, on occasion, dismissed from employment.

Nurses generally worked from 7.00am to 7.30pm each day with one day per week and every second Sunday off; an average of 66 hours per week. However, days off could be cancelled at short notice if there was a shortage of staff, and nurses were expected to stay on duty late in the evenings if there was a problem with a patient or a night nurse did not turn up.

Accounts of nurses' work and living arrangements provide a strong sense of how life within the psychiatric hospital/institution proceeded for both patients and nurses. Both were confined within the hospital and their daily lives governed by sets of routines and rules. While the nature of the relationships between nurses and patients did not form part of this investigation, there can be no doubt that a high degree of affinity existed between them. Both nurses and patients came from the same communities and social class; they knew each other's families, had attended the same schools and churches, and some were related through family connections. In the hospital they worked side by side, undertaking the work of the institution jointly; and their close connections were maintained over prolonged periods of time. Given these connections, there can be no doubt that close relationships existed between nurses and patients: whether these relationships were therapeutic within the current meaning of that concept is as yet to be discovered. However, what is likely is that nurses entered into close association with patients, providing caring, comfort and companionship.

1970 to 2000 — The Move Away from Custody

The changes in society and psychiatric services and psychiatric nursing that were taking place in Western Europe began to impact on psychiatric practice in Ireland during the 1970s. The move away from the predominantly 'introspective' nature of Irish society and psychiatric nursing was to a large extent facilitated by Ireland's accession to the European Economic Community (EEC) in 1973. For Ireland, accession to the EEC brought with it the commitment of the Irish Government to bring its policies into line with those already established in the community of Europe and this necessitated far-reaching changes in social, health and employment legislation. The publication of the report *The Psychiatric Services: Planning for the future* in 1984 marked the explicit commitment of the Government of Ireland to achieve a re-orientation of psychiatric services away from an institutionally based system to a community based service and to meet the terms of membership of the EEC. The main purpose of the report was to draw up an outline plan of the best service for people in need of psychiatric help and in so doing to take account of the successes and failures of existing services, advances in knowledge and understanding of mental illness and availability of resources, having regard to the competing demands of other public services (DoH 1984). The practice of psychiatric nursing in the three decades between 1970 and 2000 identified the move away from 'custodial care' as the most significant change in the role of psychiatric nurses during that period.

The concept 'custodial' was used by nurses to reflect the physical structure and organisation of the institution as well as the prevailing system of care provision within its confines: not simply the containment aspect of the institution. While containment was a dominant feature of the nurses' role, the term 'custodial' was used to describe a complex system that focused predominantly on maintaining the system and processes of the institution and was seen as a rigid, routinised and almost prison-like environment. Within this 'custodial' system nurses identified that the focus was on the 'place' not the 'person'; the environment within which patients were cared for was rigid, with 'all the beds in a straight row, chairs around the walls in certain places, and mats put down correctly'. The custodial system was one in which wards were locked and overcrowded; ward hygiene was poor and there were little or no recreational facilities for patients and very few medications used (Sheridan 2004, 2005).

By the 1980s, while some nurses still referred to the institutional and task-based nature of their role, the majority described being engaged in individualised patient care, based on identifiable psychiatric nursing skills. The primary skills identified were interpersonal in nature, and responses were infused with language that was uncommon in responses from earlier decades. The identified changes in the pattern of nurses' activities associated with the movement of psychiatric services from a custodial approach to a community-focused one, coupled with an increased emphasis on professionalisation of the psychiatric nursing role, and including changes in pre- and postgraduate education, resulted in an increase in the scope of practice. This increased scope of practice led to greater accountability and autonomy for nurses whereby autonomy was associated with having control over the content and structure of daily work, making decisions about the type of interventions and care to be delivered, and an expanded scope of practice.

Increased autonomy was also very strongly associated with the setting in which nursing practice took place. Nurses working in a community setting were identified as having a greater degree of autonomy than those practising in an in-patient setting. The differences in autonomy between practice settings were strongly associated with the structures existing within each setting. In-patient settings were seen to be organised around a medical approach to care with the consultant psychiatrist as the leading professional. Decisions about treatment were seen as medically orientated, with the prescription and administration of medication as the predominant approach.

Preparation

Nurses who registered during the 1980s and 1990s identified that the nature of preparation for the role of psychiatric nurse, in contrast to previous decades, was concerned with preparing students to occupy the position of registered psychiatric nurse, regardless of location. These changes in the preparation of psychiatric nurses are reflective of a number of concurrent changes in which psychiatric nursing practice began to be influenced by external factors including the emergence of community-based services and the scaling down of large institutions, as well as the impact of European policies and directives on psychiatric care in general and on nursing in particular, and the increasing need to base Irish practice in the context of international best practice models.

The major revision and implementation of the psychiatric nursing curriculum in 1986 and subsequent revisions in line with EC directives and the implementation of the diploma programme during the 1990s and the bachelor's degree in 2002 also had a significant impact on preparation for practice.

Recent Events

The report that has had the most immediate and far-reaching impact on the profession of nursing in Ireland in recent years is that of the Commission on Nursing (1998). Its recommendations and their subsequent implementation have had a significant effect on both the nature and the pace of change in the Irish nursing profession in the years since its publication. With regard to the role and practice of psychiatric nurses, the Commission on Nursing recommendations have had a number of significant impacts. First, in terms of clinical career pathways, a total of 487 psychiatric nurses have been approved as Clinical Nurse Specialists (according to figures from the National Council of Nursing and Midwifery (NCNM 2006)) and one Advanced Nurse Practitioner post has been approved, with more in the process of development. These changes in the clinical career pathways of psychiatric nurses have also impacted on the development of post-registration educational programmes and have necessitated the development of a range of programmes with the key imperative of supporting nurses in the development of clinical practice.

Conclusion

This chapter has shown that since the inception of public provision of care for the mentally ill in Ireland psychiatric nursing has and continues to be central to the delivery of psychiatric services. While the pace of change and development in the psychiatric services has been slow, prevailing social, political, economic and religious circumstances converged to influence the nature and pace of change. Psychiatric nursing in Ireland entered the second half of the twentieth century in a very similar situation to its counterparts in other countries, in a broadly custodial caring role. However, the priorities of the government of the new Irish state (creating a nation that was Irish and Catholic and concentrating on essential services) meant that the profession remained relatively static over this time period. Given the innately traditional or conservative nature of Irish society at that time, and the natural acceptance of authority, the segregated and custodial nature of Irish asylums became deeply ingrained and the practice of psychiatric nursing restrictive, and restricting on the nurses themselves. Thus when the mental health reform movement reached Ireland in the late 1960s, not only was there no model nursing system proposed, but there was no appreciation of the nursing role as practised or of the duties that were undertaken.

During the last two decades, while attempting to achieve the level of progress desired within psychiatric services, the majority of the asylums have either been closed or are nearing closure, and new mental health services have been established in communities and general hospitals. Similarly, nurse education has been subject to equally rapid change, from the traditional hospital-based certificate programme to an honours degree programme fully integrated into the third-level education system.

In conclusion, psychiatric nursing can be seen to have emerged as a product of the socio-political and socio-institutional context within which it is based, and in Ireland its practice continues to be determined by these factors.

Reflective Questions

1. How does the study of historical accounts of psychiatric nursing practice contribute to contemporary practice?
2. How may the political and economic systems in Ireland continue to impact on the education and practice of psychiatric nursing over the coming decade?
3. Identify the key changes in the role of psychiatric nurses over the past three decades and consider how these may progress into the future.
4. With reference to the historical study of nursing practice, discuss how the dominant ideology of an organisation impacts on nursing care and the role of nurses.

References

Barton, R. (1959) *Institutional Neurosis*. Bristol: J. Wright and Son.

Department of Health (1984) Report of the Commission on Nursing: *The Psychiatric Services: Planning for the future*. Dublin: Stationery Office.

Digby, A. (1984) 'The changing profile of a nineteenth-century asylum: the York Retreat', *Psychological Medicine* 14, 739–48.

Finnane, M. (1981) *Insanity and the Insane in Post Famine Ireland*. London: Croom Helm.

Goffman, E. (1961) *Asylums*. New York: Anchor.

Government of Ireland (1998) Report of the Commission on Nursing: *A Blueprint for the Future*. Dublin: Stationery Office.

Henry, H. (1989) *Our Lady's Psychiatric Hospital Cork*. Cork: Haven Books.

Hensey, B. (1988) *The Health Services of Ireland*. Dublin: Institute of Public Administration.

Jones, M. (1953) *The Therapeutic Community*. New York: Basic Books.

Malcolm, E. (1989) *Swift's Hospital: A History of St Patrick's Hospital, Dublin,*

1746–1989. Dublin: Gill and Macmillan.

Nolan, P. (1991) 'The founding of psychiatric nurse training and its aftermath'. *British Journal of Psychiatry*, 159, 46–52.

Nolan, P. (1993) *A History of Mental Health Nursing*. London: Chapman and Hall.

Nolan, P. and Sheridan, A. (2001) 'In search of the history of Irish psychiatric nursing'. *International History of Nursing Journal*, 6(2), 35–43.

Reynolds, J. (1992) *Grange Gorman: Psychiatric Care in Dublin since 1815*. Dublin: Institute of Public Administration in Association with Eastern Health Board.

Robins, J. (1986) *Fools and Mad: A History of the Insane in Ireland*. Dublin: Institute of Public Administration.

St Brendan's Hospital: Male and Female Case Book Records for 1891–1950. Dublin: St Brendan's Hospital.

St Brendan's Hospital: Patient Case Records 1957–69. Dublin: St Brendan's Hospital.

Sheridan, A. (1999) 'Letting the past illuminate the future: a focus on Irish psychiatric nursing' in D. Ryan, A. Jacob and M. Kirwan (eds), *Reflection and Rejuvenation Issues for Irish Psychiatric Nursing into the Millennium*. Kilkenny: Association of Psychiatric Nurse Managers.

Sheridan, A. J. (2000) 'Psychiatric Nursing', in J. Robins (ed.), *Nursing and Midwifery in Ireland in the Twentieth Century*. Dublin: An Bord Altranais.

Sheridan, A. J. (2004) 'An analysis of the activities of psychiatric nurses practising in Ireland 1950–2000'. *Psychiatric Nursing*, 4(1), 19–22.

Sheridan, A. J. (2005) 'Being a Psychiatric Nurse in Ireland in the 1950s', in G. Fealy (ed.), *Care to Remember: Nursing and Midwifery in Ireland*. Cork: Mercier Press.

Sheridan, A. J. (2006) 'The impact of political transition on psychiatric nursing: a case study of twentieth-century Ireland'. *Nursing Inquiry*, 13 (4), 289–99.

World Health Organisation (1956) *Technical Report Series No. 105. Expert Committee on Psychiatric Nursing, First Report*. Geneva: WHO.

2

Concepts of Psychiatric/Mental Health Nursing

Mary Farrelly

Mental health problems exist within society and have been recognised, understood and dealt with in a variety of ways at different periods in history. Where once mental disorder was viewed as a moral issue, it is now perceived by many as an illness. The development of the welfare state has seen the establishment of statutory services for people with mental health problems, which has occurred in the context of exclusion on a large, formalised scale. Psychiatric/mental health nursing also exists within the overall context of society, healthcare and services for people experiencing mental health problems. Understanding this context is important as it provides insight into the way mental health problems are dealt with by society and illuminates the factors that contribute to our understanding of mental health and illness. This chapter addresses core concepts related to psychiatric/mental health nursing, including how health, illness, mental health and mental illness are defined and determined in society. Classification systems for mental illness and the ideological basis of psychiatry and mental healthcare are explored through a consideration of the biological, social and psychological perspectives of mental illness.

DEFINING MENTAL HEALTH

The World Health Organisation (WHO 2001a:1) defines mental health as:

> ... a state of well-being in which the individual realises his or her own abilities, can cope with the normal stresses of life, can work productively and fruitfully, and is able to make a contribution to his or her community.

This definition emphasises the individual's ability to function and be self-determinant.

Concepts of mental health generally include subjective well-being, self-efficacy, autonomy and self-determination, competence, intergenerational dependence and achievement of one's emotional and intellectual potential (WHO 2001a).

CLASSIFICATION OF MENTAL ILLNESS/DISORDER

In medicine, specifically in psychiatry, sophisticated systems of classification for mental illness/disorder have been developed to characterise this complex phenomenon.

In its broadest sense, diagnosis is the analysis of the cause or nature of a symptom, condition or problem; however, the practice of diagnosis has come to be synonymous with biomedical models. Since there are no objective, specific, sensitive biological markers definitively to diagnose mental illness, diagnosis or identification of mental illness is made based on a set of behavioural criteria. Two main classification systems have been developed, the International Classification of Mental and Behavioural Disorders (ICD-10) (WHO 1992), which is the system most widely used in Europe, and the Diagnostic and Statistical Manual of Mental Disorder Fourth Edition (DSM-IV-TR), published by the American Psychiatric Association (APA 2000), which is used in the USA.

ICD-10 categorises mental and behavioural disorders into ten categories, which are subdivided into sub-categories, and guidelines are provided on clinical features to assist diagnosis.

Figure 2.1 ICD-10 Major categories of mental and behavioural disorder

F00-09	Organic, including symptomatic disorders
F10-19	Mental and behavioural disorders due to psychoactive substance use
F20-29	Schizophrenia, schizotypal and delusional disorder
F30-39	Mood (affective) disorders
F40-48	Neurotic, stress-related and somatoform disorders
F50-59	Behavioural syndrome associated with physiological disturbances and physical factors
F60-69	Disorders of adult personality and behaviour
F70-79	Mental retardation
F80-89	Disorders of psychological development
F90-98	Behavioural and emotional disorders with onset usually occurring in childhood and adolescence

The DSM-IV-TR uses a multiaxial or multidimensional approach which facilitates a more holistic, comprehensive approach to assessment and diagnoses. It assesses five dimensions:

Axis I: Clinical Disorders and Other Conditions
- The typical disorders that are diagnosed as mental illness (depression, anxiety disorder, schizophrenia).

Axis II: Personality Disorders and Mental Retardation
• Disorders which are first evident in childhood.
• Disorders of personality that have an enduring quality and encompass the individual's way of interacting with the world.

Axis III: General Medical Conditions
• Medical conditions that have an impact on the development, continuance, or exacerbation of Axis I and II Disorders.
• Physical conditions that can result in symptoms of mental illness.

Axis IV: Psychosocial and Environmental Problems
• Events that impact on the disorders listed in Axis I and II.

Axis V: Global Assessment of Functioning
• Clinician's assessment of the individual level of functioning.

Such detailed diagnostic criteria frameworks are useful in that they provide:
• a common classification for describing the problems that people experience, which facilitates communication across a wide variety of groups
• a means of organising information about mental distress which provides information that guides treatment options
• a common basis for collection of statistical information nationally and internationally that facilitates the development of public health response to mental health issues
• a basis for education of mental health professionals
• help in facilitating research into aetiology and interventions.

However, over-reliance on such systems as a means of explaining a person's experiences and distress has been criticised for offering 'little more than a simplification of a complex reality and thus being profoundly disempowering and stigmatising' (Bracken 2002:2). The increase in the number of diagnostic categories (from 106 in DSM 1, 1952 to 357 in DSM-IV, 1994) has been seen as indicative of a move to medicalise everyday problems, e.g. diagnosing shyness as 'social anxiety disorder' (Double 2002). Behavioural indicators for disorders such as 'attention deficit hyperactivity disorder' overlap with behaviours seen in children who are bored, anxious, frustrated or otherwise stressed, and the increase in the diagnosis of this condition can be seen by some as an 'easier' way to deal with this phenomenon than to deal with the underlying psychological and social issues that may contribute to the situation.

Systems of classification describe the phenomena of mental disorder but offer little in the way of explanation for its aetiology or causation. An exploration of models of mental health/illness offers an insight into frameworks for understanding theories of causation and corresponding treatment or care strategies. It is important that nurses understand the current state of knowledge in relation to causation of mental illnesses, e.g. schizophrenia, as aetiology will impact on the selection of therapeutic interventions and supportive strategies offered to families and significant others (Gournay 1996).

MODELS OF MENTAL HEALTH/ILLNESS

Mental health and illness can be considered from a variety of different perspectives. Modern approaches to health have been primarily based on an illness model that views health and illness as relating to physical factors (Giddens 1993). While the medical model has been the most pervasive in determining how the mentally ill are treated in modern society, this 'dominance should not be confused with conceptual superiority' (Pilgrim and Rogers 1993:4). Biological, psychological and social are the main models that have been used to define describe and understand mental health problems.

Biological Model

The biological model views mental illness as having a biological basis and care is focused on diagnosis and prescription of treatment, usually a physical treatment such as medication. Neuroscience is the branch of science that deals with the anatomy, physiology, biochemistry and molecular biology of the nervous system. Advances in neuroscience provide us with a greater understanding of how the brain functions and what impact variations in structure and functioning of the brain can have on human emotions and behaviour and therefore mental health. The biological model characterises mental illness as a disorder of neural communication leading to abnormal cognition, emotion and behaviour which is derived genetically or acquired.

Genetic Factors

Brain formation in the foetus is determined genetically but can be influenced by environmental factors such as nutrition of the mother or substance abuse. The basis of genetic theory is that mental illness is caused by one or more genes and can therefore be inherited. This is researched through family, twin and adoption studies. Examination of families does not exclude the possibility that environment may play a role, as members of a family will share the same environment to some extent. As expected, monozygotic twins (who share 100 per cent of genes) have a higher rate of concordance of a genetically influenced disorder than dizygotic twins (who share 50 per cent of genes). Studying twins who have been reared in different environments (through adoption) allows for the influence of environmental factors to be distinguished from genetic factors. Such studies have provided major evidence for the role of genetics in numerous psychiatric illnesses including obsessive-compulsive disorder, panic disorder, major depressive disorder, bipolar disorder, schizophrenia and Alzheimer's disease (Cardno et al. 1999; Shih et al. 2004).

Structural factors

The structure and functioning of the brain have been implicated in some mental disorders. The development of diagnostic technology such as computed axial tomography (CAT), magnetic resonance imaging (MRI) and positron emission tomography (PET) has greatly contributed to the ability of scientists to examine the structure of the brain and its metabolism. Previously examination of the brain was only possible at post mortem, when any abnormalities found could be attributed to the effects of medication. Studies have found ventricular and cortical sulci enlargement in schizophrenia sufferers (both in individuals who have received treatment and those who are first episode and have never been medicated) with corresponding lower cortical volume (Lewis and Lieberman 2000). This supports the view that schizophrenia is at least in part caused by abnormality in brain structure.

Neurochemical factors

Neurochemical imbalances in the neurotransmitters dopamine and glutamate have been implicated in the causation of schizophrenia but this evidence has been generally based on the clinical efficacy of antipsychotic drugs (which moderate dopamine activity) to alleviate symptoms and the ability of dopamine to produce psychotic symptoms in otherwise unaffected individuals (Lewis and Lieberman 2000). Increased D2 receptors have been found on post mortem and in PET scanning in the brains of individuals affected by schizophrenia, both those who have been treated with antipsychotic medication and those who have not (Wong *et al.* 1986), suggesting that the cause of psychotic symptoms may be abnormalities in the storage, transport, release or uptake of dopamine (Lewis and Lieberman 2000).

In the 1950s the discovery that tricyclic antidepressants and monoamine oxidase inhibitors were effective in the treatment of depression suggested that chemical changes in the brain might be implicated in producing symptoms of depression (Nestler *et al.* 2002). The neurotransmitters implicated in depression are monoamines such as serotonin (5-hydroxytryptamine, or 5-HT) and norepinephrine.

The use of enhanced technology and the development of a more sophisticated understanding of the complexity of neurological functioning have led to an acknowledgement that mental illness cannot be explained simply by biology but is more likely a complex interaction of biological features and environmental issues that impact on that vulnerability (Lewis and Lieberman 2000).

In summary, the use of the scientific or biological models that underpins the medical model has contributed significantly to the advancement of knowledge about mental illness. While the aetiology of many mental illnesses remains unknown, investigation into biological aspects of human behaviour and psychology has identified some biological determinants, thus leading to the discovery of many physical treatments that have alleviated distress and suffering. The most recent development in identifying a genetic cause for schizophrenia is being undertaken in the USA by the Schizophrenia Genome Project. This project is attempting to identify genes that predispose to and/or protect from schizophrenia (MIND Institute and NCGR 2006).

PSYCHOLOGICAL MODELS

During the past 150 years a range of different psychological theories of human development have been proposed, offering insight into how mental health is maintained or how mental illness develops. This has led to a vast range of different types of counselling and psychotherapeutic interventions, based on a range of psychological perspectives. Key psychological theoretical positions about the causes of mental health problems dominate the psychological field of study, including psychoanalytic, cognitive and behavioural theories.

Psychoanalytic Theory

At the end of the nineteenth century Sigmund Freud put forward a theory of the unconscious, which emerged from his engagement in clinical work with people who were experiencing mental distress. This and his notion of the importance of transference in the therapeutic alliance were significant in the development of psychoanalysis both as a treatment and a way of understanding the human condition. In Freud's theory of the mental structure the mind is divided into the id (which represents infantile urges or desires that require immediate gratification), the ego (a sense of self), and the superego (the conscience, developed through interaction with parent figures) (LaPlanche and Pontalis 1988).

According to Freud the mind is divided into three systems, the conscious, preconscious and unconscious (LaPlanche and Pontalis 1988). The developing infant represses affective material that emerges from its relationship with its parents, which can be attached to later life experience and cause mental distress and illness. Material in the unconscious system is kept in place by a process of repression which holds traumatic experiences at bay. These are maintained in the unconscious by coping strategies that manifest as mild symptoms which do not interfere with the normal functioning of the individual or cause undue distress. The dynamic structure of the unconscious ensures that there is a constant revision of how material is interpreted and understood by the individual and a stressful event can lead to a failure of repression, leading to repressed feelings emerging as mental distress. The resolution for the symptom is to be found in recalling the memory of the trauma and revival of the associated affect, a process described as remembering, repeating and working through.

Behavioural Theory

Behavioural theories developed from learning theories of human behaviour and particularly from the work of Pavlov and Skinner. Pavlov, on the basis of his experiments with dogs, described a process of classical conditioning in which a neutral stimulus is used to condition an animal into giving a certain response:

ringing a bell when food is provided conditions the animal to salivate at the sound of a bell only. Skinner described operant conditioning in which an animal's behaviour could be conditioned by reward or punishment: rewarding rats for pressing a lever by giving them food resulted in them pressing the lever more frequently (Norman and Ryrie 2004).

Behavioural models claim that human behaviour (adaptive and maladaptive) is learned and that mental distress occurs when an individual learns to behave in a maladaptive way (Antai-Otong 2003). Behaviour therapy has developed on the basis of this theory and uses techniques such as systematic desensitisation and response prevention to treat people who experience anxiety disorders such as phobias and obsessive compulsive disorder.

A model of social or observational learning proposed by Bandura suggests that an individual learns patterns of behaviour (both adaptive and maladaptive) not just through conditioning but as a result of observing others. This has contributed to our understanding of violent and aggressive behaviour and techniques of modelling to reinforce adaptive behaviour patterns.

Cognitive Theory

Cognitive theories emphasise the importance of the mental processes involved in knowing, and their effect on the emotions, behaviour and physiology of the individual. These theories are based on the work of Aaron Beck, Albert Ellis and Jean Piaget, among others (Antai-Otong 2003). Beck identified cognitive structures (schemata) which are patterns of belief, values and assumptions, which if distorted can result in symptoms of psychological disorder (Antai-Otong 2003). The goal of cognitive therapy is to examine the individual's beliefs and the effect they have on their feelings and behaviour, challenging cognitive distortions and reframing them to be more adaptive.

The multitude of different approaches towards the practice of talking therapies is problematic, and many specific approaches have not been carefully investigated. However, research has broadly found counselling and psychotherapy to be effective (Asay and Lambert 1999). In about seven out of ten cases, individuals with psychological or behavioural problems who receive therapy make appreciable clinical improvements when compared with individuals with similar presenting difficulties who receive no counselling or psychotherapy (Bergin and Garfield 1994). Neuro-imagery studies have shown critical changes in brain activation patterns following psychotherapy, leading to recent debates that psychotherapy may make neuro-anatomical changes in the brain through altering gene expression (Fonagy 2000; Roth and Fonagy 2005).

SOCIAL MODELS

Social models of mental illness consider factors in society and the context in which the person exists within society as being important in defining mental illness.

Social Causation

Social causation theory, which originated in the 1930s, accepts conventional diagnoses but also recognises that factors in the social environment cause stress and thus can contribute to the creation of a mental illness in the individual (Pilgrim and Rogers 1993). For example, a study carried out in the 1930s found a greater incidence of mental illness (particularly schizophrenia) among poorer people (Faris and Dunham 1960). Such studies led sociologists to suggest that conditions that prevailed within society were powerful in contributing to the creation of mental illness in those already predisposed.

Emile Durkheim, a major contributor to sociological theory in relation to mental illness, investigated patterns of suicide and concluded that those who belonged to a community were less likely to die by suicide (Durkheim 1952). A study carried out in south-east London discovered the prevalence of depression among working-class women was three times that of middle-class women. This study identified factors such as class, having three or more children aged under 14 living at home, lack of an intimate, caring relationship, not having full- or part-time work and having lost a mother before the age of 11 as being vulnerability factors associated with an increased incidence of depression (Brown and Harris 1978).

Critics of social causation theory would argue cause and effect, e.g. that mental illness frequently renders people unable to work and therefore the mentally ill are more likely to be poor and to slide down the social scale (known as the 'social drift'). Therefore, people are poor and isolated because they are mentally ill and not mentally ill because they are poor and isolated (Goldberg and Morrison 1963). While social causation theory acknowledges the interaction of the individual with the society in which she/he lives and the role that the particular individual's social circumstances play in the production of mental illness, it continues to locate the problem with the individual.

Mainstream psychiatry has accepted the premises of social causation theory and incorporated it into treatment modalities and service strategies. For example, the role that family dynamics play in the creation and exacerbation of mental illness is now widely accepted and has led to family therapy services being provided as part of statutory, mainstream psychiatric services. The importance of role, occupation and employment is also recognised in relation to mental illness and this has led to the development of occupational therapies and vocational services being provided within and in conjunction with the psychiatric services. This acceptance of social causation theory may be because this way of understanding mental illness is less challenging than other sociological approaches and one which can be most easily incorporated into the mainstream while maintaining the status quo.

Labelling

Labelling theory puts forward the notion that mental illness is a label placed by society on those who fail adequately to abide by the explicit or implicit rules or norms that are laid down by society. This is closely linked to the notion of deviance, which is a term used to describe behaviour that departs from what most people would consider normal or acceptable (Taylor and Field 1993). Scheff (1966) has suggested that mental illness can be understood as residual rule breaking. Residual norms are rules that govern everyday life and are implicit, e.g. looking at a person when talking to them (Giddens 1993). According to Scheff schizophrenia is simply a violation of these norms. Once an individual is thus labelled they are expected to continue to behave in the manner that places them in the category, and any attempt they make to change is strenuously opposed by the social group in which they live, thus perpetuating the label of mental illness that has been allotted to them. This theory was most famously tested in a study carried out in America in the 1970s in which eight researchers gained admission to a psychiatric hospital by complaining of hallucinations and thereafter behaved normally (Rosenhan 1973). They continued to be viewed as mentally ill by the professionals and given discharge diagnoses of 'schizophrenia in remission'. However, their duplicity was, interestingly, noted by their fellow patients who accused them of being journalists sent to check out the hospital.

Labelling theory does nothing, however, to explain the initial incident or behaviour that led to the subsequent labelling (Taylor and Field 1993) and therefore it is incomplete as an explanation for the aetiology of mental illness.

Szasz (1972), a noted anti-psychiatrist, believed that mental illness was a myth. It did not exist other than in the subjective reality of individuals, and was in essence nothing more than a form of social deviance. He viewed those engaged in professional psychiatry as agents of social control, citing the institutionalisation and segregation of the mentally ill as evidence of their work. Anthropologists have investigated cross-cultural notions of mental illness and have found that mental illness is defined differently in Third World and developing societies (Warner 1996). In some of these societies, those who display psychotic symptoms are considered to be of high status and are treated accordingly. In other countries, in contrast to the segregation experienced in the West, people who are psychotic are reintegrated into their family group and their symptoms improve very rapidly (Warner 1996). Therefore the 'reality' of mental illness can be said to be socially and culturally negotiated and not a definitive entity that endures regardless of social environment. The social construction theory can be criticised for underestimating the effectiveness of modern psychiatry, overestimating the social control function and also for failing to offer alternative solutions to the difficulties that arise for both the individual and society as a result of the phenomena of mental illness (Taylor and Field 1993).

Family Factors

Research carried out in the 1970s demonstrated a link between family factors and the rate of relapse of people who suffered serious psychotic or depressive illness. It was shown that negative attitudes of emotive criticism and intrusiveness were highly predictive of a relapse in these individuals (Leff and Vaughan 1985). This phenomenon came to be known as 'expressed emotion', with negative factors being termed 'high expressed emotion' and positive factors 'low expressed emotion' (Falloon 2003:20). Bebbington and Kuipers (1994), in an analysis of studies linking expressed emotion (EE) with schizophrenia, found the association of EE with relapse was overwhelming, and was maintained whatever the geographical location. While high contact with a high EE relation increased the risk of relapse, the opposite was true in low EE households. This has led to the development of a range of psycho-educative/psychosocial therapeutic interventions for use with families of people with serious mental health problems, with the aim of reducing the impact of environmental stresses on the individual through developing effective communication strategies. Family interventions have been shown to reduce relapse, decrease hospitalisation and improve compliance with treatment regimes for suffers of schizophrenia (Pharoah *et al.* 2003).

STRESS VULNERABILITY MODEL

The stress vulnerability model attempts to synthesise wisdom from other models to provide a way of explaining the aetiology of schizophrenia (Zubin and Spring 1977). It puts forward the notion that each person has a degree of vulnerability that under particular circumstances could express itself in, for example, an episode of schizophrenia. The individual's vulnerability is determined by internal factors such as genetic inheritance, neuropsychological processes and acquired factors such as the influence of traumas, diseases, perinatal complications, family experiences, life events and interaction with others in society. The delicate balance between mental health and illness is determined by how the individual adapts to endogenous (biochemical or neurophysiological) or exogenous (life events) 'challengers'.

Response to life event stressors is unique to the individual and may be influenced by the perceived severity of the life event stressor, the individual's perception of its stressfulness, the capabilities of the individual, the coping efforts that they incorporate and the vulnerability of the individual. Failure to adapt to stressors may result in transient or temporary disruptions to the equilibrium of the individual (Zubin and Spring relate this to a bad day or a bad week, which is familiar to us all). On the other hand, relatively minor stressors can in vulnerable individuals lead to episodes of mental illness that are far more disruptive and devastating to the individual life, which require professional assistance and care and which may become more enduring.

INFLUENCES ON THE DEFINITION OF MENTAL ILLNESS/DISTRESS

Each of the various approaches to mental disorder seems to provide only a partial answer and theories of the causation of mental illness have tended to follow the general trend of thought characteristic of a particular period of time (Zubin 1972: Zubin and Spring 1977). The separation of biological, psychological and social factors in the causation of mental illness has proved an obstacle to the development of our understanding of mental illness (WHO 2001b). Critics of biological approaches to mental illness highlight the reductionist nature of this approach, which conceptualises mental illness as a discrete entity occurring in individuals independent of their social context (Moncrieff 2003). The fact that not every person responds to medication lends support to the notion that mental illness is a complex phenomenon that needs to be viewed from a variety of perspectives in order to understand the person's unique experience and develop interventions to alleviate their distress.

Studies carried out in the USA and Europe on the relative benefits of drug-free therapeutic environments versus conventional acute in-patient treatment for people experiencing psychosis have identified that non-conventional approaches were as or more effective than traditional hospital care in short-term reduction of psychopathology and in longer-term social readjustment (Mosher 1999).

Concepts of mental health/illness cannot be considered independently of the society in which they are conceived. Mental illness has been and is conceptualised according to the cultural, political and economic environment and social and religious mores that prevail. Some would view the medicalisation of mental illness and its inculcation into healthcare as an emancipation from the guilt-burdened, moralistic approach that had previously prevailed (Romme 1998).

Other reasons offered for the predominance of biological explanations of mental illness have been that they deflect 'blame' from the family, as suggested by some social theorists such as R. D. Laing, or that they are simpler to understand than metaphysical considerations of meaning (Double 2005). However, the 'medical colonisation of everyday life' and 'the commercial incentive to promote disease and sell pills', which 'changes our view of what it is to be human', needs to be viewed for what it is and the interests — vested and otherwise — examined in context (Moncrieff 2003:16). To view mental illness simply as biological phenomena obscures the effects of social factors (Moncrieff 2003). If these societal issues are not seen as important to mental health, their influences will not be debated and considered in strategies to promote mental health and alleviate mental distress.

It is generally agreed that psychiatry as a discipline has its origins in the European Enlightenment and the movement's concern with reason and the individual subject (Bracken and Thomas 2001). Modernism is a trend of thought in society that emphasises the importance of scientific knowledge, technology and experimentation to understand phenomena. Conceptualising mental distress as being derived from biological causes, psychological causes, social interaction, or a combination of these, and as being amenable to scientific measurement can be viewed as a reflection of modernist trends in society. The association of mental illness with medicine coincided with the large-scale institutionalisation of the mentally ill into houses of industry and subsequently asylums in Europe. This was perceived by Michel Foucault and others as social exclusion rather than a medical necessity. In Ireland the scale of institutionalisation was such that in 1900, 21,000 people defined as lunatics were housed in district asylums in the 32 counties of Ireland, representing 0.5 per cent of the population (Walsh and Daly 2004). The consequences of this is that emotional distress has been defined in terms of the disordered individual rather than the context in which they exist, that technical explanations prevailed as the way of conceptualising mental distress, and that the power of coercion has been vested in the profession that controls the definition of mental distress, namely psychiatry (Bracken and Thomas 2001).

While biological or medical models tend to prevail in the organisation of services for people with mental health problems, aspects of philosophy that are concerned with the interpretation of human experience, e.g. phenomenology, are increasingly influencing psychiatry through the description and interpretation of service users' experiences and the development of services from a more sociological perspective (Thomas *et al.* 2004). The term 'postmodern psychiatry' has been used (Bracken and Thomas 2001) to describe a way of thinking about psychiatry that reflects the postmodern movement in society, which is characterised by the notion that there is no such thing as objective facts (relativism) and that reality may have many meanings (Muir Gray 1999). Postmodern psychiatry puts forward a way of thinking about mental distress that emphasises the importance of considering social, political and cultural contexts when providing services and help for those experiencing mental distress, emphasises the importance of an ethical, value-based approach to mental health that considers the meaning attached to mental distress, and questions the power of psychiatry to coerce and detain people (Bracken and Thomas 2001).

CONCLUSION

The concept of mental illness is a product of the society and the period in history in which the individual lives. Biological, psychological and social models have provided explanations for the phenomenon of mental illness and contributed to our understanding of mental distress. The current prevailing model of mental illness in the western world, including Ireland, is the biomedical model, and psychological and social models have been absorbed to a greater or lesser extent into the biomedical approach. Philosophy can offer frameworks for understanding the human condition and provide new ways of thinking about the concept of 'mental illness'.

Reflective Questions
1. Identify the biological, psychological and social factors that contributed to the distress and current situation of a patient/client you recently cared for.
2. With regard to the service you work in, reflect on what care is offered and the interventions that are provided for clients. What ideology is revealed in this care?
3. What internal and external resources have you drawn on when you were stressed and how did they enable you to work through the experience?
4. Think of a client you cared for who heard voices. What did the voices say and how could this have related to their life situation?

References

American Psychiatric Association (APA)(2000) *Diagnostic and Statistical Manual of Mental Disorders* (DSM-IV-TR) (4th edn). Washington DC: APA.

Antai-Otong, D. (2003) *Psychiatric Nursing: Biological and Behavioral Concepts.* New York: Delmar Learning.

Asay, T. P. and Lambert, M. J. (1999) 'The empirical case for the common factors in therapy', in M. A. Hubble, B. L. Duncan and S. D. Miller (eds), *The Heart and Soul of Change: What Works in Therapy?* Washington, DC: American Psychological Association.

Bebbington, P. and Kuipers, L. (1994) 'The predictive utility of expressed emotion in schizophrenia: an aggregate analysis'. *Psychological Medicine*, 24(3), 707–18.

Bergin, A. E. and Garfield, S. L. (eds) (1994) *Handbook of Psychotherapy and Behaviour Change* (4th edn). New York: John Wiley and Sons.

Bracken, P. (2002) 'Depression, psychiatry and the use of ECT'. *Asylum*, 12(4), www.asylumonline.net/archive/v12_n4_26-28.htm, accessed 10 January 2006.

Bracken, P. and Thomas, P. (2001) 'Post-psychiatry: a new direction for mental health'. *British Medical Journal*, 322, 724–7.

Brown, G. W. and Harris, T. O. (1978) *Social Origins of Depression: A Study of Psychiatric Disorder in Women.* London: Tavistock.

Cardno, A. G., Marshall, E. J., Coid, B., Macdonald, A. M., Ribchester, T. R., Davies, N. J., Venturi, P., Jones, L. A., Lewis, S. W., Sham, P. C., Gottesman, I. I., Farmer, A. E., McGuffin, P., Reveley, A. M. and Murray, R.M. (1999) 'Heritability estimates for psychotic disorders: the Maudsley twin psychosis series'. *Archives of General Psychiatry*, 56(2), 162–8.

Double, D. (2002) 'The limits of psychiatry'. *British Medical Journal*, 324, 900–4.

Double, D. (2005) 'Paradigm shift in psychiatry', in S. Ramon and J. E. Williams (eds), *Mental Health at the Crossroads: The Promise of the Psychosocial Approach.* Abingdon: Ashgate.

Durkheim, E. (1952) *Suicide: A Study in Sociology.* London: Routledge and Kegan Paul.

Falloon, I. R. (2003) 'Family interventions for mental disorders: efficacy and effectiveness'. *World Psychiatry: official journal of the World Psychiatric Association*, 2(1), 20–8.

Faris, R. E. and Dunham, H. W. (1960) *Mental Disorders in Urban Areas: An Ecological Study of Schizophrenia and Other Psychoses.* New York: Hafner.

Fonagy, P. (2000) *Grasping the Nettle: Or Why Psychoanalytic Research is Such an Irritant.* British Psychoanalytic Society, www.psychoanalysis.org.uk/fonagy1.htm, accessed 10 January 2006.

Giddens, A. (1993) *Sociology* (2nd edn). Cambridge: Polity Press.

Goldberg, E. M. and Morrison, S. L. (1963) 'Schizophrenia and social class'. *British Journal of Psychiatry*, 109, 785–802.

Gournay, K. (1996) 'Schizophrenia: a review of the contemporary literature and implications for mental health nursing theory, practice and education'. *Journal of Psychiatric and Mental Health Nursing*, 3, 7–12.

LaPlanche, J. and Pontalis, J. B. (1988) *The Language of Psychoanalysis*. London: Karnac Books.

Leff, J. P. and Vaughan, C. E. (1985) *Expressed Emotion in Families*. London: Guilford Press.

Lewis, D. A. and Lieberman, J. A. (2000) 'Catching up on schizophrenia: natural history and neurobiology'. *Neuron*, 28, 325–34.

MIND (Mental Illness and Neuroscience Discovery) Institute and the National Center for Genome Resources (NCGR) (2006) Press Release: 'MIND Institute and National Center for Genome Resources to Decode Mystery of Schizophrenia Genetics', www.ncgr.org/archives/pr/SGP.pdf, accessed 13 September 2006.

Moncrieff, J. (2003) 'Is Psychiatry for Sale? An Examination of the Influence of the Pharmaceutical Industry on Academic and Practice Psychiatry', Maudsley Discussion Paper. London: Institute of Psychiatry.

Mosher, L. R. (1999) 'Sotteria and other alternatives to acute psychiatric hospitalization. A personal and professional review'. *Journal of Nervous and Mental Disease*, 187, 142–9.

Muir Gray, J. A. (1999) 'Postmodern medicine'. *Lancet*, 354, 1550–3.

Nestler, E. J., Barrot, M., Dileone, R. J., Eisch, A. J., Gold, S. J. and Monteggio, L. M. (2002) 'Neurobiology of depression'. *Neuron*, 34, 13–25.

Norman, I. and Ryrie, I. (2004) *The Art and Science of Mental Health Nursing*. Maidenhead: Open University Press.

Pharoah, F. M., Mari, J. J. and Streiner, D. (2003) *Family Intervention for Schizophrenia (Cochrane Review)*. Cochrane Library, Issue 2. Oxford: Update Software.

Pilgrim, D. and Rogers, A. (1993) *A Sociology of Mental Health and Illness*. Maidenhead: Open University Press.

Romme, M. (1998) 'Listening to voice hearers'. *Journal of Psychosocial Nursing and Mental Health Services*, 36 (9), 40–5.

Rosenhan, D. (1973) 'On being sane in insane places'. *Science*, 179, 250–8.

Roth, A. and Fonagy, P. (2005) *What Works For Whom? A Critical Review of Psychotherapy Research* (2nd edn). New York: Guildford Press.

Scheff, T. J. (1996) 'Labelling mental illness', in T. Heller, J. Reynolds, R. Gomm, R. Muston and S. Pattison (eds), *Mental Health Matters*, London: Macmillan.

Shih, R. A., Belmonte, P. L. and Zandi, P. P. (2004) 'A review of the evidence from family, twin and adoption studies for a genetic contribution to adult psychiatric disorders'. *International Review of Psychiatry*, 16(4), 260–83.

Szasz, T. S. (1972) *The Myth of Mental Illness*. London: Granada.

Taylor, S. and Field, D. (eds) (1993) *Sociology of Health and Healthcare*. London: Blackwell Scientific Publications.

Thomas, P., Bracken, P. and Leudar, I. (2004) 'Hearing voices: a phenomenological-hermeneutic approach'. *Cognitive Neuropsychiatry*, 9(1/2), 12–23.

Walsh, D. and Daly, A. (2004) *Mental Illness in Ireland 1750–2002. Reflections on the Rise and Fall of Institutional Care*. Dublin: Health Research Board.

Warner, R. (1996) 'The cultural context of mental illness', in T. Heller, J. Reynolds, R. Gomm, R. Muston and S. Pattison (eds), *Mental Health Matters*, London: Macmillan Press.

Wong, D. F., Wagner, H. N., Tune, L. E., Dannals, R. F., Pearlsoson, G. D., Links, J. M., Tamminga, C. A., Broussolle, E. P., Ravert, H. T., Wilson, A. A., Toung, J. K., Malat, J. A., Williams, J. A., O'Tuama, L. A., Snyder, S. H., Kuhar, M. J. and Gjedde, A. (1986) 'Positron emission tomography reveals elevated D2 dopamine receptors in drug-naive schizophrenics'. *Science*, 234 (4783), 1558–63.

World Health Organisation (1946) 'Preamble to the Constitution of the World Health Organisation as adopted by the International Health Conference'. Geneva: WHO.

World Health Organisation (1992) *The ICD-10 Classification of Mental and Behavioural Disorders*. Geneva: WHO.

World Health Organisation (2001a) *Mental Health: Strengthening Mental Health Promotion* (Fact Sheet No. 220). Geneva: WHO.

World Health Organisation (2001b) *World Health Report 2001*. Geneva: WHO.

Zubin, J. (1972) 'Models for psychopathology in the 1970s'. *Seminars in Psychiatry*, 4(3), 283–96.

Zubin, J. and Spring, B. (1977) 'Vulnerability: a new view of schizophrenia'. *Journal of Abnormal Psychology*, 86(2), 103–26.

3
The Mental Health Act 2001

Mary Keys

This chapter focuses on the Mental Health Act 2001, its application and the role of the mental health nurse. The nurse has various statutory powers under the 2001 Act as well as under common law (law made by judges). Additionally, each nurse must abide by the *Code of Professional Conduct for each Nurse and Midwife*, which states that 'nurses are accountable for their practice' (An Bord Altranais 2000:4). Nurses are answerable for their acts and omissions in their work. It is important, therefore, that nurses are fully aware of their legal responsibilities in relation to the key elements of patient care.

The Mental Health Commission's (MHC) *Reference Guide to the 2001 Act* (Part 1: Adults, and Part 2: Children) (MHC 2005), as well as the various codes of practice and rules, provide operational details on aspects of the 2001 Act and are of direct relevance to nursing practice. While codes of practice do not have the force of law, they are often examined in the context of court proceedings to see if the standard in the codes has been breached, perhaps resulting in an illegal act. The main source of legal powers and duties for mental health nursing is the 2001 Act, which governs the care and treatment, in approved centres, of people suffering from mental disorder. An approved centre is a hospital or other location approved for the care and treatment of people under the 2001 Act.

The 2001 Act replaces most of the Mental Treatment Act 1945. The primary purpose of the 2001 Act is to provide a modern framework for the admission and treatment of children and adults with mental disorders. The second purpose of the Act is to put in place structures for monitoring, inspecting and regulating standards in mental health services. These new structures are the Mental Health Commission, Mental Health Tribunals and the Inspector of Mental Health Services.

This chapter will focus primarily on specific powers and duties pertaining to the admission and treatment of adults with mental disorders.

NEW STRUCTURES — MONITORING BODIES

The Mental Health Commission is the main body dealing with mental healthcare and has overall responsibility for ensuring good practice in the delivery of mental health services and for protecting the interests of those detained under the Act. An important function is the publication of codes of practice to guide staff in mental health services. Other functions include appointing members of tribunals and establishing a panel of consultant psychiatrists (CPs) to carry out independent examinations.

Mental Health Tribunals are another innovation of the Act. They provide for the review of detention orders, the examination of proposals for psychosurgery, and transferring patients to the National Forensic Service. A review will take place after each decision to detain and renew an order. Tribunals comprise three people: a consultant psychiatrist; a lawyer; and a layperson. Nurses may be expected to appear before the tribunal when appropriate.

The Inspectorate of Mental Health Services has responsibility for visiting and inspecting all places where mental health services are provided. The Inspectorate has extensive powers and must ascertain whether the provisions of the Act are being complied with and in particular whether the various codes and regulations are being observed.

PRINCIPLES

The 2001 Act sets out certain principles that underline other practices under the Act. These principles provide that:

- The best interests of the person must be the principal consideration in any decision about his/her care and treatment, including a decision about admission, as well as having regard to the interests of others at risk of harm if the decision is not made.
- In any proposal about an admission, renewal order, or treatment, as far as is practical, the person is entitled to notification and to make representations in relation to the issue and consideration must be given to these representations before the decision is made.
- In all decisions under the 2001 Act, regard must be had for the need to respect the right of the person to dignity, bodily integrity, privacy and autonomy.

These principles apply to all patients, compulsory and voluntary, and must be considered when decisions are being made about admission, care and treatment.

COMPULSORY ADMISSION

Compulsory (involuntary) admission should be limited to those who need in-patient treatment but will not agree to be admitted voluntarily. Voluntary admission is preferable to compulsory admission and the 2001 Act states that nothing in the Act should prevent a person from being admitted voluntarily for treatment. A person being compulsorily admitted must be given the option to become voluntary.

The 2001 Act provides for the compulsory admission and treatment of adults and children with mental disorder. An 'admission order' applies only to those adult patients compulsorily admitted. The first requirement for compulsory admission under the 2001 Act is the presence of a mental disorder. Mental disorder is an umbrella term and encompasses three specific categories: mental illness; severe dementia; and significant intellectual disability.

- Mental illness means a state of mind which affects the person's thinking, perception, emotion, or judgement *and* which seriously impairs the mental function of the person to the extent that he or she requires care or medical treatment for his/her own interest, or that of others.
- Severe dementia means a deterioration of the brain that significantly impairs the intellectual function affecting thought, comprehension and memory, which includes severe psychiatric *or* behavioural symptoms such as physical aggression.
- Significant intellectual disability means a state of arrested or incomplete development of mind of a person that includes three factors, all of which must be present: significant impairment of intelligence *and* social functioning *and* abnormally aggressive conduct.

The Act excludes from involuntary admission a sole diagnosis of personality disorder, social deviance, or drug and alcohol addiction, unless the person also has a mental disorder.

It is not enough to have a diagnosis of mental disorder to justify detention. The disorder must be severe and include the following factors:

- there is a serious likelihood of the person causing immediate and serious harm to him/herself, or others; *or*
- the judgement of the person is impaired and failure to admit the person could lead to serious deterioration and would prevent the administration of treatment which could only be given following admission; *and*
- the admission and treatment would be likely to *benefit* the person to a material extent.

The Act provides for one category of compulsory admission to psychiatric care. There is no difference between public and private patients under the 2001 Act.

Applications for Compulsory Admission

- An application for admission is usually made by a family member, including a spouse, parent, grandparent, brother, sister, uncle, aunt, niece, nephew or child of the person. A garda can make the application, as can 'any other person', provided the reasons are given.
- An 'authorised officer' of a health board who is of prescribed rank or grade and is authorised by the Health Service Executive can also make an application.
- Co-habitees can make an application if they have lived together for three years.

Exclusions from applications are:

- Separated spouses or spouses against whom applications or orders under the Domestic Violence Acts 1996–2002 have been made.
- Persons under 18.

- An authorised officer or garda who is related to the person or spouse of the person.
- Members of the governing body, staff or person in charge of the approved centre.
- A doctor who provides regular services to an approved centre.

The application must be made within 48 hours of the applicant having observed the person. A statement of the reasons for the application, the connection between the applicant and the person, and the circumstances of the application must be included.

Examination and Recommendation

- The application must be supported by two medical recommendations following an examination of the patient.
- The definition of 'examination' is a personal examination of the process and content of thought, the mood and behaviour of the person.
- The examination must take place within 24 hours of the application being presented to the first doctor.
- The person must be told the purpose of the examination.
- These requirements apply to an examination for the purpose of the recommendation for admission, an admission order at the hospital and the renewal of a detention order.
- The patient's general practitioner will usually be one of the recommending doctors and they can make a recommendation that the person be involuntarily admitted to an approved centre. This approved centre should be specified and the recommendation should be sent to the clinical director of the centre and a copy given to the applicant.
- Under the 2001 Act the recommendation remains in force for seven days.
- Once at the approved centre the person can be held for 24 hours for the purpose of carrying out the second examination.
- The second examination will usually be carried out by the consultant psychiatrist at the approved centre, who can make an admission order.
- The admission order lasts for 21 days initially, renewable for three months, then six months and then periods of 12 months.
- The applicant must inform the recommending doctor of any previous refusals in relation to the same application.

These requirements and time limits are important for nurses who may be involved in the removal of patients to hospital.

Removal to Hospital — Garda Power

In general, the removal of the person to the approved centre will be arranged by the applicant, clinical director or CP at the request of the recommending doctor, with the assistance of nursing staff, if the applicant is unable to do so. Where these arrangements are not possible and there is serious likelihood of immediate and serious harm to the person, or others, the Gardai will be obliged to assist.

The Gardai have power to intervene in the community if they believe that a person is suffering from a mental disorder, and there is serious likelihood of causing immediate and serious harm to him/herself or to others. The Gardai have the power to enter a premises and to take the person into custody and immediately make an application for a recommendation for admission and remove the person to an approved centre.

Information to the Detained Patient

The CP must send a copy of the detention order to the Commission within 24 hours and give notice in writing to the patient of the order along with the information on the rights available under the Act. Information about the following must be given to the patient by the CP within 24 hours of an admission or a renewal order:

- Whether the detention is under an admission order or they are being detained under a renewal order.
- A general description of the proposed treatment.
- Entitlement to contact the Inspector of Mental Health Services.
- Entitlement to have the detention reviewed by a tribunal and to appeal against the decision to the Circuit Court.
- Entitlement to legal representation for the tribunal hearings and appeal.
- The right to choose to be a voluntary patient.

This last point is based on the principle that people with mental disorders should be treated in the same way as people with other illnesses or medical conditions. The full agreement and co-operation of the patient should be sought on this issue and the patient can be reclassified as a voluntary patient at any time. The nurse will have an important role in this aspect of practice and as a member of the care team may have to explain further the various rights as well as aspects of care and treatment for the patient.

Mental Health Tribunals

- Once the MHC receives a copy of the admission order or the renewal order they refer the matter to a tribunal for an independent review.
- An independent consultant psychiatrist reviews the patient.
- The patient is assigned a legal representative (unless he/she proposes to engage one).

The tribunal can:
- direct the consultant psychiatrist to arrange for the patient to be present at the tribunal if they wish to be
- arrange for the patient's notes to be made available to his/her legal representative
- direct any person whose evidence is required to appear before the tribunal.

The tribunal notifies the CP, the patient and their legal representative of the date, time and location of the tribunal.

- The tribunal will make arrangements for the patient and their legal representative to receive a copy of the independent medical report.
- The tribunal will hear submissions and any evidence it requires in order to make its decision.
- Once a decision is made (within 21 days unless extensions apply), the tribunal will inform the patient, their legal representative, the CP and the Mental Health Commission of its decision in writing.
- The patient can appeal this decision to the Circuit Court on the grounds that they are not suffering from a mental disorder. This appeal must be made within 14 days of the receipt by the patient or their legal representative of the decision to affirm an order.

VOLUNTARY ADMISSION

Voluntary Patients and Admission to Hospital
A voluntary patient is defined in the Act as 'a person receiving care and treatment in an approved centre who is not the subject of an admission or a renewal order'. There is no requirement under the 2001 Act to complete an admission form if that person is being admitted voluntarily. It is important to note that even though a person is being admitted voluntarily this does not mean he or she is capable of making a decision to do so. Some may be compliant and not objecting but lacking in capacity to make such a decision.

Voluntary Patients and the Holding Power
The Act provides for a 24-hour holding power over voluntary patients. While voluntary patients have the right to leave an approved centre, they may be prevented from leaving by a nurse or doctor using the statutory holding power until they are assessed with a view to either detention or discharge. The MHC *Reference Guide* states the following in relation to the holding power:
- Risk must be assessed during the period and appropriate risk management strategies put in place to reduce likelihood of harm and deterioration of mental well-being.
- All efforts should be made by the approved centre to encourage voluntary consent to remain for examination before a holding power is used.
- An examination should take place without delay and within the 24-hour period.
- The Act provides no right to treat during this period and in the absence of consent treatment is justified only under the common law doctrine of necessity and based on the best interests of the person.
- The degree of intervention should be the minimum necessary to meet safety needs of all.

The decision as to whether the person should then be compulsorily admitted is made by the CP along with an examination by a second CP who may or may not approve the admission. Otherwise, the patient must be discharged. If the patient is detained the same procedures and rights apply as to a patient admitted compulsorily.

Common Law Holding Power

Nurses should be aware that they have a common law holding power to use reasonable force to restrain and detain mentally incapacitated voluntary patients, where it is necessary and in the patient's best interests. These duties would apply if, for example, a seriously confused elderly patient was leaving the ward on a freezing cold night, where the risks are obvious.

TREATMENT FOR MENTAL DISORDER UNDER THE 2001 ACT: ADULTS

The provisions in the Act relating to treatment apply to detained patients and for mental disorder only. The definition of treatment in the Act is very broad: 'physical, psychological and other remedies relating to the care and rehabilitation of a patient under medical supervision' to improve the mental disorder. This means that it includes not only ECT and the administration of drugs and various therapy programmes, but also basic nursing and care. Individual written treatment plans are essential for all patients as part of the individual care plan supported in the Act.

Consent to Treatment

Consent to treatment should be sought from all patients. The majority of patients in psychiatric care consent to their treatment. A minority may not accept they are ill and may need treatment in their own interests and the interests of others, but may lack the capacity to make these decisions. The Act permits treatment for mental disorder to be given without consent if the patient is detained and provides rules and safeguards for particular treatments. This is done by providing for second opinions and the involvement of mental health tribunals. The second opinions are binding, not just advisory. In this way mental disorder is given special status that sets it apart from other illnesses. Common law applies to treatment for detained patients for physical illness, not related to the mental disorder). Where someone needs treatment, e.g. for a leg wound, then the ordinary legal rules that apply to consent for general medical care will apply as if the person were not detained.

Procedures for consent to treatment should be linked with the principles in the Act: best interests; right to notification; and right to respect.

- The first requirement for consent is that the patient must be given adequate information on the particular treatment in a form and language that he or she can understand about the nature, purpose and likely effects of the proposed treatment.

- Second, the consent must be freely obtained without threats or inducements and the psychiatrist must be satisfied that the patient is capable of understanding the nature, purpose and likely effects of the proposed treatment.

If the patient is not capable of grasping the information (due to the illness or for other reasons), other methods of imparting information will have to be found, for example through a third party such as a family member or independent advocate. Different rules apply to medicine for mental disorder, ECT and psychosurgery.

Consent to Treatment and Common Law

Common law applies to voluntary patients, not the provisions of the Act, which apply only to the treatment of mental disorder in detained patients. Where an adult is voluntary and lacks the capacity to consent to treatment, they may be given treatment for mental and physical disorders, as long as it is necessary and in their best interests. This applies also to people who are detained and if the treatment is not for mental disorder but for a separate physical illness.

These patients are in exactly the same position legally as patients in the general hospital in relation to consenting to or refusing treatment. Generally, patients are presumed to have capacity to make decisions unless the opposite is established. Nurses may be involved in assessing whether the person is capable of understanding the information that is being given to them in order to make a particular treatment decision.

Where the patient does not have capacity to consent or refuse treatment, treatment can legally be given where it is believed to be necessary and in the patient's best interests. Best interests are assessed according to what the professional body of doctors or nurses would regard as being in the best interests in those circumstances. The notion of *best interests* is recognised as broader than medical best interests, to include emotional and welfare issues. The Irish courts held in *In re a Ward* (1995) that where capacity is not present, the person's right to consent is not lost but operates in a different manner.

The guidance on capacity to make medical treatment decisions has been outlined by the English courts in *Re C (Adult Refusal of Treatment)* (1994) concerning a man diagnosed with paranoid schizophrenia who had been advised to have a below the knee amputation due to gangrene. He applied for an order preventing the amputation then or in future without his consent. The test used by the court to establish capacity to consent to medical treatment was divided into three stages:

- the patient understands the relevant treatment information;
- the patient believes the relevant information;
- the patient weighs the information in the balance to arrive at a decision.

The relevant question in such cases is whether it is established that the patient's capacity is so reduced by his mental illness that he does not fully understand the nature, purpose and effects of the treatment.

Pharmacological Treatment for Mental Disorder

This is the most commonly used treatment. The patient's consent should be sought for each treatment and the principles in the Act should be applied. If the patient is unable or unwilling to consent, treatment can be given for the first period of three months without consent or a second opinion. After this period, the patient must give consent to further treatment or the patient's CP must seek the approval of a second CP. Where the second opinion approves the treatment, medications for mental disorder can be given to a patient for a further period of three months and thereafter for periods of three months. Otherwise the treatment cannot be imposed.

Electroconvulsive Therapy

Under the 2001 Act the administration of ECT requires the patient's written consent to the treatment. If the patient refuses or is unable to give consent, the therapy must be approved by the patient's CP and authorised by a second opinion, also given by a CP. The appropriate form must be filled in, placed in the patient's clinical file and a copy sent to the MHC.

The *Rules Governing the Use of ECT* (MHC 2006c) refer to a programme of ECT as no more than 12 treatments, prescribed by a CP. These rules require that the patient must be presumed capable of giving informed consent for ECT, unless there is evidence to the contrary. The capacity of the patient to consent is assessed by the CP under the following guidelines.

Capacity to consent to ECT must ensure that the patient:

* can understand the nature of ECT and why it is being proposed;
* understand the benefits, risks and alternatives as well as consequences of not having it;
* retain the information in order to make a decision to receive or not receive ECT;
* make a free choice and communicate that choice to consent.

It is useful for nurses to be aware of these requirements as they are often asked additional questions by patients.

Informed Consent to ECT

Appropriate information about ECT must be given to the patient by the CP to enable informed consent. This must include information on the nature, process and purpose of the treatment. It must include the likely benefits as well as the likely adverse effects, including the risk of short-term cognitive impairment. Information on alternatives and the possible consequences of not having treatment must be given. Information must be provided in both oral and written forms and be clearly and simply written. It must be available in other languages if necessary, and an interpreter must be provided, including Irish sign interpreters for any patient who is deaf. Depending on urgency, the patient may be given 24 hours to reflect on the information and must be informed that he or she may have access to an advocate of his/her choosing at any stage and an opportunity for questions.

The *Rules* include many additional requirements relating to consent, some of which are:

- A written record of assessments of capacity to consent must be kept in the patient's clinical file.
- Consent for each programme of ECT must be obtained in writing without coercion or threats.
- The patient must be aware that he/she can refuse and withdraw consent at any time.
- No relation, carer or guardian can give consent for ECT on behalf of the patient.

The Nurse and the Administration of ECT

The *Rules* require a minimum number of three registered nursing staff in the ECT suite to safely meet the needs of the patient at all times. Additional rules provide the following:

- One of these nurses must be trained in ECT and shall be known as 'a designated ECT nurse'.
- All registered nurses involved in the administration of ECT treatment must be trained in professional CPR.
- The designated ECT nurse is responsible for ensuring that before the treatment emergency resuscitation equipment is tested and checked in the ECT suite, and the emergency drugs tray has been recently checked and stocked. All such checks should be recorded.
- The designated ECT nurse must be present while ECT is being administered.

It is essential that nurses have a complete knowledge of the *Rules*, as they have a key role in ECT application and monitoring.

Psychosurgery

Psychosurgery is defined in the 2001 Act as 'any surgical operation that destroys brain tissue for the purposes of ameliorating a mental disorder'. The Act provides that psychosurgery cannot be performed on a patient unless two conditions are met: the patient gives written consent; and psychosurgery is authorised by a mental health tribunal. The tribunal will sanction the treatment if it is satisfied that it is in the best interests of the health of the patient, otherwise it will refuse to authorise it. Psychosurgery can only be given to detained patients who are capable of consenting; a court order may have to be sought in relation to patients who are not capable.

Emergency Treatment Without Consent

In emergency situations, treatment can be given to the patient without consent, where:

- the patient, by reason of his or her mental disorder, is incapable of giving consent; *and*

- the treatment is necessary to safeguard the life of the patient, to restore his or her health, to alleviate his or her condition, or to relieve his or her suffering.

In this instance the treatment cannot include psychosurgery or ECT.

Seclusion and Restraint
Seclusion
The MHC *Rules Governing the Use of Seclusion and Mechanical Means of Bodily Restraint* define seclusion as 'the placing or leaving of a person in any room alone, at any time, day or night, with the exit door locked or fastened or held in such a way as to prevent the person from leaving' (MHC 2006d:11). The definition excludes people in the National Forensic Service who are locked in rooms at night for security reasons.

The Act provides that a patient cannot be placed in seclusion unless two conditions are met:
- it is necessary for the purposes of treatment or to prevent the patient from injuring himself or herself or others; *and*
- the seclusion or restraint complies with the rules laid down by the Commission.

The definition of 'patient' includes both voluntary adults and children under a detention order. Seclusion is a form of deprivation of liberty and when used on voluntary patients consideration must be given to whether it is more appropriate to compulsorily admit such patients. The *Rules* provide that seclusion must only be used in the best interests of the patient and only when the patient poses a threat of serious harm to him/herself or others. The key principle underpinning the use of seclusion and/or mechanical means of bodily restraint is that they must only be used as a last resort and must not be prolonged beyond what is necessary.

Special consideration must be given to seclusion of a patient with a known psychosocial/medical condition in which close confinement would be contraindicated. While these are not made explicit they may include psychological conditions such as severe claustrophobia or past traumas that have involved restraint or seclusion. The MHC does not consider seclusion a therapeutic treatment intervention.

In addition, the *Rules* contain other provisions, relating to the facilities, recording of seclusion and training of staff in relation to seclusion. Training for staff involved in seclusion and mechanical bodily restraint should be mandatory and be updated as required. It is essential that all nursing staff have a sound knowledge of the rules for seclusion and restraint.

Seclusion, Crisis Situations and the Nurse
Specific rules regarding seclusion apply in a crisis situation, including the following:
- Seclusion may in addition be initiated by a registered nurse or care officer (National Forensic Service (NFS)).

- If a registered nurse or care officer (NFS) initiates seclusion, a registered medical practitioner must be notified immediately.
- A seclusion register is a book in which is entered details concerning those who are secluded and restrained. It will contain: personal details and all details relating to the seclusion; date and time of seclusion or mechanical restraint; who initiated it; who ended it; any alternatives to such action. The section of the seclusion register relating to crisis situations must be completed by the doctor, registered nurse or care officer who initiated the seclusion.
- Where there is uncertainty about continuing seclusion it can be discontinued following discussion with nursing staff, and entered into the register.

The Patient and Seclusion
- The patient must be informed of the reasons for and the likely duration of seclusion unless it would prejudice his/her mental or emotional well-being.
- As soon as is practicable, and with the patient's consent, the patient's next of kin or representative must be informed of the seclusion and a record kept of such communication in the patient's clinical file: if they are not informed, the reasons for this must also be recorded.
- Where the patient lacks capacity and cannot consent next of kin should be informed as above.
- A patient in seclusion must wear clothing in so far as is practicable otherwise the reasons must be documented in the individual care and treatment plan. The respect principles must be observed.

Bodily searches must respect the right of the patient to dignity, bodily integrity and privacy.

Monitoring Seclusion – Nurses
The requirements in relation to monitoring include:
- The patient must be under direct observation by a registered nurse for the first hour following initiation of a seclusion episode.
- The patient is kept under continuous observation by a registered nurse for the duration of the seclusion.
- Following a risk assessment, a nursing review must take place every two hours unless there is a high risk of injury to the patient. A minimum of two staff, one a registered nurse, must enter the room and directly observe the patient with a view to ending seclusion.
- A medical review must be carried out every four hours.
- Specific rules apply where a patient is sleeping, and clinical judgement must be applied on whether it is appropriate to waken the patient:
  - nursing reviews must continue every two hours without waking the patient;
  - medical reviews may be suspended when the patient is asleep but a doctor must be on call if needed.
- The patient's individual care and treatment plan must address the assessed needs of the patient in seclusion with the goal of ending the seclusion.

Ending Seclusion

- Seclusion may be ended at any time by the registered nurse in charge or care officer in charge (NFS), in consultation with a doctor, following discussion with the patient.
- A doctor may end seclusion on his or her own authority following discussion with the nursing staff and/or care officers (NFS) in the approved centre.
- The reason for ending seclusion must be recorded in the patient's clinical file and the patient given an opportunity to discuss the episode with the multidisciplinary team.

Restraint

Mechanical Bodily Restraint

Mechanical restraint is defined in the *Rules Governing the use of Seclusion and Mechanical Means of Bodily Restraint* as the 'use of devices or bodily garments for the purpose of preventing or limiting the free movement of a patient's body' (MHC 2006d:19)

Many of the requirements that apply to seclusion apply, where appropriate, to the use of such restraint.

Mechanical Bodily Restraint and the Nurse

Some of the requirements in the *Rules* that apply directly to nurses are as follows:
- Where such restraint is initiated by a nurse, a doctor must be notified immediately of the fact and it must be recorded in the patient's file. The doctor must examine the patient within three hours.
- Approved centres must have a policy regarding who can carry out such restraint and a designated member of staff must be responsible for leading such restraint.
- It must be under the direct supervision of a doctor or nurse.
- The patient must be continually assessed to ensure safety. Any specific requirements or needs of the patient in relation to such restraint, including 'advance directives' in the individual care and treatment plan, must be considered.
- The use of devices to inflict pain is prohibited.

Physical Restraint

Restraint is defined in the *Code of Practice on the Use of Physical Restraint in Approved Centres* as the 'use of physical force (by one or more persons) for the purpose of preventing the free movement of a resident's body' (MHC 2006b:8). Many of the factors that apply above to seclusion and mechanical restraint apply also to physical restraint.

Physical Restraint and the Nurse

Similar rules apply to the use of physical restraint. They include:
- Where the restraint has been initiated by the nurse a doctor should be notified immediately of the fact and it should be recorded in the patient's clinical file.

- The patient should be examined by the doctor within three hours.
- The application should be under the direction of the doctor or nurse.

CHILDREN

The Act provides for the voluntary and compulsory admission of children. A child is defined in the Act as a person under 18, unless he or she is or has been married. Most children in need of mental health services will receive outpatient treatment. Where in-patient care is needed parental consent will apply in most situations. It is essential that nurses are fully informed of the *Code of Practice Relating to the Admission of Children under the Mental Health Act 2001* (MHC 2006a) as it provides important practice and operational details regarding children in in-patient care.

The Act provides for compulsory admission of children on the basis of mental disorder. The principles in the Act — of best interests, notification and respect — apply also to children in decisions about admission and treatment. It is not within the remit of this chapter to provide a detailed account of the process of compulsory and voluntary admission to an approved centre for children. Further information on these processes and on compulsory treatment of children can be found in the Act and in the aforementioned code.

INDIVIDUAL CARE PLAN AND OTHER RIGHTS OF RESIDENTS

A resident is defined in the Act as a person receiving care and treatment in an approved centre and this means all persons, children and adults. The Mental Health Act Approved Centres Regulations (2006) define the important individual care plan as a:
- Documented set of goals developed, regularly reviewed and updated by the resident's multidisciplinary team, so far as is practicable in consultation with each resident.
- The individual care plan shall: specify the treatment and care required (which shall be in accordance with best practice); identify necessary resources; *and* specify appropriate goals for the service user.
- For a resident who is a child, his or her individual care plan shall include appropriate educational requirements and services in accordance with his or her needs and age as indicated by his or her individual care plan.
- The care plan is recorded in one set of documentation.

Provision of Information to all Residents
There is a specific requirement in the Act that the approved centre ensures that patients and residents are informed of their rights under the Act. This requirement will have to take into account many issues such as language, literacy, inability to understand due to illness or other factors, as well as changing capacity to understand the information.

The regulations on approved centres require that the following information is provided to each resident in an understandable form and language, in addition to the requirements regarding information to detained patients:

- Details of the resident's multidisciplinary team.
- Housekeeping practices, including arrangements for personal property, mealtimes, visiting times.
- Oral and written information on the resident's diagnosis, unless the provision of such information might be prejudicial to the resident's mental or emotional health.
- Details of relevant advocacy and voluntary agencies.

Nurses are in a position to ensure that in all instances the required information is imparted directly or indirectly to patients and residents.

COMPLAINTS PROCEDURES

The regulations on approved centres require policies and procedures relating to all aspects of complaints about any aspects of service, care and treatment and must ensure that all residents are aware of these, as soon as possible after admission.

DISCHARGE

The Act provides for a formal approach to discharge where an order is made ending the admission and the patient is discharged. The Act requires that the patient is not inappropriately discharged and is detained only for as long as is reasonably necessary for proper care and treatment. The duty of care in discharge planning arose in *Healy v. North Western Health Board* (1996) where the health board was negligent for failure to have a proper pre-discharge assessment on a suicidal patient. Nurses will have a key contribution to make to this pre-discharge assessment, in which consultation with family or carers is often an important aspect.

CONCLUSION

The legal requirements of the 2001 Act regarding admission and treatment of adults are addressed in this chapter. The Act has brought many changes to the practice of mental health nursing, including new legal duties and responsibilities for nurses. Nurses must have a sound knowledge of the provisions of the Act along with the requirements in the MHC's various codes of practice, rules and regulations in order to understand the new legal context in which they are working. Such knowledge will enable a more confident approach to practice and eliminate the possibility of acting in a way that is illegal or unethical. Nurses have a duty of care to their patients to avoid any injury to them through wrongful acts or omissions. Knowledge, therefore, must be kept up to date to ensure lawful, safe and effective practice. The promotion of the dignity of the individual is a core principle in human rights and the role of patient as partner in care is recognised in many aspects of the 2001 Act and various codes, such as recognition of the right to consent, empowerment through information, co-operation in the individual care plan and the acknowledgement of advance directives.

Reflective Questions
1. The overarching human right is the right to respect and dignity for the person. How might this value be advanced in mental healthcare and practice?
2. What is your role as a nurse in the development of individual care plans for residents?
3. How might the establishment of the new structures and monitoring bodies enhance a person's dignity and rights?
4. What type of information will be given to residents under the 2001 Act and how might you as a nurse provide this?

References
An Bord Altranais (2000) *The Code of Professional Conduct for each Nurse and Midwife*. Dublin: An Bord Altranais.

Mental Health Act 2001.

Mental Health (Approved Centres) Regulations 2006.

Mental Health Act (Authorised Officers) Regulations 2006.

Mental Health Commission (2005) *Reference Guide to the 2001 Act*. Dublin: Stationery Office.

Mental Health Commission (2006a) *Code of Practice Relating to the Admission of Children under the Mental Health Act 2001* COP-S33(3)/01/2006.

Mental Health Commission (2006b) *Code of Practice on the Use of Physical Restraint in Approved Centres* COP-S33 (3)/02/2006.

Mental Health Commission (2006c) *Rules Governing the Use of ECT*, R-S59 (2)/01/2006.

Mental Health Commission (2006d) *Rules Governing the Use of Seclusion and Mechanical Means of Bodily Restraint*, R-S69 (2)/02/2006), 1 November 2006.

Further Reading
Bartlett, P. and Sandland, R. (2003) *Mental Health Law: Policy and Practice* (3rd edn). Oxford: Oxford University Press.

Keys, M. (2002) *Mental Health Act 2001*. Dublin: Thompson Round Hall Press.

O'Neill, A. M. (2005) *Irish Mental Health Law*. Dublin: First Law Limited.

4

Professional and Ethical Challenges in Mental Health Nursing

Suzanne Denieffe, John Wells and Margaret Denny

In everyday life, people face situations that have ethical implications. This chapter will explore ethical principles, theories and decision-making frameworks that you as a mental health nurse need to think about, along with the many other issues that you will confront in everyday practice. In this chapter, an exploration of the relationship of ethics to morality and how contexts can affect what mental health nurses view as ethical will be reviewed. The chapter will then examine particular ethical theories and frameworks used in healthcare and relate these specifically to contemporary mental health nursing practice.

ETHICS AND MORALITY

Ethics is viewed as one of the main branches of moral philosophy and is concerned with evaluating human action (Rumbold 1993). Mental health nursing, by its nature, is concerned with actions/interactions between a nurse and a person who is in need of help with their mental health, referred to variously as a patient, client or user (Peplau 1988). Inherent in mental health nursing is the need to evaluate actions/interactions and interventions aimed at assisting such a person. Ethics provides a frame of reference with which to examine the moral thinking that lies behind such actions and the morality of the actions themselves.

DISTINGUISHING ETHICS AND MORALITY

Ethics and morality are terms that are often used interchangeably. Ford (2006) distinguishes ethics (what is right or wrong based on reason) from morals (what is considered right or wrong behaviour based on social custom). Morality comprises values and duties that people consider fundamental to their daily lives. Morals are the 'shoulds' and 'oughts' of professional practice, whereas ethics are the reasons why. Ethics looks at the meaning of such words as *right, wrong, bad, good, ought* and *duty* (Rumbold 1993). Ethics is therefore thinking and reasoning about morality and the actions that are taken in the practice of mental health nursing (Basford and Slevin 1995).

ETHICS AND NURSING

Nursing ethics is generally described as normative ethics (Beauchamp and Childress 2001). This is the framework of reference that tells people how they should act or what they should do in a situation. Normative ethics can provide a guiding framework to mental health nurses in that almost anything one does in nursing practice may cause good or harm. While defining good or harm may appear simple, difficulties can arise from diverse perceptions of what constitutes good or harm that are dependent on group and individual value systems.

The personal values that mental health nurses hold impact on their practice. It is therefore important that you, as a mental health nurse, are aware of the values that you personally hold. At a fundamental level, this focuses on what it means to be a 'person'. This is an important consideration because how we behave toward the people we care for, and therefore the boundaries/limits we set for our actions/interactions, depends on our understanding and interpretation of *personhood* (Dooley and McCarthy 2005).

Values develop from childhood and are influenced by sources such as parents, society, religion and legislation (Ford 2006). Nursing values are influenced by nurse education, legislation and codes of professional conduct. In Ireland, nurses are statutorily governed in their actions by the *Code of Professional Conduct for each Nurse and Midwife* (An Bord Altranais 2000). Membership of the nursing profession implies acceptance of the values, beliefs and attitudes of the profession incorporated within its code (Kaldjian *et al.* 2005). Nurses are required to conduct themselves in accordance with these professional values and principles (Severinsson 2001). As a mental health nurse, you are required to be fully aware of the An Bord Altranais *Code of Professional Conduct* (2000) and how it relates to your practice. It is also imperative that you are aware of your own values and the values of the nursing profession. However, this value system is also affected by the environment and context in which you practice.

CONTEXTUAL INFLUENCES ON MORAL CHOICE IN CLINICAL PRACTICE

Contexts are a significant determinant of what is seen as ethical or unethical in terms of nursing. It may be argued that this is particularly the case in mental healthcare, which often has a dimension of social and political control within clinical practice. Consequently, it is important that the mental health nurse who wishes to develop an ethical practice 'mindset' should explore the influence of context on what he or she is asked to do in practice and whether or not he or she does it. For example, in the nineteenth century it was perfectly acceptable to use a range of physical restraints on patients because the role of the nurse at that time was to keep good order in institutions (Russell 1997). However, today such nursing 'practices' of using physical restraints as standard interventions would be seen as morally unacceptable.

One might argue, therefore, that mental health nursing practice is based not on appeals to ethical absolutes alone but also to what is judged as acceptable in the social, political and professional environment of the time. It is often the case in mental healthcare that all three interact to change the way in which mental health nurses engage with their clinical role. This can lead to compromised professional values that at their worst provide a rationalisation for unethical behaviour. Two examples illustrate and shed light on such behaviour.

The last few years have seen an increased interest in the role of the psychiatrist and mental health nurse in Germany during the Nazi era (1933–45); in particular, their involvement with what was known as the T4 euthanasia programme — the extermination of people with chronic mental illness or intellectual disabilities. In the past, a general perception of Nazi healthcare atrocities was that they were a direct product of that movement's political ideology and Adolf Hitler's personal obsessions (Kershaw 1999, 2000). Healthcare professions, including nursing, were seen as passive and compliant actors (BenGershôm 1990).

However, a closer examination of psychiatry during this time reveals that the Nazis' policy towards the mentally ill was inspired and initiated by an established discourse in German psychiatric medicine on the pointless existence of people with chronic mental illness. The professional discourse referred to such patients as 'useless eaters' and 'life unworthy of life' – *lebensunwerten Lebens* (McFarland-Icke 1999). It was argued that such people were an economic drain on the nation's resources and a threat to its long-term health. This discourse was not confined to Germany; similar views were also held and discussed in other countries, such as Sweden, between the two world wars (Engwall 2005).

People with enduring mental illness and intellectual disabilities were thus characterised in Germany as 'lesser beings' than ordinary citizens. This view was reinforced by the experience of physical deprivation during the First World War (1914–18), in which German mental hospitals' and nurses' duty of care for the patient became subservient to the needs of the 'Fatherland' to conserve resources such as food and energy (McFarland-Icke 1999). As a result, many psychiatric patients were deliberately denied food, leading to malnourishment and, in some cases, death.

This *weltanschauung* (world view) of people with long-term mental illness made it easier for nurses to accept, once the Nazis came to power in 1933, a euthanasia programme (T4) that aimed to exterminate the mentally infirm. As this programme developed and was implemented, mental health nurses became the primary murderers of patients; either by deliberately withholding food from them or by leading them into the hospital gas chambers and administering the poison gas (Benedict and Kuhla 1999). Indeed, the brightest and best nurses — the identified leaders of the profession — were sent to a special training school to be educated in the political, economic, racial and eugenic principles underpinning this eugenics programme (Channel 4 2000).

Mental health nurses were educated to rationalise this approach to 'care' as a merciful intervention to end incurable suffering and a professional obligation to obey the orders of the State, which set the parameters for their actions and of which they were employees (Benedict and Kuhla 1999; McFarland-Icke 1999). Indeed, even when some mental health nurses were tried for these crimes in the 1960s, a number of the accused continued to argue that their performance of these duties was ethically and professionally acceptable because of such obligations. In all, it is estimated that from the late 1930s to 1945 nurses directly murdered at least 10,000 patients on the T4 programme (Benedict and Kuhla 1999).

The second example is set within an Irish context. In the past, the dominance of Catholic values and institutions in social welfare and healthcare shaped the ethos of nursing practice in Ireland (Fealy 2006). While this system had some benign elements, it also meant that nursing values in Ireland were often subordinate to Catholic teaching and institutions. Indeed, there is evidence to suggest that healthcare services in Ireland, including mental health services and mental health nurses, colluded with the concealment of physical abuse perpetrated in Church-run welfare institutions, or at least failed to challenge such acts as abuse when they became apparent (Finnegan 2001).

It would be comforting to think that such rationalisations and complicities on the part of mental health nurses are a thing of the past or only possible in totalitarian regimes. However, this would be an erroneous belief. In recent times, governments in a number of countries have become concerned both to contain the costs of mental health services and to allay public fears about perceived risks posed by people with mental health problems living in the community (Mechanic and Bilder 2004). This has led to a greater political willingness to interfere directly with clinical practice to ensure that the mentally ill in the community are 'policed' by clinicians. This approach has focused particularly on mental health nursing, with its traditional role of observing patients and mental health nurses' more regular contact with patients day-to-day compared with other clinical professions (Bean 2001; Buchanan-Barker and Barker 2005).

Just as in the example of Nazi Germany, this 'political project' is achieved by 'capturing' the mindset of practice through changing its language. Terms such as 'risk assessment', 'resource consciousness', being 'efficient and effective' all serve to change the language through which mental health nurses articulate what they do and thus serve to reorientate their 'world view' (*weltanschauung*) as to what is important to achieve in clinical practice. For example, in the United Kingdom the containment of risk and resource management are now principal practice considerations for mental health nurses when engaging with patients, even though some may feel uncomfortable with this reorientation (Wells 2004).

Political and social contexts confront mental health nurses with a fundamental professional choice that has a moral dimension. Wells (1998) poses the question: how far should mental health nurses adjust their practice values to policy demands with which they may disagree? In exploring and resolving such a dilemma the mental health nurse needs to reference their decision through an ethical framework. However, they also need to critically assess how the ethical framework was developed — in other words, how context shaped it. A framework is a tool;

it does not absolve the individual mental health nurse from their responsibility for making a moral choice.

ETHICAL THEORIES AND APPROACHES

It is important to understand that theories and approaches to ethics provide reasoned answers—though without definitive conclusions—to ethical issues in mental health nursing (Rawlins *et al.* 1993). Their value lies, therefore, in initiating a process of thinking about what one does.

Ethical Theories

Within normative ethics, Tschudin (2003) identifies teleology and deontology as the two broad schools of thought that shape contemporary ethical thinking. For a mental health nurse to understand ethical reasoning, they need first to understand the principles of these schools of thought.

Teleology

Teleology (Greek for 'logic of ends'), or consequentialism, is concerned with consequences or outcomes (Thompson *et al.* 2003). This thinking arises from the philosophers Jeremy Bentham (1748–1832) and John Stuart Mill (1806–73). A subgroup of teleology is utilitarianism. Utilitarianism as an ethical theory claims that what makes behaviour right or wrong depends entirely on the consequences. It affirms that what is important about human behaviour is the outcome or results of the behaviour and not the intention a person has when they act. In utilitarianism an action is right in so far as it tends to produce the 'greatest happiness for the greatest number' (Tschudin 2003:48). If an action produces an excess of beneficial effects over harmful ones, then it is right, otherwise it is not. Fundamentally, the consequences of a given action determine its rightness or wrongness, not the motive from which it was done.

Rumbold (1993) identifies two additional aspects of teleology. These are *act utilitarianism* and *rule utilitarianism*. Act utilitarianism considers whether an act is good or bad according to whether it serves the principle of greatest happiness. Rule utilitarianism tries to establish rules that are capable of producing the greatest happiness for the greatest number and the rules established are universally binding. There are fundamental differences between these two views. In act utilitarianism an act may be right or wrong depending on the situation. In rule utilitarianism, if an act should not be done, then it is never justified whatever the circumstances. For example, in a unit for older adults with mental health problems, all patients are put to bed after the nine o'clock news. This could be viewed as rule utilitarianism, if every patient is put to bed with no consideration of individuality. A lack of individual patient care is itself an ethical issue.

Using a utilitarian approach to care in mental health nursing, that is, attaining the greatest happiness for the greatest number, may in fact be problematic. One reason for this might be because people perceive pleasure and happiness in different ways. Additionally, the mental health nurse, in attempting to maximise happiness for the greatest number, may in fact ignore the needs of other people.

Deontology

Immanuel Kant (1724–1804) is regarded as a key philosopher of deontological theory. Actions of any sort, he believed, must be undertaken from a sense of duty dictated by reason, wherein individuals and their welfare were seen as ends in themselves and not as means to an end. Therefore, actions such as murder are always wrong because they do not facilitate an individual's welfare. In this context, Kant argued that for an act to be considered moral, the *actor* has to decide whether they were willing for their proposed course of action to be applied as a principle to everyone's welfare, including their own; that is to *universalise* the act. If the actor was unable to universalise their action in this way, Kant believed the act was morally impermissible.

Kant's idea of the principle underpinning actions is referred to as the *categorical imperative*. It is a deontological theory because Kant stated it should always be followed as the rule of action since its very nature was a good in itself, not a means of achieving some other purpose. It consists of four precepts:

- Act toward others as you would have others act towards you.
- Treat people as ends in themselves and not as a means to an end.
- Respect peoples' autonomy.
- Act as you would have all others act (Dooley and McCarthy 2005).

The following scenario helps to illustrate the categorical imperative in practice.

> Ann has been a patient in your unit for seven weeks. She has a diagnosis of paranoid schizophrenia and is mentally unwell now. She continuously asks 'Can I go home?' Your response is 'You will be going home soon.'
>
> Has Ann's autonomy been respected? If you were Ann in this situation, how would you feel if you got that response? Is this how you would like to be treated as a patient?

One of the weaknesses of Kant's categorical imperative, however, is that there appears to be no provision made for exceptions. Applying a deontological approach, truth telling may be seen as a vital obligation in treating people who present with mental health problems. However, it could be said that keeping a promise in a situation may be wrong or telling a lie may be right. In such situations, consideration of ethical implications should be undertaken using an ethical framework.

ETHICAL PRINCIPLES

Together with deontological and teleological theories, knowledge of ethical principles is important for mental health nursing practice. Tschudin (2003) offers a good analogy as to how ethical principles can help nursing practice. She proposes that they function like a compass, providing a direction rather than serving as a road map.

Beauchamp and Childress (2001) state that the commonly accepted ethical principles for healthcare include:

- respect for autonomy
- beneficence
- non-maleficence
- justice.

Of these four, Gillon (2003) contends that autonomy should be regarded as the *primus inter pares* (first among equals) because it should be seen as an integral component of the other three principles.

Respect for Autonomy

The term autonomy is derived from the Greek words *autos* meaning self and *nomos* meaning rule (Breeze 1998). In healthcare ethics, persons are considered rational, self-conscious and autonomous beings; they possess liberty and the right to choose for themselves (Fu-Chang Tsai 2001). Consequently, people have the right to be treated equally and with respect. The autonomous person is someone who is capable of making important decisions about their own life based on their own beliefs and values. This involves *self-determination* and *self-governance*. Self-determination incorporates the individual's ability to carry out plans, desires and wishes in order to determine the course of his/her own life. Self-governance involves possessing self-determination, yet also possessing the capability of placing rules governing self and others above one's own desires.

In mental health nursing a person's autonomy may be constrained by his or her mental health problem, e.g. if they suffer from dementia. In these instances, a distinction needs to be made between possessing autonomy and making autonomous choices (Beauchamp and Childress 2001). This is to guard against an assumption that a person possesses no autonomy. For that reason, it is the nurse's responsibility to ensure that, as far as possible, a person who may not possess full autonomy is enabled and supported to make autonomous choices. For example, choices should be offered regarding diet, recreation activities and bedtimes to someone with dementia.

Paternalism

Autonomy cannot be discussed without considering the concept of paternalism. The axiom 'Father knows best' can be used to describe paternalism. Beauchamp and Childress (2001:178) write, 'A professional has superior training, knowledge and insight and is thus in an authoritative position to determine the patient's best interest. From this perspective, a healthcare professional is like a loving parent with dependent, often ignorant, children.' The justification for paternalism is a moot point in healthcare. The distinction between weak and strong paternalism is perhaps relevant here. Weak paternalism limits the freedom of substantially non-autonomous individuals, that is, those individuals whose capacity to be autonomous is compromised in some way (Dooley and McCarthy 2005). Strong paternalism limits the freedom of autonomous people and demands far more stringent justification for its use. For example, Dr White and Nurse Green discuss Mr O'Hara's progress in the high-support hostel. After the meeting, the nurse informs Mr O'Hara that he is doing well, and is to be transferred to a medium-support hostel. This could be seen as a situation in which Mr O'Hara's autonomy is limited by an act of strong paternalism.

Beneficence and Non-maleficence

Beneficence means doing good for others (Ford 2006). The principle of non-maleficence requires that mental health nurses do not intentionally create a needless harm or injury to the patient. The *Code of Professional Conduct* (An Bord Altranais 2000) states that the aim of the nursing profession is to give patients the highest possible standard of care. Providing nursing care that avoids or minimises the risk of harm is supported not only by the principles of beneficence and non-maleficence but also by the laws of society (Dooley and McCarthy 2005). These two principles should be primary considerations for the mental health nurse. Nurses have a duty to benefit the patient, as well as to take positive steps to prevent and to remove harm from the patient. These principles are applied both to individual patients and to the good of society as a whole.

The mental health nurse provides beneficent care through a multiplicity of means. One such means is through the maintenance of confidentiality, for example, in mental health nursing practice, when a patient tells the nurse in confidence that she intends to kill either herself or her mother. This could be seen as a 'conflict of duty' in that the patient's autonomy and your duty of care are in conflict. In this instance, an ethical dilemma for mental health nurses arises when the requirement to maintain confidentiality may have to be breached; the duty to preserve life comes into conflict with the duty to maintain confidentiality (Ford 2006). Beauchamp and Childress (2001) endorse the breaking of confidentiality only when a higher obligation needs to be followed.

The Principle of Justice

'Justice in healthcare is usually defined as a form of fairness' (Rawls 1971:12) or, as Aristotle said, 'giving to each that which is his due' (1947). This implies that there must be fair distribution of healthcare in society with equal treatment for all. Petifor (2001) advises that service users with mental health problems may be vulnerable to distributive injustice in healthcare provision. They may be over-regulated in relation to their experience of clinical services, or they may not receive an appropriate share of resources because they are considered a lower priority than other groups (for example physically sick children) in a healthcare system in which resources are finite. The involvement of the service user and their advocates in this context therefore becomes a moral imperative in terms of safeguarding equitable distribution of resources within a competing healthcare dynamic. Thus, commitment to equality of esteem and involvement of users in service planning, encapsulated in such policy guidelines as *Quality in Mental Health: Your Views*, becomes a professional duty (MHC 2005).

ETHICAL DECISION-MAKING IN MENTAL HEALTH NURSING

Every day in mental health nursing practice, nurses are required to make decisions, some of which are moral decisions. Not all these moral decisions need be associated with crisis; they may have to be made in everyday situations. In mental health nursing, we may not always reflect critically on what we are doing when we make such decisions. Thompson *et al.* (2003) outline situations in which the nurse is challenged to reflect on moral decision-making. For example: when entering unfamiliar territory; when faced with greater than usual responsibility; when the consequences of a decision may be far-reaching or irreversible; or a situation where there is a conflict of duties or equally unacceptable moral outcomes. In these situations, nurses may be required to reflect and provide reasons for their decisions and actions not only to themselves but also to others.

When confronted with a situation that has a moral aspect, a mental health nurse should be able to recognise the ethical issues involved, consider the alternative actions available to them and think about the likely consequences of each alternative. This very act of thinking makes their decision ethical. Once they have made a decision and experienced its outcome a further ethical process of thinking is required. This involves reflecting upon the decision once implemented in order to learn from its outcome and to change where necessary.

This reflection on the decision-making process, both before and after an action has taken place, is greatly assisted if the mental health nurse engages in a conscious planning effort through reference to frameworks of ethical decision-making. A variety of these are available. For example, Thompson *et al.* (2003) describe a model for ethical decision-making based on the systematic approach to care, namely assessment, planning, implementation and evaluation. Alternatively, Purtillo (1999) developed a model comprising six steps of ethical reasoning:
1. Gather the relevant information.
2. Identify the type of ethical problem.
3. Use ethical theories or approaches.
4. Explore the practical alternatives.
5. Complete the action.
6. Evaluate the process and outcome.

Another model, developed by Ford (2006), is particularly appropriate in a mental health nursing context (see Figure 4.1). This model provides a comprehensive framework to allow the mental health nurse to explore situations fully in terms of their ethical aspects, a process Ford (2006) calls meta-ethical deliberation. Meta-ethical deliberation considers specific ethical duties related to ethical theories.

Meta-ethical discussion explains the origins of specific ethical duties. An example will illustrate how this works.

Figure 4.1 Ford's (2006) model of the ethical decision-making process

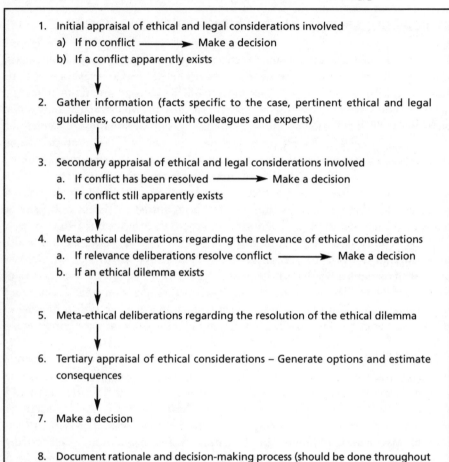

1. Initial appraisal of ethical and legal considerations involved
   a) If no conflict ———→ Make a decision
   b) If a conflict apparently exists

2. Gather information (facts specific to the case, pertinent ethical and legal guidelines, consultation with colleagues and experts)

3. Secondary appraisal of ethical and legal considerations involved
   a. If conflict has been resolved ———→ Make a decision
   b. If conflict still apparently exists

4. Meta-ethical deliberations regarding the relevance of ethical considerations
   a. If relevance deliberations resolve conflict ———→ Make a decision
   b. If an ethical dilemma exists

5. Meta-ethical deliberations regarding the resolution of the ethical dilemma

6. Tertiary appraisal of ethical considerations – Generate options and estimate consequences

7. Make a decision

8. Document rationale and decision-making process (should be done throughout the process)

Ford's Model and Informed Consent

Ford's model of ethical decision-making is explored using the following scenario (see Figure 4.2):

Tom Woolley is a 22-year-old who was admitted following a psychotic episode. He has a partner, Gail, with whom he lives. He has been prescribed a medication, which may cause sexual difficulties. He is almost fully recovered from his psychotic episode. The psychiatrist and his parents are concerned about his compliance and want the explanations of the possible side effects of the medication kept to a minimum. Tom asks you if there are any side effects that will affect his life.

Figure 4.2 Using Ford's model of ethical decision-making

1. Initial appraisal of ethical and legal considerations involved a) If no conflict Make a decision b) If a conflict apparently exists	• Has Tom a legal entitlement to full information on his medication? • Is Tom an adult with full autonomy and therefore the right to self-determination? • Has Tom currently the full mental capacity for autonomy? • Is there a conflict between your duty to care for Tom and the wishes of his psychiatrist and parents?
2. Gather information (facts specific to the case, pertinent ethical and legal guidelines, consultation with colleagues and experts)	• Ascertain the Irish law regarding informed consent and medication • What are the ethical issues in this scenario: autonomy, beneficence, non-maleficence, paternalism • Check the Code of Conduct • Speak to the psychiatrist and nursing team
3. Secondary appraisal of ethical and legal considerations involved a) If conflict has been resolved Make a decision b) If conflict still apparently exists	• Can a decision be reached about information Tom should be given?
4. Meta-ethical deliberations regarding the relevance of ethical considerations a) If relevance deliberations resolve conflict b) Make a decision c) If an ethical dilemma exists	• Reconsideration by the nurse of the ethical issues above and discussion with the multi-disciplinary team/parents/next of kin in order to assess relevance of ethical approaches/theories to Tom's situation. • Make the decision • A decision cannot be reached, and the dilemma still remains.
5. Meta-ethical deliberations regarding the resolution of the ethical dilemma	• Using the information considered above
6. Tertiary appraisal of ethical considerations — Generate options and estimate consequences	• Identify all possible options and outcomes
7. Make a decision. Document rationale and decision-making process (should be done throughout the process)	• At this point a reasoned decision will be arrived at following full consideration of all issues • This last step is important because accurate records are essential in mental health nursing care and a follow-up evaluation of the outcomes of the decision is also required.

Working through this model's seven stages of ethical decision-making enables the mental health nurse to arrive at a reasoned decision/action in the context of the situation. Applying the model to an ethical dilemma ensures that a collaborative decision is made that involves patient, family, healthcare practitioners and significant others. Failure to use such a framework may result in an ill-informed decision or key elements being overlooked, for example, in the scenario above, a failure to consider Tom's legal entitlements.

CONCLUSION

Changes in societal values and morally dependent social custom inevitably impact on mental health nursing practice, in terms of both context and application, because ultimately definitions of behaviour, mental health and mental illness are socially determined. The fluidity of social change and its relationship to the psychiatric context demonstrates the importance of ethical reflection and self-criticism in mental health nursing at both the macro- and the individual level. A chapter of this length can only briefly address all the issues involved in ethical decision-making in mental health nursing. Ultimately, it gives some indication to you, the reader, of the importance of the path you need to follow in order to be a reflective ethical mental health nurse.

Reflective Questions
1. All of us have a value system. Can you remember what values you had as a child? How do you think you acquired these values? Have they changed? Why might they have changed?
2. What value changes might occur in Ireland in the future that could influence your practice?
3. Identify what you believe are people's rights. Do people who present with mental health problems have different rights?
4. How can you as a mental health nurse apply the principle of justice in the care you provide?

References

An Bord Altranais (2000) *The Code of Professional Conduct for each Nurse and Midwife*. Dublin: An Bord Altranais.

Aristotle (1947) *Nicomachean Ethics* (trans. H. Rackham), revised reprint of 1926 edn. Cambridge, MA/London: Harvard University Press/William Heinemann.

Basford, L. and Slevin, O. (1995) *Theory and Practice of Nursing: An Integrated Approach to Patient Care*. Edinburgh: Campion Press.

Bean, P. (2001) *Mental Disorder and Community Safety*. Hampshire: Palgrave.

Beauchamp, T. L. and Childress, J. (2001) *Principles in Biomedical Ethics* (5th edn). Oxford: Oxford University Press.

Benedict, S. and Kuhla, J. (1999) 'Nurses' participation in the euthanasia programs of Nazi Germany'. *Western Journal of Nursing Research*, 21(2), 246–63.

BenGershôm, E. (1990) 'From Haeckel to Hackethal: Lessons from Nazi medicine for students and practitioners of medicine'. *Holocaust and Genocide Studies*, 5(1), 73–87.

Breeze, J. (1998) 'Can paternalism be justified in mental healthcare?' *Journal of Advanced Nursing*, 8(2), 260–4.

Buchanan-Barker, P. and Barker, P. (2005) 'Observation: the original sin of mental health nursing?' *Journal of Psychiatric and Mental Health Nursing*, 12(5), 541–9.

Channel 4 (2000) *Hitler's Biological Soldiers: Science and the Swastika*. Darlow Smithson Productions: Channel Four Television Corporation.

Dooley, D. and McCarthy, J. (2005) *Nursing Ethics: Irish Cases and Concerns*. Dublin: Gill and Macmillan.

Engwall, K. (2005) 'Starved to death? Nutrition in asylums during the world wars'. *Scandinavian Journal of Disability Research*, 7 (1), 2–22.

Fealy, G. M. (2006) *A History of Apprenticeship Nurse Training in Ireland*. London: Routledge.

Finnegan, F. (2001) *Do Penance or Perish: A Study of Magdalen Asylums in Ireland*. Piltdown: Congrave Press.

Ford, G. G. (2006) *Ethical Reasoning for Mental Health Professionals*. London: Sage Publications.

Fu-Chang Tsai, D. (2001) 'How should doctors approach patients? A Confucian reflection on personhood'. *Journal of Medical Ethics*, 27, 44–50.

Gillon, R. (1986) *Philosophical Medical Ethics*. New York: Wiley.

Gillon, R. (2003) 'Ethics needs principles — four can encompass the rest — and respect for autonomy should be "first among equals"'. *Journal of Medical Ethics*, 29, 307–12.

Kaldjian, L. C., Weir, R. F. and Duffy, T. P. (2005) 'A clinician's approach to clinical ethical reasoning'. *Journal of General Internal Medicine*, 20 (3), 306–11.

Kant, I. (1964) *Groundwork on the Metaphysic of Morals* (trans. H. J. Patton). New York: Harper and Row. (Original work published 1785.)

Kershaw, I. (1999) *Hitler — Hubris*. New York: Norton and Co.

Kershaw, I. (2000) *Hitler — Nemesis WW*. New York: Norton and Co.

McFarland-Icke, B. (1999) *Nurses in Nazi Germany: Moral Choice in History*. New Jersey: Princeton University Press.

Mechanic, D. and Bilder, S. (2004) 'Treatment of people with mental illness: a decade-long perspective'. *Health Affairs*, 23(4), 84–95.

Mental Health Commission (2005) *Quality in Mental Health: Your Views. Report on Stakeholder Consultation in Quality Mental Health Services*. Dublin: Mental Health Commission.

Peplau, H. E. (1988) *Interpersonal Relations in Nursing*. New York: Macmillan Education.

Petifor, J. L. (2001) 'Are professional codes of ethics relevant for multicultural counselling?'. *Canadian Journal of Counselling*, 35, 26–35.

Purtillo, R. (1999) *Ethical Dimensions in the Health Professions* (3rd edn).

Philadelphia: Saunders.

Rawlins, R. P., Williams, S. R. and Beck, C. K. (1993) *Mental Health – Psychiatric Nursing* (3rd edn). London: Elsevier.

Rawls, J. (1971) *A Theory of Justice*. MA: Harvard University Press.

Rumbold, G. (1993) *Ethics in Nursing Practice*. Edinburgh: Balliere Tindall.

Russell, D. (1997) *Scenes from Bedlam: A History of Caring for the Mentally Disordered at Bethlem Royal Hospital and the Maudsley*. London: Bailliere Tindall.

Severinsson, E. (2001) 'Confirmation, meaning and self awareness as core concepts of the nursing supervision model'. *Nursing Ethics*, 1, 36–44.

Thompson, I., Melia, K. M. and Boyd, K. M. (2003) *Nursing Ethics*. Edinburgh: Churchill Livingstone.

Tschudin, V. (2003) *Ethics in Nursing, The Caring Relationship* (3rd edn). Edinburgh: Butterworth Heinemann.

Wells, J. S. G. (1998) 'Severe mental illness, statutory supervision and mental health nursing – meeting the challenge'. *Journal of Advanced Nursing*, 27, 698–706.

Wells, J. S. G. (2004) 'Community mental health policy in the 1990s: a case study in corporate and street level implementation' (unpublished PhD thesis). King's College, University of London.

5

Care Planning: Assessment, Models of Care/Care Frameworks

Liam McGabhann

Care planning is an element of nursing that is introduced at an early stage of nurse training. The process of care planning is usually associated with a cyclical approach to care, e.g. *assessment*, *planning*, *intervention* and *evaluation*, often in association with a model of nursing. Nurses' understanding and perception of the usefulness of care planning is often at odds with the nursing literature, which in turn may be at odds with the realities of practice. In an attempt to avoid some of these pitfalls, this chapter will concentrate on the process of care with an emphasis on matching evolving care with relevant documentation, regardless of what framework or model nurses are required to follow. Models of nursing as care frameworks will not be discussed here: they are covered in depth elsewhere, e.g. Meleis (2005). The aim of this chapter is to enable the integration of the service user and nurses' experience of nursing care with a visible process of care that is meaningful and conducive to documenting for the purpose of continuity. More specifically, this chapter will explore the place of evidence-based assessment in nursing care and examine more inclusive approaches to service users and other healthcare professionals.

PROCESSES OF ASSESSMENT AND CARE

The Nursing Process
The 'nursing process' (Lewis 1970; WHO 1977) was a strategy born out of a need for nurses to articulate the care they as practitioners were providing for patients. It was an attempt to provide an evidence-based approach to nursing care (Marriner 1975) underpinned by a particular model of nursing. As a vehicle for change, the nursing process promised to be a perfect method for framing nursing care. The cyclical repetitive approach is similar to other effective models of change in healthcare (e.g. Schon 1983). The problem solving process includes variations of *assessment* — *planning* — *intervention* — *evaluation*, with scope for repeat cycles as necessary, and it is as relevant today (Bishop and Ford-Bruins 2003) as when it first evolved. It is worth reiterating at this point that the 'nursing process' is simply a vehicle for demonstrating nursing care within a care plan. If this plan has no meaning within the reality of the nurse's practice then the process will stand still. And worse, the time taken up with writing meaningless care plans will

take away from time spent with patients and clients. If Mulhearn's (1989) and Savage's (1991) accounts of the nursing process serving as a means to achieving improved medical practice are also considered, then clearly there can be incongruity as to whether a care plan becomes a nursing process or a medical action plan. An incongruous example might look like Figure 5.1.

Figure 5.1 Care plan: an incongruous example

Presenting problem	Goals of care	Interventions/Action
Admitted due to relapse of schizo-affective disorder	(a) Return to optimum level of functioning	(a) Develop a therapeutic relationship
	(b) Administer prescribed medication	(b) Monitor effects of medication

Assessment————————Planning——————————Intervention——————————Evaluation

This is not to say that the example might not be applicable to nursing interventions, though one would hope that the plan would be framed differently if this were the case. Chenitz and Swanson (1984) discuss the concept of surfacing the nursing process. This is where the nurse brings to the surface exactly what she/he is doing with a client, what information is identified and how she/he is eliciting it; then what actual skills and/or approaches are being used (e.g. brief interventions, supportive counselling, social skills training). 'Surfacing' the nursing process gives life, meaning and achievable possibilities to a care plan. Consider the example in Figure 5.2, where particulars of the care plan are more specific and articulate (though, for the purpose of illustration, not comprehensive).

This is an example of a person admitted to an acute psychiatric admission unit. Depending on the context of care the plan, process and documentary format will differ.

Focus of Nursing Care

The utilisation of interpersonal relationships has always been central to the focus of mental health nursing (Peplau 1952; Altschul 1972; Barker 2001). Subtle changes in how nurses engage with interpersonal processes have emerged over time, and an emphasis on 'doing to or for' the patient has been replaced by the more collaborative notion of 'doing with' the person in distress. Health policy has embraced the concept of 'service user involvement' in all aspects of service delivery from individual practitioner involvement to organisational provision (DoH (UK) 1999; Government of Ireland 2001, 2006). The long unheard voices of service users are slowly seeping into the realities of collaborative daily practice (Diamond et al. 2003). Although not without difficulty, the service user is becoming acknowledged as 'lay expert' by experience, alongside the 'professional expert' (Prior 2003). The recognition of service user as central to the process of care offers hope for the often fragmented continuum of care associated with different professional perspectives in service provision. To date the service user is often the only constant in the care continuum and as such is in a perfect position to piece together the fragments of service provision.

Figure 5.2 Care plan

Presenting problem	Goals of care	Interventions/Action
Crisis admission for John, who is reported as experiencing acute psychotic symptoms	(a) Assess John's mental state and level of social functioning prior to admission (b) For John to feel safe in hospital (c) To help alleviate John's present distress	(a) Engage in collaborative discussions with John in relation to his experiences, offering reassurance where possible (b) Carry out mental state assessment interview* (c) Complete Social Functioning Scale* with John (d) Discuss John's attitude to taking medication and any issues he might have with it (e) Review problem and goals once initial engagement and assessment period is over (within one week).

Assessment————————Planning——————————Intervention———————————Evaluation

* These are specific assessment tools

Recent health policy (Government of Ireland 2001 and 2006) denounces individualistic uni-professional approaches to care in favour of multidisciplinary care. This need not necessarily be problematic as long as there is overall cohesiveness and integration of care. Individualistic introspective approaches that do not encompass wider influences, such as family, social factors and patient preferences, will have limited impact on overall care. An example from clinical practice might be where a person is admitted to an acute admission ward due to 'non-compliance with medication'. The care plan may focus on compliance with medication through the safe, observed administration and observation of effects. It may even offer education on the importance of taking medication. Of course the outcome will be positive, i.e. the person will be compliant when on the ward. Then to the surprise of some, the same person is admitted with the same problem a short time after discharge. Clearly the single professional perspective and approach does not work here and, importantly, the nurse(s) may become despondent about the negative impact of their nursing care. But the care plan could be more meaningful if the Community Mental Health Nurse (CMHN) and/or the family or significant others were incorporated into the process of care. In addition, a more collaborative approach to working with the patient and their attitude to medication may have longer-term benefits, e.g. moving from a stance of 'compliance' to one of 'concordance'. Particular aspects of this type of intervention could begin at ward level and transfer into the community via the patient, CMHN and family member. This more integrated care planning approach would offer greater satisfaction to all concerned and improve the usefulness of the nursing process for in-patient and community nurses.

Because nurses often see care planning as a simple documentary procedure they can often overestimate their knowledge and skills in relation to care planning and overlook the wider implications. Parsons and Barker (2000) identified this tendency when evaluating a mental health practitioner educational programme. Nurses' overestimation of their care planning skills was not borne out when assessed in practice. The importance of nurses 'surfacing' their care plans, being cognisant of the location of care in relation to the care continuum, and aware of the need to integrate it into multidisciplinary care planning, is key to effective practice.

THE PRACTICE OF ASSESSMENT AND CARE PLANNING

The key to the practice of assessment and care planning appears to be the process of engagement in therapeutic relationships. Mental health nurses are in a prime position to capitalise on this, as their core activity is purported to be the development of a therapeutic relationship. Therefore, while surfacing the particular skills and interventions that they might employ in care planning is important, it may not be necessary to have a plethora of therapeutic approaches to hand, as long as the process is meaningful to the context of care. Assessment lies at the heart of effective care planning. Most nurses bring an ethos of care to their practice and for mental health nursing this involves a desire to rescue people from their mental distress. This trait, though laudable, often deters nurses from carrying out a comprehensive assessment of people in distress. Instead nurses can latch onto first impressions and presentations that they can deal with. Barker (2004:6) defines mental health nursing assessment as 'the decision making process, based upon the collection of relevant information, using a formal set of ethical criteria, which contributes to an overall evaluation of a person and his circumstances'.

Although nursing, medical or other diagnosis is an important element of assessment, in itself it is narrow and does not encompass the breadth of a person's experience that led to and may perpetuate their distress. The collection of information is part of a two-stage process of assessment. The second part is the use of that information to identify patient needs, plan interventions and sometimes aid the evaluation of intervention outcomes. The scope of assessment is probably infinite, hence the importance of setting some parameters for the purpose of this chapter. Barker (2004) lists levels of people's lives that may need to be assessed, adding the caveat that this method is not entirely possible because parts of the whole lived experience cannot be assessed in isolation:

- **The physiological self** is the very basic biochemical level of functioning and in reality we cannot be sensitive to this essential level of functioning.
- **The biological self** is more easily consciously felt: it refers to working organs and the musculoskeletal system, where changes, e.g. pain, can be felt and assessed.
- **The behavioural self** is how we think, feel and act depending on the situation. Here our thoughts and feelings have a significant effect on how we behave.
- **The social self** involves our relationship with the people who make up our world, such as family friends and others that impact on our selves.
- **The spiritual self** is where our hopes, dreams and beliefs reside. It is here where we experience views of ourselves and our world that are all too often impossible to define or capture in assessment.

A perhaps less 'humanistic', more descriptive summary of areas warranting assessment prior to formulating a care plan is offered by Gamble and Brennan (2006):

- Risk.
- Physical and mental health status.
- Social needs and functioning.
- Symptomatology and coping skills.
- Quality of life and its effects on others.
- Housing and money.
- Social support.
- Medicine and its effects.
- Work skills and meaningful daily activity.

Both examples offer a broad scope for assessment and, depending on the practice or experience of life context, either, both or a combination of the two might be appropriate. Each person will have their own perceptions and understandings of how the world and people in the world normally present themselves. They are influenced by experiences, socialisation, education and professionalisation. Therefore, when engaged in the assessment of another individual, it is important to acknowledge differences and ensure that the assessment strategy does not disadvantage the person's experience because of those differences. It is necessary to clarify what type of assessments are to be carried out and offer a rationale as to why the approach is been taken and to what ends: for example, in the interest of the patient, as an aid to further intervention and evaluation or as part of a standardised approach to everyone.

Three frequent approaches to assessment are: interviewing; observation; and use of assessment tools. Often these are integrated and there is crossover between them, for example a sleep chart can be described as an observation checklist or as an assessment tool. Likewise some mental state assessment tools (e.g. KGV 1977, *see* Figure 5.3) are also described as structured clinical interviews.

The Interview

Interviews are often structured in a particular format (e.g. initial assessment formats or mental state interviews) that is applied to all people. Depending on the flexibility of approach they may assume that all people are alike; or they may be more flexible and person-centred, such as narrative interviews in which the person is asked to relate the story of their experience and how they think they can be helped. The semi-structured interview is offered here as a form of initial assessment somewhere between a standardised and narrative format and the principles are easily understood and applied (Fox and Conroy 2006). There are two important underlying principles associated with this approach.

1. Be pragmatic — approach the interview with a clear outcome in mind, i.e. to establish what problems are currently causing the individual difficulties in their daily life and what the practical consequences are. Emphasis must be placed on the consequences rather than the cause.
2. Expectation — nurses will have expectations of the individual. It is important that they demonstrate positive assumptions about the client. This includes the assumption that the person will be responsive to the help offered and work in partnership with the nurse, allowing them to have control and responsibility. Acknowledge that this person is coping or trying to cope with their problems; that the problems are real and not just there because the person does not help themselves; and that the person is telling the truth about their problems. The principles may sound simple, though for some practitioners with traditional paternalistic belief systems there may be some difficulty employing them, but they are necessary for successful engagement with a client.

Identifying specific problems is not always easy. Various formats can help the interviewer to focus the interview on establishing these specifics and in particular drawing out components of the problem (e.g. antecedents, behaviours, consequences) that help inform resultant interventions. For a comprehensive discussion of these formats, see Gamble and Brennan (2006). Interviews are a useful assessment method for eliciting information and beginning or improving the process of engagement. Normally they will be complemented by further assessment through observation and/or use of specific assessment tools.

Observations

Observation is often second nature to nurses who spend a lot of time among healthcare professionals in contact with patients/clients. It is useful as a means to corroborate and accentuate information derived from the interview, though where possible should not be used as a stand-alone assessment. By definition an observation is taken from the perspective of the observer, and care should be taken when interpreting observations or taking action as a consequence, as perceptions can be misleading. Other sources, such as explanations by the patient/client or family member, should also be taken into the equation.

Examples of observations might depend on the context of an assessment, and the list is extensive. Pertinent examples include:

- sleep pattern
- dietary intake
- physical observations: pulse, temperature, blood pressure
- behaviours
- appearance
- odour
- interaction with others
- posture and movement
- potential side effects of medication
- speech content and form
- activity levels
- responses to environment and/or individuals.

Use of Specific Assessment Tools

Although any form of information collecting can be described as an assessment tool, increasingly specific measurement tools are being employed in mental healthcare. They are particularly useful in validating and supporting clinical judgement and decision-making and providing a measured evidence base to interventions. They are also useful for making sense of decisions made by other people involved in care. One might use a depression scale to indicate the severity of depression in an individual. Consequently, following interventions, a second score might be taken that indicates improvement. A score in itself is an indicator, but it does not tell the assessor any more about the person or their experience. It does enable the person in distress to see that improvement has been made and if the particular statements or domains making up the assessment tool are then discussed in relation to improvements, the ensuing discussion will give substance to the score.

Assessment scales are often developed as research instruments in the first instance and then adopted for use in clinical practice. The structured line of questioning can help clients and practitioners to draw out particular issues for a client that warrant further investigation. In cases where people's problems appear insurmountable and sometimes unspecific, there are tools available that will help break down the problems into measurable, observable specifics. Scales may be completed by practitioners or/and by the people themselves. Either way it is important that client and nurse discuss the implications of completed scores. This enables focused interventions to be applied. For a glossary of common scales used in mental health see Gamble and Brennan (2006). Figure 5.3 provides a brief overview of sample scales commonly used in mental health nursing.

Not all tools are subject to scrutiny through research, though they may be equally useful in clinical practice. A simple tool for practice is the scaling question: the client is asked to rate their problem, distress or degree of goal achievement on a scale of one to eight or zero to 100. The nurse may also rate these from their perspective and discuss differences and common perceptions. This method of assessment is excellent in care planning: adaptable to any documentary format used; simple to complete in any type of meeting with clients; and a useful indicator of change. It can be quite difficult to detect change at times during ongoing engagement, particularly where people have little hope for improvement. Assessment tools play an important role in capturing change and if the results are incorporated into positive discussions, there is increased potential for a person to perceive a better future. A comprehensive assessment will set out a baseline for effective care planning. It is unlikely that any one nurse or patient/client will be able to address all the needs/problems identified in the assessment, nor should they try. Assessment should not stop once care plans are developed and should play an important part in ongoing evaluation of care.

PROBLEMS AND GOALS IN CARE PLANNING

Depending on the approach nurses are taking, needs, strengths or problems may be used in care planning, though each may be framed differently. For consistency we shall discuss 'problems', while recognising that 'needs' or 'strengths' can equally be applied to the illustrated care planning process. Working towards 'goals' is common to all approaches at an individual engagement level or at an organisational level (Macpherson *et al.* 1999).

Problem Statements

Problems need to be articulated in such a way that they are conducive to resolution, otherwise there is a danger of continually refocusing on an unmovable intangible problem. Problem statements are an end product of the initial assessment process and a basis for consequent interventions in care. Useful problem statements will include a definition of the problem, the impact of the problem and the consequences for the person (see Figure 5.4). Where possible the statement should be in the client's own words, jargon-free and always agreed with them. For some nurses working in institutional settings, role ambiguity may make it difficult for collaborative problem statements in the first instance. For example, an involuntary patient may just want to get out of hospital and see no other problem. It is possible to work in collaboration with a patient on this problem, though it may be necessary to negotiate other problems that can be worked on in the meantime so that ongoing engagement is encouraged.

Figure 5.3 Assessment scales used in mental health nursing

Assessing	Assessment scale	Brief overview
Symptoms	BPRS — Brief Psychiatric Rating Scale (Overall and Gorham 1962)	A validated measure of general psychiatric symptoms including verbal reports (somatic concerns, anxiety, guilt, grandiosity, depressive mood, hostility, suspiciousness, hallucinatory behaviour and unusual thoughts) and observations by practitioner during interview. Originally had 16 items, with several adaptations over time and according to context. This is a seven-point Likert scale ranging from 'not present' to 'extremely severe'.
	KGV — Manchester Severity Scale (Krawiecka et al. 1977)	A semi-structured psychiatric assessment tool that uses a phenomenological sequence of questions to elicit symptoms and meanings of symptoms to the service user. Similar to the BPRS in that it scores both verbal responses in interview and practitioner observations. It has undergone several adaptations, most recently by Stuart Lancashire (1996), who developed a 12-point Likert scale.
	BDI — Beck Depression Inventory (Beck et al. 1981)	Measures the severity of depressive states where the person self-scores a four-point Likert scale or practitioner completes it through interview. Contains 21 items.
Global Assessment of Need	CAN — Camberwell Assessment of Need (Phelan et al. 1995)	Assesses the met and unmet needs of people with serious mental illness. The scale contains 22 items across a range of health and social care needs, scored on a four-point Likert scale. Easy and quick to complete by way of a semi-structured interview.
Health Beliefs	BAVQ — Beliefs About Voices Questionnaire (Chadwick and Birchwood 1995).	30 questions with yes or no answers, designed to elicit the feelings a person has about hallucinatory voices.

Assessing	Assessment scale	Brief overview
Social Functioning	SFS — Social Functioning Scale (Birchwood *et al.* 1990)	Assesses the aspects of a person's social functioning that are affected by their mental health difficulties. Covers seven areas of functioning (including social withdrawal, activities, independence, relationships and employment) providing a guide to goals, interventions and measurement of progress.
Medication Side Effects	LUNSERS — Liverpool University Neuroleptic Side Effects Rating Scale (Day *et al.* 1995)	A self-rating scale with 51 items that enables service users to rate the presence of side effects from neuroleptic medication. It also scores the level of distress caused by each side effect.

Figure 5.4 Impact and consequence of the problem for the person

Problem definition	Impact	Consequences
Avoids going out. Believes people say bad things about him	Stays at home in bedroom	Feels lonely and isolated

Source: adapted from Gamble and Brennan 2006

It is useful to measure the extent of problems or the level of distress they are causing the person, as this will help nurse and client to demonstrate the effectiveness of their interventions. A simple format is the scaling question that can be used to establish a baseline measure and thereafter to measure impact of the care plan. Figure 5.5 offers an example linked to the problem described in Figure 5.4 whereby the patient and nurse will rate the problem.

Figure 5.5 Rating scale

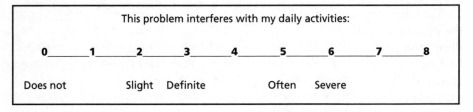

Once the problem statement is complete, the person's goals can be agreed.

Goal Statements

Goals are considered to be a positive change for the client in relation to their current problem. They normally describe behaviour that when consistently implemented will result in a reduction in the severity of the problem. They should not be finalised until there has been a discussion about how they can be achieved. Like problems, goals need to be observable and measurable, otherwise evaluation will be difficult. A useful guideline in formulating goal statements is to use the SMART approach (Specific, Measurable, Achievable, Realistic and Time-bound) (Egan 1990). An example for the above problem might be that described in Figure 5.6.

Figure 5.6 An example of a goal statement

The behaviour	Conditions	Frequency
Go out of house with family member	Walk through lightly populated areas	For half an hour three times a week

Ensure a baseline measure is taken by patient/client and nurse of goal achievement at designated intervals, as in the example in Figure 5.7.

Figure 5.7 Rating scale

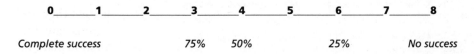

My progress towards achieving this goal:

0_____1_____2_____3_____4_____5_____6_____7_____8

Complete success   75%   50%   25%   No success

So far the processes described have not been incorporated into an overall care plan, and discrete examples offer aspects of a wider approach to care that may incorporate a variety of client and nurse interventions. Incorporating a documentary framework has been avoided to prevent pigeon-holing the care planning process into any one framework or model.

The following case study will, while avoiding a documentary framework, bring the processes together into one care plan with built-in ongoing evaluation. For illustrative purposes the care plan will centre on preventing relapse as described by Knight (2002). This can be carried out at a basic level by any nurse or more specifically by a nurse with skills training. Here the basic level will suffice. The care plan relates to in-patient and community care with the involvement of John, his family and members of the multidisciplinary team, though the care plan is initiated and processed through a nursing care plan.

Case Study

John is a 25-year-old male admitted to an acute psychiatric admission unit following a fight with a group of people sitting outside a pub. He was brought to the unit by the Gardai and his mother. They were concerned that his bizarre behaviour and aggression towards the group of people would pose a risk to himself or others. John has been admitted to the unit on four occasions, the first time when he was 19 and most recently six months ago. He has a medical diagnosis of schizo-affective disorder. John lives at home with his mother, father and two sisters. He also has a brother who lives in a flat nearby. John says he gets on okay with his family and has a particularly good relationship with his mother.

John left school after his Leaving Certificate and completed a course in technical drawing. He has had a few jobs, which he does not stay in for very long, usually leaving or being let go due to 'not getting on with them'. He has not worked since his last discharge. John used to like walking in the country, playing football, listening to bands and socialising with a couple of good friends. He has had a few short-term heterosexual relationships, though none since his last admission. For the past four months John has stopped going out with friends and playing football. He spends a lot of time in his room listening to music, only going out for brief periods with his family members when they pressurise him.

Problem statement

(John and his named nurse on the unit developed the problem statement during the first few days of admission following initial assessment and a consequent semi-structured interview.)

> 'When I am stressed and meet people out and about I believe they are calling me a pervert. I get angry and confront them, which sometimes ends up in a fight. Then I get brought into hospital where I don't want to be.'

Goal statement

(The goal statement is broader than previous examples, although step-by-step exposure to going out may form an element of the plan at a later stage once he has taken on board a strategy to try and prevent readmission. The CMHN rather than in-patient nurse will probably instigate this.)

> 'I want to be able to go out and about without getting into fights and ending up in hospital.'

Interventions

(Interventions are agreed in advance with John. See box below for stages of relapse prevention approach.)

1. John and nurse will develop a timeline of events, significant interactions and the effect of these on John's stress levels over four weeks prior to admission.
2. John to identify triggers that seem to tie in with his rising stress levels, breaking these down into feelings, behaviours and thinking. With John's permission, include his mother's or other identified family members' observations in identifying these

triggers. If necessary use cue cards for John to look through with a list of possible triggers. (*There are common triggers associated with relapse, but breaking down triggers into feelings, behaviours and thinking makes it easier to measure effects, particularly if other complementary interventions are being used.*)

3. Ask John to identify the coping mechanisms he presently employs to deal with his stress and concerns about people calling him a pervert. With John, talk about those that have a positive impact and a negative impact, encouraging further development of the positive mechanisms.

4. Discuss further coping mechanisms with John, teaching and practising these where relevant and agreed (e.g. distraction techniques, relaxation techniques at key times). If John is willing to engage with it, discuss the possible role of medication in his coping with his stress. (*If John is agreeable, this is a good time to bring his mother into the process as she might be party to helping him with coping mechanisms (e.g. going out with him for short periods). It is also an opportunity to bring his CMHN into discussions.*)

5. With John's agreement, devise a plan for John to implement if his identified triggers begin to return in the future. This could be staged according to the triggers' intensity and level of escalation. Try to ensure that John's mother and CMHN are part of the plan, i.e. if certain triggers happen they will remind him of the plan and/or by prior arrangement with John instigate an intervention (e.g. increase distraction or relaxation techniques, reduce activity, take PRN medication or arrange session with CMHN or psychiatrist). The key is for the plan to be activated before John's stress levels result in another incident that might have him admitted to hospital.

6. Arrange for CMHN to meet with John after discharge at designated intervals to go through the plan and measure the present extent of problem and goal achievement. (*It is here where the CMHN's engagement might begin to explore other problems and goals.*)

Relapse Prevention Approach: Stages of the Process
- 1 and 2 identifies relapse signature
- 3, 4 and 5 is the relapse prevention plan
- 5 involves rehearsal, monitoring and clarification of plan.

RATIONALE FOR INTERVENTIONS

A rationale must be given for any interventions, otherwise colleagues may not be aware of the approach, process and/or changes in the patient and some may not understand what is going on. Equally, the rationale and approach taken should be discussed with other professional colleagues, as the work will be impacted upon by their engagement with the process. For example, no mention was made of psychosis in the care plan, as it was not something that John entertained. At the same time it is likely that John will be treated with medication as an in-patient for psychosis. A clear rationale for interventions will go a long way to preventing miscommunications and inadvertent sabotage of the relapse prevention plan.

Note: Be prepared and flexible to adapt to changes occurring with John that do not fit the care plan. Ensure that the care plan changes accordingly. For example, relapse prevention work often engages patients in questioning their own beliefs about their experiences, and they may change these as interventions occur. Remember to go with the patient's theory and pace of change.

CONCLUSION

Today's healthcare environment requires nurses to demonstrate in practice and in writing what care they are providing. Historical influences on how we construct and implement care plans have to some extent hindered the integration of care planning with actualities of practice. This is not a justification for not doing them well. Clinically effective care plans need to give meaning and life to the experiences of people in mental distress and nurses trying to improve upon these experiences. Without this they are simply paper exercises and nurses would be better off doing something useful with their time. It is hoped that the processes and methods outlined in this chapter offer some potential for integrating the realities of practice with a documentary of care.

Reflective Questions
1. Consider the care plan of a person you have nursed. To what extent did it reflect the medical diagnosis and care as opposed to interventions agreed by the patient/client and nurse?
2. Effective assessment and care planning requires nurses to engage in a collaborative way with the lived experiences of people they care for. How could this involve a shift in your present understandings, perspective and approach to nursing?
3. Think about a person you have nursed. To what extent did their assessment and care reflect their lived experience and hopes for the future?
4. Reflect on John's case study and the processes described in this chapter. How might they be usefully incorporated into the care of someone in your practice area?

References
Altschul, A. (1972) *Patient-nurse Interaction*. Edinburgh: Churchill Livingstone.
Barker, P. (2001) 'The tidal model: developing a person-centred approach to psychiatric and mental health nursing'. *Perspectives in Psychiatric Care*, 37(3), 79–87.
Barker, P. (2004) *Assessment in Psychiatric and Mental Health Nursing: In Search of the Whole Person*. Surrey: Nelson Thornes.
Beck, A. T., Ward, C. H., Mendelson, M., Mock, J., and Erbaugh, J. (1961) 'An inventory for measuring depression'. *Archives of General Psychiatry*, 4, 561–71.

Birchwood, M., Smith, J. and Cocherane, R. (1990). 'The Social Functioning Scale: the development and validation of a new scale of social adjustment in use in family interventions programmes with schizophrenic patients'. *British Journal of Psychiatry*, 157, 853–9.

Bishop, D. and Ford-Bruins, I. (2003) 'Nurses' perceptions of mental health assessment in an acute inpatient setting in New Zealand: a qualitative study'. *International Journal of Mental Health Nursing*, 12, 203–12.

Chadwick, P. and Birchwood, M. (1995) 'The omnipotence of voices II: the beliefs about voices questionnaire'. *British Journal of Psychiatry*, 166, 11–19.

Chenitz, W. C. and Swanson, J. M. (1984) 'Surfacing nursing process; a method of generating nursing theory from practice'. *Journal of Advanced Nursing*, 9, 205–15.

Day, J. C., Wood, G., Dewey, M. and Bentall, R. (1995). 'A self-rating scale for measuring neuroleptic side effects. Validation in a group of schizophrenic patients'. *British Journal of Psychiatry*, 166, 650–3.

Department of Health (UK) (DoH) (1999) *National Service Framework for Mental Health*. London: HMSO.

Diamond, B., Parkin, G., Morris, K., Bettinis, J. and Bettesworth. C. (2003) 'User involvement: substance or spin?' *Journal of Mental Health*, 12 (6), 613–26.

Egan, G. (1990) *The Skilled Helper: A Systematic Approach to Effective Helping*. California: Brooks Cole.

Fox, J. and Conroy, P. (2006) 'Consolidating the assessment process: the semi-structured interview', in C. Gamble and G. Brennan (eds), *Working with Serious Mental Illness: A Manual for Clinical Practice* (2nd edn). London: Bailliere Tindall.

Gamble, C. and Brennan, G. (2006) *Working With Serious Mental Illness: A Manual for Clinical Practice* (2nd edn). London: Bailliere Tindall.

Government of Ireland (2001) *Quality and Fairness: A Health System for You*. Dublin: Stationery Office.

Government of Ireland (2006) *A Vision for Change: Report of the Expert Group on Mental Health Policy*. Dublin: Stationery Office.

Knight, A. (2002) 'Relapse prevention interventions in psychosis', in N. Harris, S. Williams and T. Bradshaw (eds), *Psychosocial Interventions for People with Schizophrenia: A Practical Guide for Mental Health Workers*. Basingstoke: Palgrave Macmillan.

Krawiecka, M., Goldberg, D. and Vaughn, M. (1977) 'A standardised psychiatric assessment scale for rating chronic psychotic patients'. *Acta Psychiatrica Scandinavica*, 55, 299–308.

Lewis, L. (1970) *Planning Patient Care*. Iowa: WC Brown Co.

Macpherson, R., Jerrom, B., Lott, G. and Ryce, M. (1999) 'The outcome of clinical goal setting in a mental health rehabilitation service. A model for evaluating clinical effectiveness'. *Journal of Mental Health*, 8(1), 95–102.

Marriner, A. (1975) *The Nursing Process: A Scientific Approach to Nursing*. St Louis: Mosby.

Meleis, A. I. (2005) *Theoretical Nursing: Development and Progress* (3rd edn). London: Lippincott Williams and Wilkins.

Mulhearn, S. (1989) 'The nursing process: improving psychiatric admission assessment?' *Journal of Advanced Nursing*, 14, 808–14.

Overall, J. and Gorham, D. (1962) 'Brief Psychiatric Rating Scale'. *Psychological Reports*, 10, 799–812.

Parsons, S. and Barker, P. (2000) 'The Phil Hearne course: an evaluation of a multidisciplinary mental health education programme for clinical practitioners'. *Journal of Psychiatric and Mental Health Nursing*, 7, 101–8.

Peplau, H. E. (1952) *Interpersonal Relations in Nursing*. New York: Putnam.

Phelan, M., Slade, M., Thornicroft, G., Dunn, G., Holloway, F., Wykes, T., Strathdee, G., Loftus, L., McCrone, P. and Hayward, P. (1995) 'The Camberwell Assessment of Need: the validity and reliability of an instrument to assess the needs of people with severe mental illness'. *British Journal of Psychiatry*, 167, 589–95.

Prior, L. (2003) 'Belief, knowledge and expertise: the emergence of the lay expert in medical sociology'. *Sociology of Health and Illness*, 25, 41–57.

Savage, P. (1991) 'Patient assessment in psychiatric nursing'. *Journal of Advanced Nursing*, 16, 311–16.

Schon, D. A. (1983) *The Reflective Practitioner: How Professionals Think in Action*. New York: Basic Books.

World Health Organisation Regional Office for Europe (1977) *Development of Designs in, and the Documentation of, the Nursing Process. Report on a Technical Advisory Group, Copenhagen, 7–10 June*. Geneva: WHO.

6
Mental Health and Mental Health Promotion

Denis Ryan and Christine Deasy

This chapter introduces the reader to the key concepts of mental health promotion. It begins by contextualising mental health promotion in current discourses and definitions of health and mental health. It proposes a holistic understanding of health promotion, incorporating mental health and mental health promotion as a domain of practice. It situates the practice of mental health nursing within the understanding of health and mental health promotion.

DEFINING HEALTH

To understand mental health promotion and the role of the nurse in this domain of practice, it is important to understand the concepts of health and health promotion. Health is one of the concepts that is most taken for granted once we have it. The word 'health' is drawn from an old English word (*hael*) meaning 'whole' (Naidoo and Wills 2000). Despite the World Health Organisation's (WHO) long-standing definition of health, which has remained largely unchanged since 1946, and the ancient origins of the word itself, health remains one of the concepts on which there is little consensus. In its constitution, the World Health Organisation defined health as 'a state of complete physical mental and social well-being and not merely the absence of disease or infirmity' (WHO 1946:2). An important aspect of this definition is that it refers to health as a 'state'. The WHO clarified this definition in the mid-1970s, when it reiterated that health is a 'state' but emphasised that health should not be understood exclusively as an absence of illness.

The fact that such clarifications are necessary points to a fundamental issue in terms of understanding health, i.e. there can be key differences between official definitions and popular understanding of health. While the WHO definition of health is both long-standing and broadly accepted, the popular understanding of health has tended to remain focused on its direct relationship with illness. This may well be linked with the fact that most definitions of health are offered by medical, as opposed to health, specialists. Whatever the reason, health has tended to be understood as a state in which illness is absent, rather than a state with its own distinct characteristics and conceptual elements.

The idea of health being considered a particular 'state' is also probably erroneous and unhelpful, as it suggests that health is static and unchanging. Health as experienced by an individual is in fact dynamic and changes over time. Personal understandings of health are likely to be very different among males and females (Cox 1985) or teenagers and older adults (Ryan *et al.* 2006). Social role and occupational status also influence understandings of health (Jones 1994).

In the context of such constraints, the WHO have more recently described health as:

> The extent to which an individual or group is able, on the one hand, to realise aspirations and safety needs and on the other hand, to change or cope with the environment. Health is therefore seen as a resource for everyday life, not the objective of living: it is a positive concept emphasising social and personal resources as well as physical capabilities.
>
> (WHO 1984:23)

Understanding health as a 'resource' rather than a state is closer to the understanding of well-being as proposed by Ryan *et al.* (2006:6), who argue that:

> Wellbeing refers to the person's ability to understand, accept, manage or cope with their own level of ability or functioning. It will encompass their worldview of their own situation, their perception of their health status in the context of their living arrangements and may be influenced by internal factors such as self-esteem, cognitive processes, knowledge, insight, among others.

Situating one's health status within such variables as personal ability, living arrangements, social situation and knowledge suggest a transactional understanding of health and a more holistic understanding of the concept. More important, from the perspective of mental health, it places mental health as a core component of health status. Understanding the influences on health and health status as being either influenced by multiple variables (Ryan *et al.* 2006) or determined by them (WHO 2004a) means that responsibility for promoting health, preventing illness or managing manifestations of ill health become shared responsibilities.

DEFINING MENTAL HEALTH

The same types of difficulty emerge when trying to define mental health as with the definition of health. These difficulties relate primarily to the fact that it is conceptually incoherent to adopt a reductionist approach which sub-divides mental health from health, if one assumes a holistic understanding of health. Historically, health was viewed as a holistic concept. Hippocrates, the Greek physician and father of medicine, born around 400 BC, believed health to be dependent on equilibrium between the mind, body and environment. Galen, the Roman physician and philosopher, born AD 129, had a similar philosophy.

The seventeenth-century philosopher René Descartes, whose work has continued strongly to influence contemporary thinking, is credited with crystallising the distinction between the mind and the body. This presumed dichotomy led to a separation between so-called 'mental' and 'physical health'. The separation of mental and physical health is inconsistent with a holistic view of health and of individuals, which is a fundamental assumption of health promotion. This fragmentation has not been unnoticed. Indeed, there have been calls internationally for the activities of mental health promotion to be mainstreamed with health promotion (Herrmann 2001, WHO 2001a). Mental health promotion, based on a holistic understanding of health, should be an integral part of health promotion rather than a separate entity.

Accepting that mental health is a core component of health has implications for its definition. Essentially it means that we cannot understand mental health as a discrete entity, but should rather look at it as an element of an integrated whole. Moving to this holistic understanding of health has implications for the practice and ethos of health service professions. The return to a more holistic public and professional understanding of health is emphasised in the *Green Paper on Mental Health* (European Commission 2005:4) in its assertion that 'there is no health without mental health'.

Just as physical health is more than the absence of physical illness and disease, mental health is more than the absence of mental illness. However, there is often confusion between the terms *mental health* and *mental illness* and the fact that the term *mental health* is often used interchangeably with the term *mental illness* has compounded this confusion. Brennan (2000) emphasises this point in his assertion that psychiatric services in Ireland are now referred to as mental health services and psychiatric nurses as mental health nurses.

To clarify the distinction between mental health and mental illness Ryan *et al.* (2006:85) argue that 'mental illness may be conceptually understood as the end point on a continuum of mental health within the context of a holistic understanding of health'. Interestingly, they also note that 'mental health can be seen as a continuum ranging from optimum health to minimum health (including illness states) rather than an absolute state'. In keeping with this notion of continuum, Fontaine (2003:45) argues that mental health is a 'lifelong process and includes a sense of harmony and balance for the individual, family, friends and community'.

The WHO (2001b), consistent with their idea of health as a state, describe mental health as a state of well-being in which the individual realises his or her abilities, is able to cope with the normal stresses of life, works productively and fruitfully and contributes to his or her community. This understanding of mental health can be legitimately criticised on the basis that it understands mental health as a static entity, rather than a dynamic or holistic concept that involves both the individual and the broader context in which they find themselves. Mental health must be understood as a transactional phenomenon that involves an integrated relationship between the individual and the broader world in which they live (Ryan *et al.* 2006). In that regard there are a number of factors that may positively and negatively influence mental health (see Figure 6.1).

Figure 6.1 Factors that may influence mental health

Positive influences	Negative influences
Social competence	Poor interpersonal relationships or social isolation
Positive self-esteem	Low self-esteem, discrimination
Good physical health	Having a physical illness or disability
Appropriate coping and life skills	Inadequate or inappropriate social and coping skills
The ability to deal with change	Inability to communicate or express feelings
Adequate resources, social and environmental structures	Unmet needs, poverty, unemployment
Having access to support services	Difficulty accessing support services

Source: Ryan *et al.* (2006)

MENTAL HEALTH PROMOTION IN THE CONTEXT OF THE OTTAWA CHARTER

Clearly, the definition of mental health as a holistic concept means that we must also understand work associated with promoting mental health within that framework. Indeed, it could be argued that the definition of health promotion, as set out in the Ottawa Charter, is the embodiment of mental health promotion. It argues that health promotion is 'the process of enabling people to increase control over, and to improve, their health' (WHO *et al.*1986:1), which suggests a facilitative process. It also argues that in order to achieve a state of well-being it is necessary for relevant individuals or groups to be able to 'identify and to realize aspirations, to satisfy needs, and to change or cope with the environment' (WHO *et al.* 1986:1). These abilities are closely allied to self-esteem enhancement, the development of coping strategies as well as the cognitive processes related to decision-making and are clearly within the realm of mental health and, by implication, mental health promotion.

Health promotion, as guided by the Ottawa Charter (WHO *et al.* 1986), involves activities aimed at: building healthy public policy; the creation of supportive environments; strengthening community actions; developing personal skills; and the reorientation of health services. Mental health promotion must also be seen in this context. This understanding is consistent with the definition of mental health promotion offered by Hodgson (1996:2), who defines it as work focused on 'the enhancement of individuals, families, groups or communities to strengthen or support positive emotional, cognitive and related experience'. This clearly advocates that mental health promotion activities should be directed at both individuals and groups. Ryan *et al.* (2006) propose that mental health promotion should therefore focus on two key 'capacity' issues; namely supportive actions and empowerment approaches. Supportive actions enhance the factors that contribute to optimal health and simultaneously reduce factors that lead to illness conditions, while empowerment approaches focus on helping individuals and groups identify and respond appropriately to factors that negatively impact on health status. Where the focus of these actions or interventions are directed towards individuals or families, they can be considered to be occurring at a micro level, while actions directed towards communities or policymakers can be said to be taking place at a macro level.

MENTAL HEALTH PROMOTION IN THE CONTEXT OF IRISH HEALTH ACTIVITY

From a macro level perspective, examination of the mental health service in Ireland demonstrates how health promotion principles have underpinned policy and service developments since at least 1984 when the national policy document entitled *Psychiatric Services: Planning for the Future* (Government of Ireland 1984) was published. This document set out a framework for the reorientation of mental health services. It also set the agenda for the restructuring of the organisational arrangements for mental health services. The principles set out in this policy document were clearly embedded in a philosophy of community empowerment and development. In more recent times other manifestations of this approach include the enactment of the Mental Health Act 2001, the establishment of the Mental Health Commission and the publication of the strategy *A Vision for Change* (Government of Ireland 2006), in which there was a strong emphasis on principles of social inclusion and a recognition of changing demographics and the need for awareness of ethnic diversity in multicultural societies. Therefore, while not explicitly stated, the ethos of the Irish mental health services has been embedded in principles of health promotion for more than a quarter of a century — at least at a policy level.

From a micro level perspective there are a number of strategies that are used to promote the mental health of individuals. These include working with individuals in areas such as: skills building to increase life skills, social skills and coping skills; enhancing self-esteem and self-acceptance; advocacy; and empowerment. While these approaches are shared among many occupations working in mental health fields, they are very common interventions in mental health nursing. There are also a number of national programmes operating to promote mental health, examples of which are presented in Figure 6.2.

Figure 6.2 Examples of national programmes operating to promote mental health

Programme	Organised by	Focus
Mental Health Matters	Mental Health Ireland	A mental health resource pack for secondary schools aimed at addressing the issue of mental health in a realistic, relevant and age-appropriate manner for 14–18-year-olds
National Public Speaking Project	Mental Health Ireland	Schools Mental Health Awareness and Public Speaking Project aims to promote awareness among young people of the importance of positive mental health and to reduce negative attitudes and prejudices associated with mental illness
Cool School	North Eastern Health Board's child psychiatric services	Anti-bullying programme and support targeted at the Irish second-level schools service
Relationship and Sexuality Education (RSE)	Department of Education	School-based programme that aims to develop responsible attitudes, values and beliefs about sexual identity, personal relationships and intimacy in pupils at junior cycle level
Social and Personal Health Education (SPHE)	Department of Education	School-based programme at junior cycle level, in post-primary schools. Focus is on promoting physical, mental and emotional health and well-being, developing skills for self-fulfilment and living in communities, promoting self-esteem, self-confidence and responsible decision-making
Community mothers programme	HSE	Evidence-based community programme, which is targeted at disadvantaged first and second time parents of children under the age of two. Experienced mothers from the local community are trained to visit families to provide necessary support
Fás Le Chéile	HSE (formerly North Western Health Board)	Promotes positive relationships between parents and young children. Parent group leaders are trained to run courses for parents, in conjunction with their local primary school

Programme	Organised by	Focus
Le Chéile and Art in Mind	Mental Health Ireland (Limerick)	Le Chéile aims to provide a supportive and relaxed meeting place for those who have experienced difficulties in coping with their families and their friends. This is run in conjunction with a creative arts programme
Mental Health Days	HSE (former NWHB) Health Promotion Service in partnership with Mental Health Service, Regional Child and Family Service, Psychology Service, Youth Service and the voluntary and community sector	School-based events for senior cycle students, teachers and parents. The aim is to promote positive attitudes to mental health, introduce students and teachers to positive coping skills and provide an opportunity for students, teachers and parents to meet with the service providers
Go for Life	Age and Opportunity initiative funded by the Irish Sports Council	Aims to involve older adults in all aspects of sport and physical activity

APPLYING THE PRINCIPLES OF MENTAL HEALTH PROMOTION

It is accepted that mental health promotion in its broadest sense refers to any action to enhance the mental health of individuals, groups or communities (Ryan *et al.* 2006). In practice, however, some difficulties arise in relation to a poor distinction between health promotion and illness prevention. Examples of this can be found in the Suicide Prevention Strategy (HSE *et al.* 2005), which incorporates elements of health promotion principles, but clearly both the title and legitimate remit of the strategy is directed to the prevention of self-harm. While there can and probably should be an overlap between these domains of practice, health professionals are sometimes not clear on the distinctions between promoting mental health and preventing mental illness, but they should be, as this type of ambiguity contributes to the misunderstanding.

Distinguishing Mental Health Education and Promotion

Much of the work of health professionals who engage in 'health promotion' activities involves making information available to service users and interpreting that information for them. For example, public talks, workshops and seminars on 'health' topics are intended to educate those who attend on how to manage their illnesses or those of their relatives. Although these are an important element of an empowerment approach, they are limited. While the intention of such an approach is to facilitate the empowerment of individuals or families, through education, its focus is normally specifically related to illness conditions as opposed to health promotion from a holistic perspective, yet they are frequently referred to as health promotion activities. It is imperative that health professionals are aware that health promotion incorporates a wider approach than this. Health education, a legitimate activity aimed at empowerment, is distinct from health promotion. Whitehead (2001) proposes that nurses frequently fail to conceptualise the differences between both as distinct processes and argues that what nurses refer to as health promotion would often be more appropriately called traditional health education.

Mental Health Promotion in Irish Mental Health Services

Most mental health nurses in Ireland operate in secondary and tertiary services, where their practice is primarily focused on supporting individual clients in the management of their own illness conditions. Within that context, it is also crucial that mental healthcare is delivered in an empowering, participatory and collaborative manner. The requirement to base practice on principles of empowerment is enshrined in the *Code of Professional Conduct* (An Bord Altranais 2000), which emphasises the role of the therapeutic relationship in empowering clients to make life choices. Similarly, Peplau (1994) asserts that the changes clients need to undertake occur within the context of such specific helping relationships. While such sentiments clearly place empowerment (one of the core concepts of health promotion) in a position of centrality within the role of the mental health nurse, they do so almost exclusively on an individual level.

Centrality of the Client

The importance of client participation was brought to the fore by the World Health Organisation's claim that people have the right and duty to participate individually and collectively in the planning and implementation of their healthcare (WHO 1978). However, there is some evidence to suggest that for health service users, genuine participation, based on principles of partnership and equality in healthcare, while desirable, is not always a reality (Anthony and Crawford 2000). Authors such as Zauszniewsky (1997) assert that patients could better employ their health-strengthening resources, assume more responsibility and have greater control over their life situation if allowed to take a participatory role. Nutbeam (1998) further argues that people have to be at the centre of health promotion action and decision-making processes for them to be effective. Research investigating mental health nurses' perceptions of user involvement in care planning found that while mental health nurses value the concept, many factors conspire to inhibit user involvement in care planning, including perceptions of both nurses and service users and their personal characteristics and beliefs, conflicting roles and responsibilities and organisation constraints (Anthony and Crawford 2000).

MENTAL HEALTH PROMOTION AGENTS

Mental health is central to building a healthy, inclusive and productive society (WHO 2005:2). 'Mental health promotion increases the quality of life and well-being of the whole population, including people with mental health problems and their carers' (WHO 2005:1). Therefore mental health promotion enhances mental well-being for all.

It is perhaps somewhat ironic that increased awareness of the economic and personal consequences of mental health problems has led to a greater emphasis on promoting population mental health. Mental ill health affects one in four of the EU population, with anxiety and depression being the most common disorders (European Commission 2005). Between 15 and 20 per cent of adults and 15 and 22 per cent of those aged under 18 suffer some form of mental health problem (European Commission 2003). It is also estimated that in excess of 58,000 EU citizens die from suicide every year (European Commission 2005, citing Eurostat). In an Irish context there has also been an unfortunate upward trend in terms of suicide since the 1980s, with a mortality rate of approximately 12.9 per 100,000 of the population, which is approximately equivalent to other European Union countries (HSE *et al.* 2005).

Much mental health promotion activity, as argued, has tended to focus on those with existing or identified mental health problems. This is understandable, insofar as it is recognised that those with mental health problems often do not experience equal opportunities because of discrimination caused by stigma. Another possible explanation relates to the recognition that 'resources available to mental health are often inadequate and inequitable compared to those available in other parts of the public health sector' (WHO 2005:10). This has meant in reality that resources have been focused on treatment management and perhaps illness prevention rather than health promotion. Mental health promotion through the activities of capacity building, support and empowerment has a role to play in preventing some types of mental illness, improving the quality of life for those with mental health problems and preventing suicide.

Where health promotion or at least its ethos has proved particularly beneficial is in the area of advocacy and empowerment of mental health service users. Advocacy and empowerment are both central to health promotion. The WHO suggests that 'the lack of empowerment of mental health service users and carers organisations and poor advocacy hinder the design and implementation of policies and activities that are sensitive to their needs and wishes' (WHO 2005:3). The WHO network of Health Promoting Hospitals, in its task force on Health Promoting Psychiatric Services, has identified models of good practice for mental health promotion in psychiatry and is working on developing standards for mental health promotion. This work is indicative of a change in attitude towards the centrality of health promotion within mental health and is a welcome development.

There is a now a growing research base supporting the development of health promotion practice in the context of mental health. Systematic reviews and meta-analyses on specific mental health topics suggest that significant gains can be achieved from promoting mental health and preventing ill health, including improvements in mental health and a reduction in the risk of mental disorders, as well as social and economic benefits (see Jane-Llopis *et al.* 2005; WHO 2004a; WHO 2004b).

Some of the potential benefits of mental health promotion are:

- Strengthening the capacity of individuals and communities.
- Assisting those with mental health problems in recovery and enhancing quality of life through supportive and empowering interventions.
- Improving physical health and well-being.
- Reducing the stigma and discrimination experienced by those with mental health problems.
- Reducing the structural barriers to mental health.
- Early recognition of mental health problems and early intervention.
- Preventing or reducing the risk of some mental health problems.
- Improving the health of workers has the potential to increase productivity and creativity and to reduce days lost through illness.
- Promoting the mental health of children may increase their resilience and in turn reduce their potential for mental health problems in adulthood.
- Empowers individuals, groups and communities to meet their own needs.

(Adapted from Ryan *et al.* 2006)

The Focus of Mental Health Promotion

Taylor (1998) describes the aim of mental health promotion approaches as threefold, namely to:

- enhance protective factors;
- decrease risk factors for poor mental health; and
- reduce inequities among populations.

This tripartite model is consistent with the suggestion of capacity building, support and empowerment (Ryan *et al.* 2006). Strategies to promote mental health are diverse and can range from developing the personal skills of individuals to reducing structural barriers to health. A summary of mental health promotion strategies (approaches) is provided in Figure 6.3.

Figure 6.3 Strategies for promoting mental health

Advocacy

Capacity building of individuals and communities

Reducing inequalities and other structural barriers to health

Targeting select populations and at risk groups

Increasing understanding and awareness of mental health and mental illness

Reducing stigma/ discrimination and promoting recovery for those with ongoing mental health problems

Contributing to health policy and healthy public policy

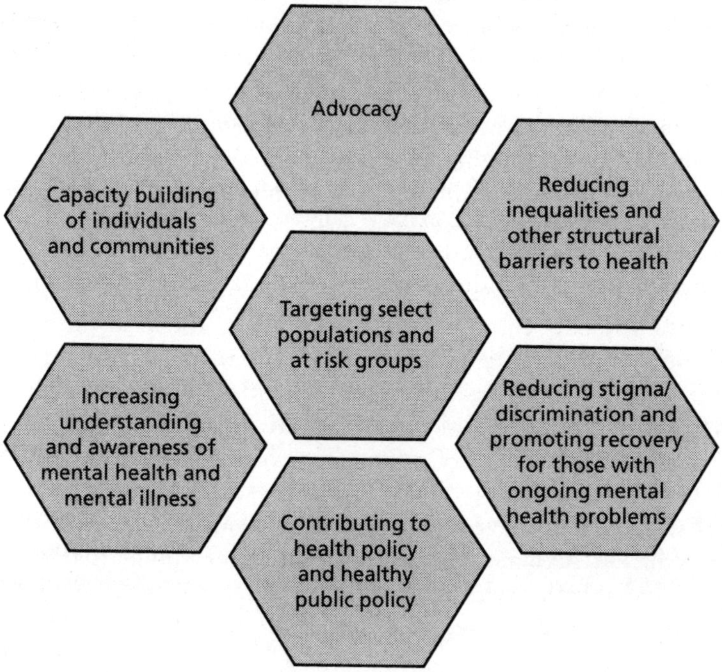

Source: adapted from Ryan *et al.* 2006

RESPONSIBILITY FOR MENTAL HEALTH PROMOTION AND MENTAL HEALTH NURSING

Historically, mental and physical health promotion developed as separate entities, largely because of the influence of the medical model. Traditionally in this country mental health promotion has been the responsibility of the health sector and the mental health service in particular. This has resulted in health practitioners in tertiary mental health services being more associated with mental health promotion than health promotion practitioners. This in itself is problematic, given that the focus of most mental health services is on the management of illness conditions and their association with traditional methods of treatment.

Giving sole or primary responsibility to the mental health service for promoting mental health is also problematic when we consider the factors that influence mental health. It is evident that many of the factors outlined in Figure 6.3 above are outside the sphere of activity of the mental health service. These can only be comprehensively addressed through a synchronised, multi-sectoral approach that focuses on whole populations, individuals at risk, vulnerable groups and those with existing mental health problems. This requires shared vision, strategic planning, resources, and a partnership approach across a range of sectors, disciplines, organisations, agencies and departments (Ryan *et al.* 2006).

While there is now a greater appreciation of the reciprocal or interactional relationship between physical and mental health, this is not adequately reflected either in health service provision or in health promotion activities, which suggests that a health promotion/mental health promotion dichotomy continues today. However, there is some evidence that the artificial boundaries between mental health promotion and health promotion may be changing. In 2006, for example, the All Ireland Health Promoting Hospitals Conference and the International Health Promoting Hospitals Conference both had mental health promotion elements, which was a welcome development.

Mental health promotion is central to the role of the psychiatric nurse (An Bord Altranais 2005). However, the focus of psychiatric/mental health nursing practice has traditionally concentrated on the care of the ill at the expense of health promotion and illness prevention (Ryan 2003). Deasy's (2005) research found that that while mental health nurses in Ireland were engaged in promoting the mental health of their clients, most were not involved in promoting the mental health of the wider community or politically active in addressing the broader determinants of mental health. Many of the nurses in Deasy's (2005) study perceived that they could have a greater role in creating awareness of mental health and reducing stigma. This reiterates the earlier point that traditional practice at an individual level, rather than at the macro level, remains both a strong influence and a challenge in terms of altering mental health nursing practice.

These findings also point to the potential for mental health nursing. While practice has tended to be focused on individuals rather than at a macro level, the potential for mental health nurses to have an involvement at health promotion, preventative and primary care level is clear. However, it means moving from areas of traditional practice to new frontiers and outside familiar organisational arrangements. Such a move would also require a change in the preparation of practitioners, with a greater emphasis on interdisciplinary education and a shift from reductionist to holistic models.

At a broader level, Irish mental health nurses should be aware that an Irish mental health promotion strategy is planned but has not yet been published. It is hoped that this strategy will provide a strategic, synchronised and targeted approach to mental health promotion in Ireland in the coming years (Ryan *et al.* 2006). However, it is argued that mental health promotion would be best embedded within an overall health promotion strategy. It is important to note that many of the previous national strategy documents have highlighted the need for promoting mental health, including the *Health Promotion Strategy: Making the Healthier Choice the Easier Choice* (Department of Health 1995).

There is also recognition of the increasing need to address mental health to improve overall health for the island of Ireland. Indeed, a study published by the Centre for Cross Border Studies and the Institute of Public Health in Ireland, *Promoting Mental Health and Social Well being: Cross-Border Opportunities and Challenges'* (Barry *et al.* 2002) called for the establishment of an all-island Mental

Health Promotion Steering Group to develop mental health promotion in a co-ordinated fashion that would avoid unnecessary duplication. Mental health nurses need to be able to rise to the challenge of such an approach if they are to be able to contribute to health promotion within this type of holistic framework.

CONCLUSION

Health promotion has emerged as an important domain of health practice in the latter part of the twentieth and early part of the twenty-first century. It has become a dominant philosophy that has influenced both policy and practice nationally and internationally. Mental health promotion is a central and inextricable component of health promotion, in the same way that health and mental health cannot be considered separately. Mental health nursing is continually evolving as a professional endeavour. Perhaps more than many healthcare occupations, mental health nursing practice has mirrored the changes in practice in the care and management of those with mental health difficulties. Since it emerged from the asylum system, mental health nursing practice has shifted from an occupation strongly influenced by a medical model of training to one that has embraced holistic concepts of care. This chapter has argued that mental health nursing is ideally placed to continue this paradigm shift to its next logical situation. It is proposed that mental health nursing should be centrally placed in the wider health promotion domain across all levels of health practice, including primary, secondary and tertiary care. In keeping with the ethos and principles of health promotion, this evolution should form part of an integrated approach, involving all key stakeholders.

Reflective Questions
1. What are the differences between health promotion and mental health promotion?
2. How does nursing contribute to mental health promotion as an area of practice?
3. Discuss the distinctions between health education and health promotion.
4. Discuss the distinctions between illness prevention and health promotion in a mental health context.

References

An Bord Altranais (2000) *The Code of Professional Conduct for Each Nurse and Midwife* (2nd edn). Dublin: An Bord Altranais.

An Bord Altranais (2005) *Nursing: A Career for You*. Dublin: Nursing Careers Centre.

Anthony, P. and Crawford, P. (2000) 'Service user involvement in care planning: the mental health nurse's perspective'. *Journal of Psychiatric and Mental Health Nursing*, 7(5), 425–34.

Barry, M. M., Friel, S., Dempsey, C. and Avalos, G. (2002) *Promoting Mental*

Health and Social Well-being: Cross-Border Opportunities and Challenges. Armagh: The Centre for Cross Border Studies.

Brennan, D. (2000) 'A consideration of the mental health promotion policies and programs in the Eastern Health Board region, in the context of a developed theory of mental health promotion' (unpublished MEd thesis). Trinity College Dublin.

Cox, S. (1985) 'Women's work: women's health'. *Occupational Health: a Journal for Occupational Health Nurses,* 37 (11), 504–13.

Deasy, C. (2005) 'Health promotion in mental health nursing: an exploratory study of the perceptions of mental health nurses in one geographical region' (unpublished MA (Health Education Promotion) thesis). University of Limerick.

Department of Health (1995) *A Health Promotion Strategy: Making the Healthier Choice the Easier Choice.* Dublin: Stationery Office.

European Commission (2003) *The Health Status of the European Union–Narrowing the Health Gap.* Luxembourg: European Communities.

European Commission (2005) *Green Paper – Improving the Mental Health of the Population: Towards a Strategy on Mental Health for the European Union.* Brussels: Health and Consumer Protection Directorate-General.

Fontaine, K. L. (2003) *Mental Health Nursing* (5th edn). New Jersey: Prentice Hall.

Government of Ireland (1984) *Psychiatric Services: Planning for the Future.* Dublin: Stationery Office.

Government of Ireland (2001) *Mental Treatment Act.* Dublin: Stationery Office.

Government of Ireland (2006) *A Vision for Change – Report of the Expert Group on Mental Health Policy.* Dublin: Stationery Office.

Health Service Executive, National Suicide Review Group and Department of Health and Children (2005) *Reach Out – National Strategy for Action on Suicide Prevention: 2005– 2014.* Naas: Health Service Executive.

Herrman, H. (2001) 'The need for mental health promotion'. *Australian and New Zealand Journal of Psychiatry,* 35(6), 709–15.

Hodgson, R. J. (1996) 'Mental health promotion' (Editorial). *Journal of Mental Health,* 5(1), 1–2.

Jane-Llopis, E., Barry, M., Hoisamn, C. and Patel, V. (2005) 'Mental Health Promotion Works: A Review'. *IUHPE – Promotion and Education,* 2, 9–25.

Jones, L. J. (1994) *The Social Context of Health and Health Work.* Basingstoke: Palgrave.

Naidoo, J. and Wills, J. (2000) *Health Promotion: Foundations for Practice* (2nd edn). London: Balliere Tindall.

Nutbeam, D. (1998) 'Evaluating health promotion — progress, problems and solutions'. *Health Promotion International,* 3(1), 27–44.

Peplau, H.E. (1994) 'Psychiatric and mental health nursing: challenge and change'. *Journal of Psychiatric and Mental Health Nursing,* 1(1), 3–7.

Ryan, D. (2003) 'The person who is paranoid or suspicious', in P. Barker (ed.),

Psychiatric and Mental Health Nursing: The Craft of Caring. London: Arnold, 305–11.

Ryan, D., Mannix McNamara, P., and Deasy, C. (2006) *Health Promotion in Ireland: Principles, Practice and Research*. Dublin: Gill and Macmillan.

Taylor, L. (1998) *Mental Health Promotion in Canada: Working Towards a National Plan of Action for Promoting the Mental Health of Canadians*. Birmingham: Clifford Beers Conference.

Whitehead, D. (2001) 'Health education, behavioural change and social psychology: nurses' contribution to health promotion'. *Journal of Advanced Nursing*, 34(6), 310–21.

World Health Organisation (1946) *Constitution*. Geneva: WHO.

World Health Organisation (1978) *Report of the Primary Healthcare Conference: Alma Ata*. Geneva: WHO.

World Health Organisation (1984) *Health Promotion: A Discussion Document on the Concepts and Principles of Health Promotion*. Copenhagen: WHO.

World Health Organisation (2001a). *The World Health Report 2001: Mental Health – New Understanding, New Hope*. Geneva: WHO.

World Health Organisation (2001b) *Strengthening Mental Health Promotion* (Fact Sheet no. 220). Geneva: WHO.

World Health Organisation (2004a) *Prevention of Mental Disorders: Effective Interventions and Policy Options, Summary Report*. Geneva: WHO.

World Health Organisation (2004b) *Promoting Mental Health: Concepts, Emerging Evidence, Practice: Summary Report*. Geneva: WHO.

World Health Organisation (2005) 'Mental health action plan for Europe: Facing challenges, building solutions', www.euro.who.int/document/mnh/edoc07.pdf., accessed 14 January 2007.

World Health Organisation, Canadian Public Health Association and Health Welfare Canada (1986) *Ottawa Charter for Health Promotion*. Presented at the International Conference on Health Promotion, 17–21 November. Ottawa.

Zauszniewsky, J. A. (1997) 'Teaching resourcefulness skills to older adults'. *Journal of Gerontological Nursing*, 23(2), 14–20.

7
Community Care and Rehabilitation

John McCardle

Community care is about delivering comprehensive services to clients as close as possible to their home environment. This chapter will focus on the major components of community mental health nursing care and rehabilitation in Ireland today and into the future. It will briefly consider the main historical factors that have taken mental health service provision to its current point and identify the philosophy and principles that will impact on future practice as well as the new mental health policy framework which will be implemented over the next decade. Dominant approaches to care and therapeutic interventions that nursing will have to embrace if community care and rehabilitation is to be delivered effectively to clients are also addressed.

HISTORICAL PERSPECTIVES OF COMMUNITY CARE

While the health service in Ireland developed in parallel with the health service in Britain throughout the eighteenth, nineteenth and early twentieth centuries, it has developed its own direction for most of the twentieth century. Until the 1960s the activities of psychiatric nurses in Ireland were based in hospitals. The Commission of Inquiry on Mental Illness issued their report in 1966 (Department of Health (DoH) 1966) and recommended that mental hospitals should be seen not as centres of custodial care but rather as centres of rehabilitation with an aim of returning clients to the community. While more and more patients were discharged into the community, the nature of psychiatric nursing care, however, did not change much until the mid-1980s, in comparison with the United Kingdom where it happened almost a decade earlier.

Under the Health Act (DoH 1970) eight boards were set up, each comprising a body corporate with the authority to enter into arrangements with other bodies, such as voluntary hospitals and private hospitals, to provide services on their behalf. The Health Boards allowed services to develop separately to meet local needs with broad guidance from a number of national documents. The result of this practice has been that different areas offered a slightly different service, staffed in a slightly different way and with different grades of nursing staff. The White Paper *Planning for the Future* (DoH 1984) set out a blueprint for the implementation of community-based psychiatric care in Ireland. This report emphasised a planned sectorised service with a comprehensive provision of healthcare for a population of known size within defined geographical boundaries and by a multidisciplinary psychiatric team based in each sector. While some of this plan has been delivered, the medical and nursing professions deliver much of the care in many sectors with minimal support from other disciplines.

The Report of the Commission on Nursing (DoHC 1998) reviewed all aspects of nursing and supported the seamless psychiatric service that was in place covering acute centres, day hospitals, high-support hostels and community services. It also reinforced the view that psychiatric nurses should be able to function comfortably within all of these different aspects of the service. The Commission on Nursing did, however, recognise the need for the development of specialist aspects of the traditional CPN service and recommended this new grade of specialist to be titled Community Mental Health Nurse (CMHN). The report also identified the need for educational programmes to underpin the new roles, particularly in the delivery of health promotion and suicide prevention to encompass a population health perspective that included visiting schools and accessing potentially vulnerable groups.

CURRENT AND FUTURE COMMUNITY CARE STRUCTURES

The Health Service Executive (HSE) was set up in January 2005 as a unified structure for health service delivery. It is divided into four geographical areas and care delivery is organised through three main branches: the Hospitals Network; Primary, Continuing and Community Care (PCCC); and Population Health.

Historically, Ireland has relied on hospitalisation, and to some extent this is still true: admission rates remain high and many admission units are still institutionally based (DoHC 2006). Community care in most areas is delivered through a combination of generic Community Mental Health Nurses (CMHNs) and medically led outpatient clinics. A collaborative model of intervention is delivered between the nursing and medical professions with varying input from other paramedical professions depending upon the geographical area. CMHNs in Ireland currently carry large caseloads, averaging over sixty clients, resulting in low levels of psychosocial intervention delivered to clients (McCardle 2003).

Currently the mental health service is in a period of transition as a new model of service provision has been outlined in the report of the expert group on mental heath policy, *A Vision for Change* (DoHC 2006). A timeframe of seven to ten years has been placed on the implementation of this new structure. It is proposed that care will be delivered through multidisciplinary teams that will offer a wide variety of specialist services to populations of between 50,000 and 400,000. Furthermore, there will also be increased involvement of service users at every level of the service, with increased emphasis on and utilisation of advocacy services for all users.

PHILOSOPHY AND PRINCIPLES OF COMMUNITY CARE AND REHABILITATION

The philosophy and principles that underpin the service of community care and rehabilitation must guide the approach to care, choice of intervention and mode of practice of the mental health nurse. Figure 7.1 identifies the key philosophical concepts and principles that mental health nurses must consider or hold.

Figure 7.1 Key community care philosophical principles

Life in the community	This refers to the belief that the client with mental health difficulties has the same right to be an integrated member of the community as anyone else. Where some form of residential in-patient setting is required it should be the least restrictive possible.
Partnership	The client has the greatest capacity to influence his/her own healthcare and as such should be a partner in that process with the health service provider. A philosophy of partnership between the nurse and the client leads naturally to choice, involvement, inclusion, equity and empowerment.
Person-centred	Consideration of this philosophy will deliver a service that targets and prioritises the individual's needs. Individual assessment and care planning should be the focus of nursing care.
Promote recovery	This philosophy will focus on providing the opportunity for the client to retain self-control, build self-esteem and achieve a sense of belonging in their life.
Best interests of the client	This principle requires that the interventions delivered are the most likely to deliver a positive health outcome for the client.
The client should be treated with dignity and respect	There are some common themes when clients' opinions are sought about the service. This requires the maximum involvement of the client in the decision-making process with adequate information to be able to participate in that process to the fullest extent possible.
Embrace a holistic model of intervention	This will impact directly on the role of the nurse and the focus of nursing practice. The client's needs must be the objective of nursing intervention in every aspect of his/her life. The service must adapt to meet the client's needs rather than fit the client into the services on offer.

PRINCIPAL COMMUNITY CARE INTERFACES

The Community Mental Health Team (CMHT) cannot deliver mental healthcare in isolation from other health service providers or other community services. While caring for every client's individual needs will require interfacing with a large range of services, it is important to consider the key interfaces and the impact that these will have on the care received by the client. Primary healthcare is the main point of access for the majority of people in the community.

Primary care teams provide most of the help that individuals with mental health problems need, but some will need referral to CMHTs. These clients should be able to access services that are responsive, timely and effective. The CMHT's services should be sensitive to cultural needs, including the needs of people from ethnic minority communities. This interface needs to have an open two-way channel of communication in which information is shared between service providers and moves with the client from primary care to the CMHT and back again to primary care. In some cases where the client has enduring mental illness this interface needs to operate on a partnership or shared care level with each service providing care for the client over a prolonged period of time.

The CMHT will also be required to interface with the National Hospitals Network as some referrals will come from the emergency departments or wards in the general hospitals. Such referrals will have to be assessed and either referred on or offered a care package from the mental health service. Where a mental health liaison nurse is available to triage general hospital referrals and offer an initial assessment, these referrals will be more streamlined. In services where a mental health liaison nurse is not available, the response from within the CMHT will also have to be timely and effective. Clients accessing the CMHT from this entry point will also have a primary healthcare boundary that must also be considered.

While all the mental health service will be managed from the PCCC division of the HSE, the acute in-patient units will, for the most part, be placed in general hospitals. A small proportion of the CMHT caseload will require admission to allow care to be delivered in a more intensive therapeutic environment with higher levels of supervision. Essentially this is an internal mental health interface and the client needs to be able to perceive this interface as an extension or optional alternative of the CMHT. However, it is important that many of the CMHT members continue to play a part in the overall treatment plan during hospitalisation to ensure effective, efficient reintegration to the home environment on discharge.

APPROACHES TO COMMUNITY CARE

The dominant focus of mental healthcare in Ireland has concentrated on the seriously mentally ill. The following approaches will provide structures to deliver therapeutic interventions within CMHTs.

The Case Management Approach

The case management approach to community care was developed in the USA and has more recently produced positive care outcomes in the UK when used within CMHTs (Morgan 2003). While there are a variety of adaptations, it essentially involves designating one member of the CMHT to co-ordinate and plan an individual's care requirements. The role of the case manager includes the identification of people in need, the system for referral, the assessment of care needs, delivery of care, monitoring the quality of care and reviewing the clients' needs. Wright and Giddey (1993) suggested that no one individual healthcare worker was required to undertake all these functions but might be required to ensure that they were completed, thus ensuring accountability. As such, the case manager needs to have a manageable caseload and be knowledgeable about the resources available in their area. This method aims to ensure that the clients receive the support required to live independently with the minimum intervention or duplication of care offered. In some models of case management the case manager provides a client advocate role to ensure the client's needs are met and their rights are respected.

Assertive Community-Based Treatment

The approach to care known as assertive community-based treatment is aimed at clients with enduring mental illness who cannot or will not engage with the service. Currently many services in Ireland are only developing this approach to care and many areas have not moved beyond maintaining clients in the community through hostels and generic CMHN support. The government policy *Vision for Change* (DoHC 2006) indicated that assertive outreach will be a principle strategy employed by rehabilitation teams as they are developed.

This approach is essentially a combination of evidence-based, therapeutic interventions that are targeted specifically at service users requiring intensive service input. The interventions are provided by a team with a low staff–client ratio (approx 1:10–12) and occur in the least restrictive setting possible (Morgan 2003). The onus is generally placed on the team to maintain contact and offer support, as the nature of the client's condition is such that he/she will not seek help and will be likely to relapse as a result. In this respect the service is needs-led as opposed to demands-led and is provided for as long as intervention is required.

Key principles that underpin this method to care delivery include flexibility, person-centeredness, choice, practical support, advocacy, specific key worker allocation, and liaison with other agencies. There is a wide range of evidence-based interventions that can be included and strategies are constantly evolving as new evidence becomes available (Fleet 2004).

Core outcomes of assertive community-based care include engagement, assessment, medication concordance, family inclusion, education, risk management, cognitive-behavioural strategies and empowerment. Marshall and Lockwood (2001) concluded that clients receiving this approach to care experienced reduced hospitalisation, increased service contact, increased satisfaction with the service, and increased likelihood of independent living and employment.

Rehabilitation/Recovery Process

Rehabilitation and recovery are concepts that have come to be associated with clients experiencing enduring mental illness. While this is true it is also limiting, as these are important concepts to be considered in relation to any individual with mental illness that requires intervention from a health professional. While these concepts are closely related they are not the same thing. Mental health policy differentiates them as follows:

> Recovery reflects the belief that it is possible for all service users to achieve control over their lives, to recover their self-esteem, and move towards building a life where they experience a sense of belonging and participation.
>
> (DoHC 2006:105)
>
> Rehabilitation describes a facilitative process that enables disadvantaged individuals to access as independent a life as possible in social, cultural and economic terms.
>
> (DoHC 2006:104)

These definitions highlight differences in these concepts in line with many other aspects of the literature on this area. While rehabilitation is a process that involves health professionals engaging with the individual to facilitate increased independence, recovery is the personal experience of the individual as they adjust to a positive sense of self with mental illness.

The underlying message from these definitions moves the focus of care from a medical model towards a social integration model. Performance indicators that traditionally focus on admission and discharge levels or symptom reduction must concentrate more on the level of independence that the individual has achieved. From a holistic perspective, symptom reduction is not a pre-requisite of recovery. Traditionally, mental health services have tried to fit the client into the services that are on offer rather than offering a service that is tailored to meet the client's needs. Mental health nurses need to consider this change of philosophy and refocus their nursing practice so that greater flexibility and adaptation are offered while delivering a more individualised nursing care package in the client's home environment.

In order to promote the opportunity of recovery through the provision of rehabilitative care programmes, CMHTs must reconsider the boundaries of the nursing role. During acute episodes of mental health problems the client may require either crisis intervention, a short stay in an in-patient service, or assertive community-based support in the home. This challenge will involve the nurse delivering a more client-centred, individualised care plan that emphasises a holistic approach, assisting the client with personal development, medication management or social and personal relationships. Other interventions may also be required to focus on accommodation, employment or education. If nursing interventions are to be truly holistic nurses need to consider what they can offer the client in every aspect of their life. It is only then that the rehabilitative process can provide the platform that will offer the client the opportunity for recovery.

Figure 7.2 Concept map of client care pathways in the mental health nursing service

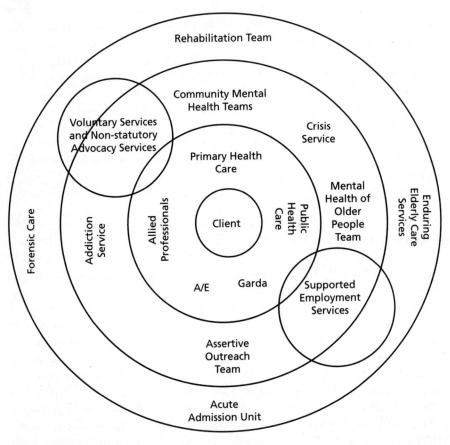

The Care Pathway
The client may need to avail of a range of services to meet an individually tailored care plan. The concept map set out in Figure 7.2 allows a variety of care pathways to be considered in relation to any individual. This map places the client at the centre. The first point of care for the individual will be a service or services identified in the next tier of the model. These form the first stage of the referral pathway and should collaborate to provide an initial assessment of and response to the client's needs. Where these services are unable to meet the client's needs, he or she should be referred to a service on the next tier of the model as appropriate to their needs. The services at this level will be able to offer a more comprehensive

range of assessment and treatment options. The complexity of the client's needs will determine whether or not he/she will be referred to a service or services in the outer tier of the model. Furthermore, a number of services will provide support to the client in conjunction with the mental health service across a number of different spheres such as advocacy services or supported employment services.

The following vignette illustrates the pathway through the tiers and the involvement of other support services.

> Joe is a 49-year-old man who lost his job ten months ago and has since experienced marital difficulties. Joe's brother has become concerned about his increased isolation and general disinterest in life. He has brought Joe to the GP, who feels that Joe is depressed and refers him to the CMHT. The CMHT co-ordinator arranges an assessment and the CMHN or other CMHT member undertaking the assessment concludes that Joe has active suicidal ideation with a plan to harm himself. The CMHN organises admission to hospital. Following a period of treatment in hospital Joe returns home with support from the CMHT and an advocate from the local advocacy network. After receiving cognitive behavioural intervention the CMHT involves the supported recovery services as part of Joe's ongoing rehabilitation treatment plan and shortly after Joe is discharged back to the ongoing care of the primary care team.

THE ROLE AND PRACTICE OF THE CMHN

The nursing staff who deliver nursing care in the community environment have a number of intervention models to influence and guide their practice. Traditionally the medical model has largely influenced the approach of nursing, as much of nursing practice has been determined by the client's medical diagnosis. However, nursing practice has produced a wide variety of nursing models that equip the nurse to organise and deliver care. Alternatively, CMHNs that operate within a social model tend to place an emphasis upon the social systems that influence the clients' life, such as family, friends and working environment.

The role and practice of CMHNs encompass a wide range of issues and these two facets of the CMHN service are inextricably linked. The main roles of the CMHN are assessor, therapist, consultant, clinician, educator, and manager (Carr et al. 1980). While these roles have been moulded and expanded, they are still valid and broadly reflected in the literature relating to the role of the CMHN. The practice within these roles has been heavily influenced by the education and training of the CMHN and the relationship with the other health professionals with whom they work closely. Professional nursing practice within the sphere of CMHN care involves patient care, therapeutic interventions, medication management, caseload management, assessment of patients, risk management, autonomy, and the relationship with other disciplines, in particular consultants.

Assessment of the patient could be broken into first assessments, ongoing evaluative assessment, and assessment of concordance with medication.

Assessment has been reported in the literature as a role (Barratt 1989), a method of work (Adams 1996) and an essential element of practice (Johnson *et al.* 2001; Crawford *et al.* 2001). The practice of medication management includes organising prescriptions, supplying medication, supervising the patient taking medication, checking concordance, observing effects and side effects and administering depot and oral medication in the home environment. While this reflects the clinician role, the CMHN undertaking medication management can place more emphasis on educational input and compliance therapy (Gray *et al.* 2001; Jordan *et al.* 2002), which suggests that this function may fit better within a therapeutic role than a clinician role.

Within the therapeutic role, supportive counselling of a broad-based nature is used widely in conjunction with practical assistance. This may involve listening to whatever personal issues are of concern to the client and whatever emotions require expression. Other support of a practical nature entails organising links with other support systems, organising transport to social outlets, or helping to source items for the home that would enhance the patient or relation's quality of life. CMHNs tend to depend on oral contracts and agreements with clients to attend other facilities and in many cases social skills training may help to develop confidence and motivation in the patient to attend such services.

The therapeutic role of the CMHN in the United Kingdom has been expanded to include psychosocial interventions and family work. These interventions are aimed at reducing the impact of high levels of expressed emotion within family relationships. Interventions of this nature are aimed at improving communication within the family, reducing criticism, hostility and over-involvement. The approach draws on a combination of cognitive behavioural skills and techniques from systemic family therapy (Leff *et al.* 2001). While these methods have proved effective, training in psychosocial methods resulted in significant increases in the amount of time CMHNs spent with patients with schizophrenia and their families (Brooker and Butterworth 1993). In Ireland, large caseloads have prevented CMHNs becoming involved in psychosocial interventions of this nature (McCardle 2003).

Family psycho-education is another approach that has been developed in conjunction with family work. This tends to comprise professionally led programmes that are focused on the person's condition, such as a family education programme for families of clients with schizophrenia. These programmes are intended to empower families with the information and skills needed to maintain health or promote the recovery of the client. The content of the programme would include issues such as dealing with conflict, and symptom management. Some of these programmes are well established and have developed into peer-led programmes with evidence-based results (Dixon *et al.* 2004).

THE CMHN'S ROLE IN THE MULTIDISCIPLINARY TEAM

The dominant model of care delivery in Ireland to date has been a bi-disciplinary model involving the nursing and medical professions. As has already been noted, this is changing to a multidisciplinary approach within a CMHT structure. Each discipline within these teams will be required to negotiate areas of generic practice that are common to all and areas of professional practice that are discipline-specific. The CMHN will have to work collaboratively with the other disciplines and in partnership with service users and carers. This requires the CMHN to be clear about the role and scope of practice that they bring to the team and how they contribute to the overall service to the patient.

EMERGING COMPONENTS IN THE IRISH CONTEXT

The components of advocacy, risk management and the voluntary sector have played a part in service delivery to a varying degree in Ireland to date. These factors must be promoted as community care and rehabilitation increases, and become central to future models of mental healthcare practice because they have the potential to affect positively the care that the client receives.

Advocacy

The ultimate advocacy goal for any of us is to be able to self-advocate on our own behalf in relation to our needs. This should not be any different for the individual with mental illness. However, there may be times when self-advocacy is not possible and therefore other forms of advocacy may be required to ensure that the client's needs are met. People with mental illness tend to be a vulnerable group in society, so the function of advocacy should be to provide safeguards to protect their interests. It is important to have a number of different forms of advocacy available as no single form of advocacy can meet all the needs of the individual.

In Ireland there are two main advocacy organisations that operate independently of the health service. The Irish Advocacy Network is a peer advocacy organisation that offers a number of advocacy services nationally. STEER (Support Training Education Employment Research) is a community-based mental health service user initiative formed as a partnership between service users and carers/family members. It is a cross-border agency that is involved in a number of projects with the HSE North West.

The nursing profession in Ireland traditionally prided itself on being able to offer an advocacy service to the client. Many aspects of psychiatric nursing intervention, such as enabling, supporting, educating or empowering, overlap with the role of an advocate. It is particularly important for the nurse working in this new paradigm of CMHT to be conscious of holding an advocacy philosophy, as this can often be the main link between the client and the community. The advocacy role also requires knowledge of other groups that provide citizen advocacy services, such as the Money Advice and Budgeting Service or the Citizen Advice Bureau so that these can be used as required to the benefit of the client. These strategies will enable the client to have a voice and a choice in the services on offer.

Voluntary Sector

When any individual cannot access the same benefits of society (such as education, employment or housing) as others, this is known as social exclusion. This can affect the members of any vulnerable group in society and the users of the mental health service are no exception. Social exclusion can reduce the progress of the rehabilitation process and increase the benefits of maintaining the sick role. While this can be reduced through the use of equality legislation and other preventative policy strategies, these approaches have not been successful in removing it as a factor from healthcare.

Access to mainstream education, housing and employment are issues that need to be prioritised within the rehabilitation process and they must be part of the core functions of teams working in the community. The role of the nurse needs to be expanded beyond direct care delivery to include strategies to improve contact between clients and the rest of the community and increase social integration. CMHTs need to develop networks at local level with adult education institutions, housing associations and employers in the community. Such healthcare strategies are a new departure from the traditional healthcare model, but if the rehabilitation process in Ireland is to move beyond resettlement the nursing profession must embrace these methods of practice. This means that delivering healthcare in the community requires knowledge of the adult education establishments and courses on offer so that the nurse can enable the client to take advantages of opportunities on offer. It may also mean exploring supported employment opportunities that will enable clients to enter employment with extra support initially as part of rehabilitation and recovery. Socially inclusive strategies such as these need to become a central tenet in promoting recovery within mental healthcare.

Risk Management

Patient safety and observation have been part of the core culture of psychiatric nursing since the inception of the profession. Within the institutional system some of these principles were held to be more important than others, such as personal responsibility, decision making and choice. However, the process of de-institutionalisation and the establishment of community care structures have brought these other principles to the fore and consideration needs to be given to how all these principles can be accommodated without compromising client safety. Community mental health nursing staff, like all other health professionals, have a duty of care to ensure the users' safety.

Duty is the standard of care owed to a client that is created by virtue of the nurse-patient relationship. Furthermore, it means making sure that every client receives appropriate care by competent, professionally qualified staff. It is making sure the clients are properly identified, receive the correct intervention with correct procedures and receive the appropriate response when an unexpected event arises.

All strategies available to reduce risk need to be considered and evaluated in relation to the best interests of the client. A clear risk management policy is an essential tool for safe care delivery in CMHTs as it will enable the decision-making process and reduce the likelihood of reverting to hospitalisation and breaking the rehabilitation process.

The term 'risk management' usually refers to self-protective activities intended to prevent real or potential threats of financial loss due to accident, injury or medical malpractice (Kraman and Hamm 1999). Three key steps are involved: risk identification, risk analysis and risk control. Risk identification includes developing processes to identify areas in a professional practice area that have a potential to cause the client harm. Risk analysis involves not only the review of accident- and incident-screening data, but also any near-miss data to identify trends before a client injury occurs. This analysis includes evaluating the specific practice involved to determine any practice changes that will continue to improve the margins of safety. Risk control is concerned with dealing with practices or incidents that result in harm or injury to a client. Where such practices result in instances of professional malpractice or negligence there are likely to be accompanying costs. Risk management is aimed at improving care practice and reducing the accompanying costs of malpractice.

CRISIS INTERVENTION AND RESOLUTION

The purpose of crisis intervention is to reduce the impact of the current developments in any specific situation. In the field of mental health this generally involves directing resources at the client and/or family in an effort to replace or reduce the likelihood of admission to hospital. A holistic crisis service should include social workers and other professionals who can work on crisis issues in addition to mental health, so that crisis areas that could be addressed would encompass broader life issues. These might include areas such as housing, employment, benefits, emotional crises, and parenting crises. This crisis service could be incorporated into the interventions offered by CMHTs or offered through an acute home-based treatment team. Situations that would normally have led to admissions could then be responded to by the newer CMHT or Crisis Resolution Home Treatment Team services.

Ideally, this form of crisis service consists of a 24-hour home and community visiting service to provide:
- Assessment at times of crisis.
- Short-term home treatment and support when assessed as appropriate until a crisis is adequately resolved or until the care co-ordination is passed to another team.
- Access to in-patient care when assessed as appropriate.
- Access to other short-term facilities, such as a crisis house or other high-support facility.

CONCLUSION

Community care and rehabilitation will continue to be central to the developing mental healthcare environment over the next ten years. However, the focus will move from leaving the institution to promoting concepts of rehabilitation and recovery. The main driver will be a partnership between multidisciplinary CMHTs and client advocacy organisations. The CMHN will be in a position to influence the emerging healthcare environment through the delivery of evidence-based nursing care, risk management strategies and developing comprehensive care pathways that provide the opportunity for client recovery. New challenges will materialise as crisis intervention and assertive community-based treatment services become the norms of mental healthcare delivery structures. The nursing profession must position itself to play a key role in a modern mental health service with the capability to offer the client whatever is needed in their home environment.

Reflective Questions
1. This chapter has indicated that the scope of nursing practice needs to evolve to embrace a broader concept of rehabilitation. What new practices need to be developed to meet this new challenge?
2. The concept of partnership, wherein the client plays a major role in their own healthcare, will provide new challenges to the current decision-making process. Can you identify these challenges? Discuss strategies that will address them.
3. Every client has an individual care pathway and corresponding care team interfaces. Choose two clients and map their care pathway.
4. Taking the same clients chosen in question three, reflect on the care team interfaces and evaluate the communication patterns between the different teams involved in the clients' care.

References
Adams, T. (1996) 'A descriptive study of the work of community psychiatric nurses with elderly demented people'. *Journal of Advanced Nursing*, 23, 1177–84.
Barratt, E. (1989) 'Community psychiatric nurses: their self-perceived role'. *Journal of Advanced Nursing*, 14, 42–8.
Brooker, C. and Butterworth, C. (1993) 'Training in psychosocial intervention: the impact on the role of community psychiatric nurses'. *Journal of Advanced Nursing*, 18 (4), 583–90.
Carr, P., Butterworth, A. and Hodges, B. (1980) *Community Psychiatric Nursing*. London: Churchill Livingstone.
Crawford, P., Carr, J., Knight, A., Chambers, K. and Nolan, P. (2001) 'The value of community mental health nurses based in primary care teams: "switching on the light in the cellar"'. *Journal of Psychiatric and Mental Health Nursing* 8, 213–220.
Department of Health (1966) *Report of the Commission of Inquiry on Mental Illness*. Dublin: Stationery Office.

Department of Health (1970) *The Health Act*. Dublin: Government Publication Office.

Department of Health (1984) *The Psychiatric Services — Planning for the Future*. Dublin: Stationery Office.

Department of Health and Children (1998) *The Commission on Nursing Report*. Dublin: Government Publication Office.

Department of Health and Children (2006) *A Vision for Change: Report of the Expert Group on Mental Health Policy*. Dublin: Government Publication Office.

Dixon, L., Lucksted, A., Stewart, B., Burland, J., Brown, C.H., Postrado, L., McGuire, C., and Hoffman, M. (2004) 'Outcomes of a peer-taught 12-week family-to-family education program for severe mental illness'. *Acta Psychiatrica Scandinavica*, 109, 207–15.

Fleet, M. (2004) 'Assertive community treatment with people experiencing serious mental illness', in D. Kirby, D. A. Hart, D. Cross and G. Mitchell (eds), *Mental Health Nursing; Competencies for Practice*. New York: Palgrave Macmillan.

Gray, R., Wykes, T., Parr, A-M., Harls, E. and Gournay, K. (2001) 'The use of outcome measures to evaluate the efficacy and tolerability of antipsychotic medication: a comparison of thorn practice and CPN practice'. *Journal of Psychiatric and Mental Health Nursing*, 8, 191–6.

Johnson, S., Coleman, M. and Bowler, N. (2001) 'CPNs and the severely mentally ill'. *Mental Health Nursing*, 21 (2), 10–15.

Jordan, S., Tunnicliffe, C. and Sykes, A. (2002) 'Minimizing side effects: the clinical impact of nurse-administered "side effect" checklists'. *Journal of Advanced Nursing*, 37 (2), 155–65.

Kraman, S. S. and Hamm, G. (1999) 'Risk management: extreme honesty may be the best policy'. *Annals of Internal Medicine*, 131 (12), 963–7.

Leff, J., Sharpley, M., Chrisholm, D., Bell, R., and Gamble, C. (2001) 'Training community psychiatric nurses in schizophrenia family work: A study of clinical and economic outcomes for patients and relatives'. *Journal of Mental Health*, 10 (2), 189–97.

Marshall, M. and Lockwood, A. (2001) *Assertive Community Treatment for People with Severe Mental Disorders (Cochrane Review)*. Oxford: The Cochrane Library 4

McCardle, J. (2003) 'The exploration of the nature of community psychiatric nursing practice and the role of community psychiatric nurses (CPNs) in Ireland' (unpublished thesis). University of Ulster.

Morgan, S., (2003) 'Case management and assertive outreach' in B. Hannigan and M. Coffey (eds), *The Handbook of Community Mental Health Nursing*. London: Routledge.

Wright, H. and Giddey, M. (1993) *Mental Health Nursing: First Principles to Professional Practice*. Cheltenham: Stanley Thomas.

SECTION 2

Therapeutic Modalities in Psychiatric/Mental Health Nursing

8

Therapeutic Communication in Mental Health Nursing

Chris Stevenson

... no matter how hard one may try, one cannot, not communicate.
(Watzlawick *et al.* 1967: 49)

We all communicate every day. So much so, that we take the process for granted. This is understandable. If we all stopped to reflect on our communication processes, how would we get on with our lives? In mental health nursing, however, communication is the medium through which we try to effect change with the person experiencing difficulties or distress. In order to communicate effectively, and thus therapeutically, we have to ensure that we have the basic communication tools and that they are in good order; and we have to pick up new tools, and learn how to use them, in order to work in specific care episodes — one size does not fit all. This chapter takes the reader from the basics in communication Do-It-Yourself to more sophisticated approaches.

HEALTH AND SAFETY WARNING

Just as with DIY, it is important to attend to the health and safety issues when undertaking to use communication as a therapeutic medium. The nuts and bolts are the basic techniques and principles in which everyone engaging in clinical practice in mental health needs to be fluent. The more advanced techniques covered in 'Screwdrivers and Spanners' and 'Power Tools' represent pieces taken from more comprehensive therapeutic approaches. They are offered here as useful tools to use in a stand-alone way, with careful clinical judgement. For the reader who has an interest in these approaches it is imperative to engage further with the literature or in further training.

NUTS AND BOLTS

'For the want of a nail, the shoe was lose [lost] ...' (Benjamin Franklin, US author, diplomat, inventor, physicist, politician and printer (1706–90)).

There are many books on the nursing, psychology, counselling and psychotherapy shelves that deal in detail with the basics or core tools in communication (in nursing, readers might want to refer to Stevenson *et al.* 2004). In this section, the 'nuts and bolts' of communication, verbal and non-verbal, most pertinent to mental health nursing will be presented. These are grouped under tools:

- for listening
- to help build meaning
- to aid exploring
- to facilitate comforting, supporting and enabling.

It is no accident that the groups are labelled by verbs — it is important to think of communication as an *active* and *dynamic* interactive process. Although the skills are grouped for convenience, these boundaries are artificial and the same skills can be used with different effect.

Listening

Even if the mental health nurse does nothing but listen, there is likely to be a therapeutic effect (also see below). People who use the health services consistently remind us of the power of listening by the nurse (Webb and Hope 1995; Kai and Crosland 2001). Effective listening is beyond merely hearing the words, phrases or sentences that people use. Active listening is effective in helping to elicit the person's mental health story. It requires full attention or presence in the encounter. This attention needs to be communicated to the person who is talking. An effective way to do this is to offer minimal encouragers, like nodding, saying 'yes' or 'mm' and, where appropriate, using touch. Egan (1998) offers a formula for listening with the acronym SOLER:

- Squarely facing the person.
- Open posture, for example, not crossing one's arms across the body.
- Leaning forward and so showing interest.
- Eye contact of an appropriate nature: that is, not 'staring the person down' but catching the person's eye frequently.
- Relaxed posture. If the person talking detects unease in the listener s/he will be inhibited.

Other important factors in active listening are ensuring that there is time to listen and that the context is right. The location where the talking and listening takes place can be varied. For some people a quiet area without interruptions helps. For others, this may be too intense and conversation while engaging in a task may be easier, e.g. while washing the dishes or going for a walk. It is important not to interrupt. Interjections often mean the listener is not listening at all but wanting to pursue her/his own agenda. It is unhelpful to judge, evaluate or advise the person. In most cases, this involves imposing one's own viewpoint and not showing respect for the person's expertise in relation to her/his life experience.

It is also critical to 'tune in' to what the person is saying. This may involve the listener 'tuning out' from their own thoughts or views. By tuning in, interest in the person is being expressed. If the person who is talking detects lack of interest from the listener, s/he is likely to stop talking and may feel quite uncomfortable. Such silences need to be distinguished from therapeutic silences. There are times when people find the telling of their story too painful and may need to pause. Even if no conversation is occurring the mental health nurse can still communicate therapeutically non-verbally by being present and attentive.

The attuned mental health nurse uses the skill of listening for content and feelings during a conversation. In relation to content, it is important not to 'go beyond' what the person has communicated. Given that we all bring our own experiences to a therapeutic encounter, it is easy to augment what we have heard. In relation to feelings, sometimes people will express these directly. At other times they will use metaphors, for example, 'I am Alice in Wonderland', or 'I am a sinking ship'. Sometimes the feelings will be communicated non-verbally, e.g. by abrupt movements, or facial expression.

Building Meaning

Therapeutic communication embodies the factor of building meaning. When we try to build meaning with a person in distress, it is important to recognise that we may be responding from a particular position. Johnson (2000) points out that most responses fit into one of the following categories:

- advising and evaluating
- analysing and interpreting
- reassuring and supporting
- questioning and probing
- paraphrasing and understanding.

In advising and evaluating, there is an attempt to guide the person. The mental health nurse is implicitly evaluating the person or the person's behaviour. Advising and giving information are different. In analysing and interpreting, the mental health nurse processes what the person has said in order to come up with a deeper meaning. S/he then offers this to the person as an interpretation, with the desire to be therapeutic. In reassuring and supporting, the mental health nurse communicates realistically, e.g., 'that must have been difficult for you' rather than falsely reassuring and supporting, e.g., 'everything will be all right'. In questioning and probing, the mental health nurse tries to gain a greater understanding of where the person is in terms of their distress. S/he asks questions that allow a more expansive response, e.g., 'what's brought you to this point?' In paraphrasing and understanding, there is an opportunity for the mental health nurse to demonstrate that s/he has listened accurately to what the person has said. This shows that the nurse is keen to gain an understanding of the person's perspective of the distress, while acknowledging that it is never possible to understand the distress itself. Only the person who is experiencing the distress is an expert in that respect.

Mental health nurses need specific skills in relation to building meaning with the person in distress.

1. **Paraphrasing** has already been mentioned. It implicitly holds the question, 'is my understanding of what you are saying the same as what you mean to say?' It checks the mental health nurse's accuracy of understanding. Paraphrasing is an important tool, but it can be frustrating for the person if the mental health nurse does nothing but paraphrasing. This is because an impression of 'stuckness' is created where the same things are said all over again, just in slightly different words.
2. **Reflecting feelings** is a means to ensure the person's emotional world is acknowledged by the mental health nurse. It is similar to paraphrasing but in the emotional domain, e.g., 'maybe you are feeling sad at being away from your daughter'.
3. **Connecting thoughts and feelings** adds depth to the mental health nurse's understanding of the person's subjective world. S/he may ask 'how do you feel when your Dad says that you are just lazy?'
4. **Summarising** is a means of reviewing the conversation that has occurred between the person in distress and the mental health nurse. It is a rounded way to bring a close to an episode of communication and creates a platform for further communication, e.g., 'so to sum up what we have talked about so far ...'

In order to build meaning, it is insufficient simply to gain understanding. It is necessary to express understanding too. Often mental health nurses do so through using empathy. Empathy is distinguished from sympathy, which may be defined as 'feeling for' another. Empathy is the ability to perceive the world from another person's viewpoint and to take on that perspective while not losing one's own. Empathy is expressed by verbal and non-verbal means, e.g., saying 'that must have been an uncomfortable position to be in' or moving closer when someone reveals their difficult experience.

Exploring

It is important to be able to sensitively explore areas that may be relevant to the person's distress that s/he has not spontaneously talked about. It assists the building of meaning as both the nurse and person in distress begin to understand together what is contributing to the total distress experience. Exploration also helps to make visible ways of dealing with the distress. There are different kinds of exploration. In planned exploration, the mental health nurse directs the search for meaning, often using specific tools (see 'Screwdrivers and Spanners', below). In spontaneous exploration, the nurse picks up and follows through on a cue offered by the person in distress (see 'The Blue Banana', below). This is important as sometimes people find it difficult to state outright what is troubling them, or to divulge personal and painful information. The person will offer a cue as a means of inviting the nurse to ask more questions to make it easier to broach the uncomfortable subject.

In the following section, some basic tools and skills of exploration are described.

Prompting Skills

The mental health nurse uses verbal prompts to start or carry on the conversation. Minimal encouragers, as discussed above, include utterances (e.g. 'uh huh'), and they simultaneously carry a message of 'I'm with you, please carry on'. The nurse may use one-word or phrase accents to encourage the person to expand, e.g., 'you *won't* be going for a walk today?' Gentle commands can be used to gain more details, e.g., 'tell me what you're thinking about right now'. Open-ended statements can be used as starter questions to introduce a topic, e.g. 'So is this your first time in hospital?' Allowing the person in distress to finish the question is a further way of gaining information, for example, 'So, you're most concerned about ... ?'

Self-disclosure

When the nurse chooses to self-disclose to a person in distress s/he closes up the power differential between them. Self-disclosure that is honest and open encourages the person to offer more about her/himself, e.g., 'I remember when my Dad died and I felt the whole world was falling in.' The level and timing of disclosure has to be thought about carefully. Self-disclosure that is too difficult for the person who is in distress to hear may be non-therapeutic and indicate that the nurse is using the session to meet her or his own needs. That is not to say that therapeutic gain is not possible for both sides in a therapy episode — therapeutic communication *is* a two-way street—but the mental health nurse should not *prioritise* her/his own agenda. Antaki *et al.* (2005:181) describe self-disclosure as a social performance which must be '*brought off* [delivered successfully]* in interaction' and requires consideration of the context and consequences for the people engaged.

Probing Skills

Questions represent probing skills. The two most basic are open and closed questions. Open questions are open-ended and encourage a descriptive or elaborative answer. Open questions often begin with words like who, what, where, when, and how, e.g. 'how was your day today?' They allow a flexible response and offer the mental health nurse an opportunity to follow through on responses that have a low level of disclosure. For example, if the person says, 'I am depressed', the mental health nurse may seek more detail by asking, 'When you are depressed, what can you not do that you would like to?'

Closed questions are defined as those to which the person can answer 'yes' or 'no' or choose from a predefined range of answers, e.g. 'Is the upset you're experiencing sadness, or anger, or disappointment?' Closed questions are useful in gaining specific information quickly. They do not work well when a more exploratory interview is needed. Some questions have limited value when probing. If using a 'why' question, the mental health nurse needs to be aware that the person may not have an answer to give and feel embarrassed or inadequate.

---

*   My addition.

Leading questions involve the mental health nurse imposing her/his interpretation on the person, as in 'You're very angry about John'. Multiple questions, e.g. 'I was wondering if you could tell me how you came to be here today, and what were the main factors and what you think needs to happen now', can simply confuse or overwhelm the person.

Comforting, Supporting and Enabling

When working with people in emotional distress, it is insufficient to simply use skills that explore the nature of that distress. Simultaneously, the nurse needs to be able to support and comfort the person and enable her/him to feel personally secure enough to be able to engage in the therapeutic encounter. There are various ways of responding that allow the person to experience comfort, support and enablement.

Morse (1992) distinguishes between caring and comforting. Caring focuses on the nurse's activity towards the person. Comforting focuses on the needs of the person in distress. Often, the most effective comforting involves the nurse speaking in a human-to-human way, e.g. asking how the person is getting along, showing interest and concern, giving information about what is happening, and being prepared to be with the person in a fully engaged way. In offering comfort the mental health nurse offers reassurance without giving false hope, e.g. 'sometimes people worry that when they come into hospital they won't ever leave. What we will do is make sure that we work hard on your problems and try and get you to a point where you feel able to manage better', rather than 'we'll have you home in no time'.

In offering support (see Ellis *et al.* 2005 for an exploration of support as a concept), the mental health nurse hopes to sustain the person and prevent her/him from 'caving in' or 'falling apart'. Wortman (1984) suggests that support is conveyed through:

- Expressions of positive regard and esteem. Positive regard involves being with the person and appreciating her/his position in a non-judgemental way. Esteem involves accepting the person in her/his own right and acknowledging her/his qualities.
- Encouragement to express and acknowledgement of feelings and points of view.
- Access to information.
- Practical and tangible assistance.
- A sense of belonging.

A further way to support the person is though identifying their resources. Often, mental health nurses dwell on the deficits and symptoms of someone in distress. The Tidal Model (Barker 2000) and solutions-focused approaches (Stevenson *et al.* 2003) differ in that they look at what resources the person has, whether in spirituality, life experience or problem-solving behaviours. These resources are elicited by asking 'strengths questions' during the assessment, e.g. by asking who are the people, things and beliefs that are important to the person, or 'what have you been able to do to make the problem seem more bearable?' or 'what was happening when the problem seemed to be less present in your life?' The nurse now opens the assessment out to consider some of the personal 'assets' or 'resources' of the person. Who and what are the people, things and beliefs that are important to the person, and that might play a part in the person's care plan?

Effective comforting and supporting are in themselves enabling is relation to the person engaging in the therapeutic encounter. Unless the person feels safe to talk s/he will be inhibited in engaging in conversation. Once the person is more engaged, however, it is important to enable full participation as far as possible. This involves a variety of communication strategies:

- Allowing the person to set the agenda, e.g., 'what do you think it would be important to talk about today?'
- Accepting the person's expertise in relation to her/his own experience, e.g. 'you have been living with the problem and must know it better than me.'
- Checking that the meaning taken is accurate, e.g., 'have I got that right?'
- Making sure the person has the information s/he needs, e.g. 'is there anything [or anything more] you need to know about X?'
- Joint care planning, e.g. 'what do you think would distract you from hearing the voice?' or 'do you think it would be helpful if we went and had a game of pool?'
- Inviting the person to evaluate the care given, e.g. 'You know our plan to spend 15 minutes writing your thoughts about losing Jennifer. How do you think it worked?'

SCREWDRIVERS AND SPANNERS

Beyond the micro skills explained earlier, there are some forms of questioning that are particularly useful in helping the person to tell their story. These help the mental health nurse 'talk to listen' rather than listen to talk. That is, the questions elicit rich responses from the person that help the mental health nurse appreciate the person's world. They are not questions that allow the nurse to demonstrate how much s/he knows, but which close down the responses available to the person. Different practitioners will have their favourite questioning tool. In this section I present those that I have found most useful in working with people experiencing distress, and also with their families. They might collectively be called 'interesting and interested questions'.

Circular Questions

Ann Rambo and her colleagues suggest that the best therapists are those who have a natural curiosity (Rambo *et al.* 1993). Being curious is a skill that can be translated into the ability to ask questions. Open and closed questioning has been discussed above. However, there are many questions of a different order which are used in working with families. These are described as circular questions. Circular questioning is a system of questioning developed by the Milan family therapy group (see Becvar and Becvar 2005) that helped them to test hypotheses generated by the team from referral information. Linking questions to hypotheses can create a purposeful and coherent interviewing pattern that reveals new information and peoples' different perceptions of the problem. It exposes 'what' is happening rather than focusing on 'why' something is happening. How this information is discussed becomes the basis for ongoing work. Circular questions are based on triads, i.e. people are asked to comment on the thoughts, behaviour and relationships of other family members. For example, the therapist might ask the mother in a family, 'since your father-in-law came to live with you, has the relationship between your daughter and son been better or worse?'

Circular questions can be grouped for convenience into six rough categories, which overlap to some extent: specific interactive sequence questions; before and after questions; attempts to solve problems; classification/ranking questions; mind-reading questions; hypothetical questions.

1. Specific interactive sequence questions involve more than one person. For example, 'When Ann (mother) is depressed, what does your father do?'
2. Before and after questions track changes in behaviour before and after a specific event. For example, Sister: 'Helen and Joanne are very close to each other.' Therapist: 'Did they get close to each other before or after your mum died?'
3. Attempts to solve problems are identified through questions that ask what worked, who helped. For example, 'When Jane became depressed before, what was helpful?'
4. Classification/ranking questions involve putting people, events and explanations in hierarchies according to specific criteria. For example, 'who in the family is most upset?' or 'Between A, B and C, who do you think is closest to D?' or 'Of the explanations given by mother, which one do you think dad agrees with most?'
5. Mind-reading questions give information on closeness in the family and reveal differences of opinion between people over important issues. For example, Therapist: 'If your sister were alive today, what do you think she would say?' Mother: 'She would say it had to happen.' Therapist: 'In a moment I'm going to ask your brother whether he agrees or disagrees with your sister's view. What do you think he will say?'
6. Hypothetical questions are about (past/current/future) situations, ideas or explanations. For example, 'Let's suppose that you got a job and would be able to afford to rent a place of your own; which of your parents would be most upset when you moved out?'

You may have noticed that some questions combine well together. The last example combines a hypothetical and a ranking question.

Other Helpful Questions

There are other important kinds of questions in working with people in mental health distress and their families: future-oriented questions; comparison questions; observer perspective; gender questions; relative influence questions. Some of these incorporate elements of circular questions.

1. Future-oriented questions. The most famous of these is the miracle question, 'If a miracle were to happen tonight while you were asleep and tomorrow you awoke to find this problem was no longer a part of your life, what would be different? How would you know that this miracle had taken place? How would other people be able to tell without you telling them?'

2. Comparison questions. For example, 'Is your parents' relationship better or worse lately?' or 'Have you felt more like a daughter or more like a wife this week?' or 'Was that always the case, or was it once different?'

3. Observer perspective. For example, 'What do you imagine he feels when he gets into this situation?' or 'How do you think your GP sees the problem?' or 'When your father gets into an argument with your sister, what does your mother usually do?'

4. Gender questions. For example, 'Do you believe that men should be sad/afraid/in need of approval?' or 'Do you believe that women should feel angry/be assertive/competitive/entitled to put themselves first?' (Asked of both genders.) Gender questions can be used to explore inter-generational beliefs about men's and women's roles, e.g., 'Did either of your parents have a hard time meeting their parents' expectations about femininity/masculinity?' or 'If your father/mother disapproved of the manner in which you are a man/woman, how would you know that?' Gender questions can combine well with some other kinds of question, e.g., in future-oriented questions such as, 'If you have a son/daughter, would you like him/her to feel differently about his masculinity/femininity?' or 'Would your parents approve if you raised your children with different ideas about being a man/woman in the world?'

5. Relative influence questions. These questions invite two different descriptions of the person's/family members' association with the problem. The first is a question about the influence the problem has in their lives (directed to all family members). For example, 'When Tom is hearing voices, how does the family find itself operating differently?' (This is passive influence.) The second is a description of the influence of family members in the life of the problem (active influence). For example, 'When Tom is hearing voices, what do the family members do to try to make the voices go away or be less of a nuisance for Tom?'

The Blue Banana

Sometimes people in distress do not feel able to talk about their problem directly. This is often the case if the problem is embarrassing or emotionally painful or draining, or the diagnosis frightening or not understood. On other occasions, the person in distress is so taken up with the problem or diagnosis the conversation is constrained. For example, the person in depression may constantly return to a statement of 'well, I can't because I'm depressed' or 'it's just the depression'. It is perfectly possible to work with people towards recovery without being constrained by the person's caution or being tied up in diagnostic knots. The blue banana technique can help the mental health nurse be therapeutic in the sense of helping him/her move forward in relation to integrating the *experience* of distress into present and future lives. This technique was explained to me by Professor Phil Barker.

Step 1: The person needs to understand that what has brought them to the current point is to be referred to as 'the blue banana'. Although this can lead to some surprise, people are usually willing and able to take the idea on board. Often, the process leads to amusement and so lifts some of the tension that is around the problem.

Step 2: The mental health nurse asks questions without trying to uncover the nature of the problem. So questions might be:
- When did the blue banana first come into your life?
- How did you first notice it?
- What was happening when the blue banana arrived?
- What does the blue banana stop you from doing?
- On a scale of one to ten (with one being no impact and ten being totally affected), how far does the blue banana influence your life?
- Who would be most keen to see the blue banana go away? Who would be next most keen?
- Who would be the least keen to see the blue banana go away? Who would be the next least keen?
- Who else is affected by the blue banana?
- If you woke up tomorrow and the blue banana was gone, what would be the very first thing that you would notice? Who would be the first other person to notice? What would you be able to do that you perhaps cannot do now?
- What kinds of resources do you have in your tussle with the blue banana? (Spiritual resources in the broadest sense, as in ideas and beliefs and values, practical resources, emotional resources, people as resources.)
- When have you been able to ignore the blue banana, or put it to one side?
- What have you been able to do to make the blue banana loom less large in your life?
- Who has the greatest influence/smallest influence over the blue banana?

Mental health nurses tend to be sceptical about the blue banana interview technique. Often, nurses are encouraged to follow a 'mining' model of understanding, that is, trying to dig deep to uncover the 'real' problem. Knowing the cause of a problem does not necessarily lead to productive therapeutic work: for example, knowing about someone's experience of trauma does not always point to how to help the person in the here and now. On the other hand, the blue banana technique encourages working to solve immediate problems that will allow the person to move on with her/his life.

POWER TOOLS

Therapeutic communication is by definition interventive. It creates a difference for the person in mental health distress. Some communication, however, is so powerful it can be seen as an intervention in its own right*. In this section the technique of 'externalising the problem' (White 1988/9) is described and explained.

Sometimes people in distress become defined by the distress or problem. They are overwhelmed by it. In these circumstances it can be difficult to believe that the problem will ever lessen, much less go away. Externalising the problem is useful when the problem is thought to be inherent to the person and is seen as very fixed, e.g. 'I'm just a sad, depressed person'. It encourages people to objectify and sometimes personify the problems they are experiencing; to take them from within to outside themselves. Externalising offers a new story that can free people from the fixed and dominant story they have about a problem. The following section sets out, step by step, the process the mental health nurse engages in if using externalisation.

Step 1
As with much therapeutic communication, there are useful questions. In the case of externalising the problem, the questions used in Step 1 are the 'relative influence' questions described in more detail above:
- What influence is the problem having on your life?
- What influence are you having on the 'life' of the problem?
- What do you do to try and make the problem go away or get less? (Sometimes what people try to do to rid themselves of the problem actually becomes the problem, for example, someone constantly trying to 'cheer up' someone describing her/himself as depressed.)

Step 2
In the second step the mental health nurse has to gain a full definition of the problem to be externalised. There are specific guidelines to follow:
1. Take the person's definition (whether specific or general) as sacrosanct. For example, 'he has tantrums when ...' or 'I have low self-esteem' or 'we have a communication problem'.
2. The definition of the problem may change over time as people struggle to describe their experience, as they move from the general to the specific. This is not the person being economical with the truth (see Reed 1996 for a postmodern exploration of lying and deception in mental health encounters). Rather, it is a process that is reliant in part on the relationship between the

---

* Although powerful, it does not mean that the person is powerless.

person and mental health nurse, in particular the building of trust and the ability of the nurse to help the person build meaning (see above).

3. Sometimes people use professional descriptions of their problems, e.g., 'I am depressed' or 'Jim is schizophrenic'. Try to find a less expert and more popular definition. The means to this end is using good questioning. For example, 'when you describe Jim as schizophrenic, what is it that he does that allows you to know that?'

4. Through this process, find a description of the problem that is mutually acceptable, and that is not located in the person. For example, voice hearing might be characterised as 'Channel 1001', linking it to TV and giving it an independence from the person.

5. If necessary, use characters/personifications. White (1988/9) famously used the personification 'Sneaky Poo' in working with Nick, who was dealing with childhood encopresis. White noted that the poo was making a mess of Nick's life, isolating him from other children and interfering with his school work and galvanised Nick and his parents to battle with the 'Sneaky Poo'.

Step 3
The mental nurse finds unique outcomes, that is, occasions when the problem has not been there or has been dealt with better than other times. It is not always easy for the person to think about when the problem is not there. Often the problem is monopolising the person's life. In this circumstance, the mental health nurse must be persistent. The following guidelines can help:

1. Start with current unique outcomes that are present as you meet with the person. For example, if the person says, 'I am always afraid of speaking about the problem', the nurse replies, 'you are here speaking with me today'. In other words, the unique outcome is identified for the person.

2. If the nurse cannot find a unique outcome in the present, search for one in the past, e.g. 'When was the last time you managed to hold off "the blues"?' followed by 'What was happening then?'

3. The person may be able to offer future unique outcomes which involve the person's plans to escape the problem. For example, the mental health nurse might ask, 'What can you do to make the future look more favourable?' This is a pre-suppositional question, which means that contained in it there is an assumption about what will happen. In this case, there is an assumption that the person can and will be able to influence her/his own future. Such questions, when used in this form, indicate to the person that there is a way forward or action that is open to her/him.

Why does externalising the problem work? When people identify unique outcomes they necessarily change their relationship to the problem. They recognise they can resist the problem. It has become external to them. They refuse to submit to the problem and its effects. The problem becomes less effective. So, through the process of communication a therapeutic effect is achieved.

CONCLUSION

In this chapter, I have tried to offer what I have found useful in my own practice, giving examples and steps to follow. I hope that I have indicated that communication does not have to be dull. The mental health nurse who uses fun and creativity will be a more effective and therapeutic communicator. I learned many of the techniques described through clinical supervision offered by multidisciplinary colleagues. Many were honed through critical review as I reflected on my own practice, often using video playback. For the developing practitioner, these processes are crucial, although sometimes painful. It is not enough to simply learn communication skills and techniques, however. They must be integrated into one's own style. Simply following a preset recipe will not help to engage with the person: it is a force to de-individualise her/him as it disregards the person's own preferences and abilities. Although I hope that the chapter is useful to mental health nurses developing their repertoire, it is neither definitive nor the only source of learning. Mental health nurses learn from being in practice. Lest we forget, in this context, people who are experiencing mental health distress are our best teachers, provided that we are open to their guidance and feedback.

Reflective Questions
1. Are good therapeutic communicators born or made?
2. What is the best example of therapeutic communication in your practice so far (we can always improve)?
3. What therapeutic communication skill would you like to develop further?
4. Which therapeutic communication skills do you find the most challenging?

References
Antaki, C., Barnes, R. and Leudar, I. (2005) 'Self-disclosure as a situated interactional practice'. *British Journal of Social Psychology*, 44, 181–99.

Barker, P. (2000) 'The Tidal Model: the lived experience in person-centred mental health care'. *Nursing Philosophy*, 2, 213–23.

Becvar, D. S. and Becvar, R. J. (2005) *Family Therapy: A Systemic Integration* (6th edn). Boston: Allyn and Bacon.

Burr, V. (1995) *An Introduction to Social Constructionism*. London: Routledge.

Egan, G. (1998) *The Skilled Helper* (6th edn). Pacific Grove, CA: Brooks/Cole.

Ellis, D., Jackson, S. and Stevenson, C. (2005) 'A concept analysis of support', in J. Cutcliffe and H. McKenna (eds), *Essential Concepts in Nursing*. Oxford: Elsevier.

Johnson, D. W. (2000) *Reaching Out: Interpersonal Effectiveness and Self Actualization*. Boston, MA: Allyn and Bacon.

Kai, J. and Crosland, A. (2001) 'People with enduring mental health problems described the importance of communication, continuity of care and stigma'. *British Journal of General Practice*, 51, 730–6.

Morse, J. (1992) 'Comfort: the refocusing of nursing care'. *Clinical Nursing Research*, 1(1), 91–106.

Rambo, A., Heath, A. and Chenail, R. (1993) *Practising Therapy: Exercises for Growing Therapists*. New York: Norton Professional.

Reed, A. (1996) 'Economies with "the truth": professionals' narratives about lying and deception in mental health practice'. *Journal of Psychiatric and Mental Health Nursing*, 3, 249–56.

Stevenson, C., Jackson, S. and Barker, P. (2003) 'Finding solutions through empowerment: a preliminary study of a solution oriented approach to nursing in acute psychiatric settings'. *Journal of Psychiatric and Mental Health Nursing*, 10, 688–96.

Stevenson, C., Grieves, M. and Stein-Parbury, J. (2004) *Patient and Person: Empowering Interpersonal Relations in Nursing*. Oxford: Elsevier.

Watzlawick. P., Bavelas, J. B. and Jackson, D. D. (1967) *Pragmatics of Human Communication*. New York: Norton.

Webb, C. and Hope, K. (1995) 'What kind of nurses do people/patients want?' *Journal of Clinical Nursing*, 4(2), 101–8.

White, M. (1988/9) 'The externalizing of the problem and the re-authoring of lives and relationships' in M. White (ed.), *Selected Papers* (5–28). Adelaide, Australia: Dulwich Centre Publications.

Wortman, C. B. (1984) 'Social support and the cancer patient'. *Cancer*, 53 (supplement): 2339–62b.

9

An Overview of Psychotherapeutic Approaches

Jean Morrissey

Psychotherapeutic approaches or psychotherapies are commonly used to assist individuals, families and groups to cope with difficulties in their psychological and social functioning. This chapter aims to provide the reader with an overview of the underlying principles which inform the practice of the main psychotherapeutic approaches used in mental health care, including: psychodynamic therapy; cognitive behaviour therapy; humanistic therapy; family therapy; and group therapy.

DEFINING A PSYCHOTHERAPY

Psychotherapies are psychosocial treatments which usually share a set of distinguishing characteristics. Psychotherapy is defined as 'an interpersonal process designed to bring about modifications of feelings, cognitions, attitudes and behaviour which have proved troublesome to the person seeking help from a trained professional' (Strupp 1978:3). The characteristics of psychotherapy include 'the presence of a client–therapist relationship, the interpersonal context of the psychotherapies and implied notion of training and professionalism as well as the sense that therapies are conducted according to a model that guides the therapist's actions' (Roth and Fonagy 2005:5). Each psychotherapy or psychotherapeutic approach provides a model of human behaviour as well as a focus for the level to which an intervention is addressed. Psychotherapy may be offered to individuals, couples, families or groups across the life span for relatively short or long periods of time and may be independent of or combined with pharmacological treatments. The format of the psychotherapeutic approach treatment may also differ in terms of its intensity and setting, for example it may be offered five times weekly or monthly in a community-based or in-patient setting. Notwithstanding this, psychotherapeutic approaches of all orientations believe in the fundamental importance of a good client–therapist relationship.

The increased awareness of psychotherapy as a treatment for helping individuals with psychological problems has led to a greater acceptance of psychotherapy as a treatment modality for mental health problems (Department of Health (UK) 2001). However, as psychotherapy has become more fully established, questions have been raised concerning its efficacy, particularly in light of the growing demand for evidence-based practice. Hence there is an increasing demand for a systematic and balanced evaluation of the current status of all major psychotherapeutic approaches. This is problematic, however, given the multitude of different approaches within the practice of talking therapies, many of which have not been investigated. Nevertheless research has broadly found the practice of talking therapies, i.e. counselling and psychotherapy, to be effective (Asay and Lambert 1999). For further detailed coverage on what works best for persons with different mental health problems see Roth and Fonagy (2005).

Mental health nurses may be exposed directly or indirectly to various psychotherapeutic approaches and/or interventions throughout their clinical placements, for example participating in an anxiety management group, teaching a client to use distraction techniques or observing a family therapy session. Having an understanding of the principles that inform different psychotherapeutic approaches can assist nurses in their therapeutic work when working with individuals, families or groups. For those who have an interest in a particular approach it is imperative to engage further with the literature and/or to undertake further training.

PSYCHODYNAMIC THERAPY

Psychodynamic therapy is the oldest of the modern therapies and is informed by psychoanalytic theory, based on the theories first formulated by Sigmund Freud. Psychodynamic therapy focuses on the unconscious processes as they are manifested in a person's present behaviour. A psychodynamic approach enables the client to examine unresolved conflicts and symptoms that developed early in life and that are at least in part unconscious. It is one of several mainstream therapies that focus on aspects of the personality and it is used to treat a variety of conditions, such as depression and personality disorders. According to Freud, instincts drive and direct behaviour and constitute the dynamics of personality. There are many instincts but they are grouped into two basic ones; Eros and Thanatos. Eros is the life instinct — the instinct for the preservation of the self and of the species. Its energy is called libido. Thanatos is the death and destruction instinct and includes aggression (Jacobs 1994).

Freud's model of the mind is divided into three systems. The conscious is what we are immediately aware of at any given moment. The preconscious may be viewed as a screen between the conscious and unconscious and includes all those memories of which we are not immediately aware but which can easily be brought to consciousness. The unconscious includes repressed memories and sensations that are not so readily available, as well as more primitive impulses and fantasies. According to Freud the personality consists of three major systems: the id (consists of primitive instinctual drives or urges, with all their hereditary elements, which require immediate gratification); the ego (a sense of self); and the superego (the vehicle of the conscience and of parental and cultural values) (Sandler et al. 1997). Personality is developed in early childhood through a series of psychosexual stages of development, namely the oral, anal, phallic, latency and genital stages.

Material in the unconscious is kept in place by a process of repression which holds traumatic experiences in place. These are maintained in the unconscious by coping strategies or defence mechanisms. There are numerous defence mechanisms, including the following:

1. repression
2. sublimation
3. fantasy
4. regression
5. rationalisation
6. reaction formation
7. projection
8. conversion
9. compensation
10. identification
11. denial
12. displacement.

The development of defence mechanisms begins with the child's struggle against its sexuality during the first years of life. They can deny, falsify or distort reality. They operate unconsciously and may impede realistic behaviour (Patterson 1986).

PRINCIPLES OF PSYCHODYNAMIC THERAPY IN PRACTICE

The aim of psychodynamic therapy is to develop a relationship with the client that aims to explore his/her unconscious mind. This involves much introspection and reflection from the client. The therapist reflects on how the client is feeling — through words and behaviour—working through the client's resistance, transference and defence mechanisms. The main features of the psychodynamic approach are: 'the client's difficulties have their ultimate origins in childhood experiences, the client may not be aware of the true motives or impulses behind his/her actions and the use of techniques such as dream analysis, and interpretation of the transference relationship' (McLeod 1998:33).

Boundaries. Therapy sessions have strict boundaries to preserve the sanctity of the therapeutic relationship. Maintaining the boundaries involves insistence on sameness, e.g. of timing, date, room etc. All variables are controlled. The therapist reveals little about his/her own private life or personal views.
Setting. In classical analysis the patient lies on the couch. One reason for both the couch and the invisibility of the therapist is to help the 'patient' or 'analysand' (terms used in psychoanalysis) use the analyst (therapist) as a screen upon which to project his/her imagined perceptions of the analyst (Jacobs 1994).
Free association. The psychodynamic approach is a highly verbal talking therapy, encouraging full expression of thought, fantasy and feeling. The therapist prefers

the client to 'free associate', i.e. speak of anything that is uppermost in his or her mind. The aim is to be totally non-directive.

Transference. Use of transference is one of the most distinctive features of psychodynamic theory and practice. Transference occurs whenever emotions, perceptions or reactions based on past experiences are displaced on to the therapist. This might take the form of identifying the therapist with a parent and may be negative (hostile) or positive (affectionate) (Jacobs 2006).

Counter-transference. This occurs when the therapist unconsciously begins to transfer their own repressed feelings onto their client (Wilkins 1997; O'Kelly 1998).

Interpretation. Interpretation is a theoretical idea and a procedure that attempts to provide the client with the meaning of the material revealed in free association, reports of dreams, symptoms and transference. It is the means of relating present behaviour to its origins in childhood. Interpretation helps the client gain insight into the defence mechanisms and resistances that the ego uses to cope with repressed material and which hinders the process of therapy. The therapist interprets any transference in terms of past relationships.

Resistance. While resistance is present in all therapies, a major focus in psychodynamic therapy involves understanding and working with resistance. Resistance includes whatever the client does, deliberately or unconsciously, to prevent, circumvent or otherwise block the progress of therapy (Stark 1994). It can take many forms, for example violating rules, restricting content, being manipulative, withholding communication, etc. What distinguishes the psychodynamic approach is the recognition that resistance has to be handled by understanding the reasons for such defensiveness, for example because the client is afraid of what will emerge and of the therapist's reactions (Stark 1994).

COGNITIVE BEHAVIOUR THERAPY

Cognitive behavioural therapy (CBT) is a focused psychotherapy that is widely used to treat a number of psychiatric problems, including depression, anxiety and eating disorders. More recently, CBT has been used to reduce distress and improve functioning in clients who have severe and enduring mental health problems.

CBT is based on the idea that our thoughts (cognitions) influence our feelings (affect) and our actions (behaviours) (Westbrook *et al.* 2007). Hence our thoughts, feelings and behaviour all interact together. When people hold unrealistic and negative beliefs about themselves or their experiences an emotional upset will result, and if this negative thinking is extreme or persistent it may lead to an emotional disorder such as depression. For example, a person is unsuccessful at a job interview and thinks 'I am a failure, I can't achieve anything'. Such beliefs may have a negative impact on the person's mood, making them feel depressed. The problem may become worse if they react by avoiding applying for another job, which in turn may further reinforce their negative beliefs ('I am a total failure, I will never get a job'), resulting in the person entering into a problem cycle. It is therefore not events that produce bad feelings but the way these events are appraised by the person (Trower *et al.* 1994).

A major difference between CBT and psychodynamic therapies is the degree of importance given to exploring early childhood experiences for the origins of maladaptive patterns of thinking and behaviour. In CBT, while it can be helpful to explore early experiences to enable the client to place the problems in a historical context, this is not a major part of the therapy. The CBT view is that people are disturbed not so much by past events as by the way that these events are viewed in the present (Trower *et al.* 1994).

Variants of Cognitive Behaviour Therapy

CBT can be seen as an umbrella term for many variant therapies which share some common elements, for example:

- *Personal Construct Theory* (Kelly 1955)—the way in which the person seeks to give meaning to their world. Each of us constructs our own view of reality (schema) through a process of experimentation.
- *Rational Emotive Therapy* (RET) (Ellis 1962)—the role of irrational beliefs and the way in which they lead to maladaptive emotional responses.
- *Stress Inoculation Training* (Meichenbaum 1985)—the persistence of 'neurotic' disorders is due in part to the fact that clients engage in unhelpful internal dialogues when faced with stressful situations.
- *ABC Model* (Ellis 1977, see Figure 9.1) provides a useful tool which nurses can use to explain to clients the relationship between thinking and emotions.

Figure 9.1 The ABC model

A = activating event		work colleague fails to acknowledge the person
B = beliefs	(a) inferences	'My colleague has ignored me' 'He must be angry with me' 'He probably dislikes me'
	(b) evaluation	'It's awful if someone dislikes you'
C = emotional consequences behavioural consequences		depression future avoidance of colleague

Source: Trower *et al.* 1994

Conceptualisation of Psychological Disturbance and Health

Beck (1976) suggests that psychological health requires us to be able to use the skills of reality testing to solve personal problems as they occur. In psychological disturbance people revert back to more primitive thinking, which prevents them functioning as effective problem-solvers. This thinking tends to be global, absolute and judgemental. For example, once a person is depressed a set of cognitive distortions known as the *cognitive triad* (negative view of oneself, the world and the future) exerts a general influence over the person's everyday life (Beck 1976). Other biases in information processing also act to consolidate the depression, whereby the person exaggerates and over-generalises minor problems and selectively attends to events that confirm their negative view of self.

Behavioural factors will also serve to exacerbate the depression, e.g. reduced activity, lack of stimulation, withdrawal from life, which in turn reduces the opportunity for positive experiences. Beck identified 'logical errors' that characterise the thinking in emotional disorders. Some of the logical errors in clients suffering from emotional disorders (e.g. depression and anxiety) are:

- Arbitrary inference — 'She did not phone today … she does not love me any more.'
- Selective abstraction — 'One of the ten questions was difficult to answer.'
- Over-generalisation — 'I am always making mistakes.'
- Magnification (catastrophising) — 'Failing my driving test will be a disaster and I am bound to fail.'
- Minimisation (discounting the positive) — 'Getting a mark of eighty per cent was OK.'
- Mind reading — 'Everyone thinks I am stupid.'
- Personalisation — 'They always pick on me.'
- Absolutistic, dichotomous thinking — 'Unless I do it perfectly there's no point in trying.'

Principles of CBT in Practice

Collaborative approach. Although the therapist is directive in CBT, the client is expected to be actively engaged and the therapy is viewed as a collaborative endeavour.

Cognitive assessment. This focuses on the problems the person is experiencing in relation to:

- life/work situation, relationships and practical problems
- altered thinking, emotions, physical feelings or symptoms and behaviour.

The aim of the cognitive assessment is to identify not only the As (activating events) and Cs (consequences) but also the Bs (beliefs), i.e. the cause of the distress. The therapist structures the interview, but the client identifies the problems that concern him/her. A Socratic style of questioning is used to help patients identify, clarify and explore meaning, feelings and consequences as well as to gradually discover insight or explore alternative actions. For example:

- What exactly does this mean?
- How does this relate to what we have been thinking?
- What do we already know about this?
- What would happen if …?
- What evidence is there to support this?
- What are the advantages and disadvantages of …?

Interventions. Cognitive interventions include identifying the thoughts that impacted on mood changing in a specific situation.

Goal setting. Specific goals/changes for treatment are identified. A range of tools is used to monitor outcomes, such as questionnaires, diaries and worksheets.

Diary keeping. A diary is used to record information. Over time, typical thinking patterns will start to emerge.

CBT involves teaching the client to: ✦₴ﾟ·

- monitor their mood and the activating event
- identify maladaptive thinking and beliefs
- realise the connections between thinking, emotions and behaviour, i.e.
    - conceptualising the problem (ABC model)
    - reality testing of maladaptive thinking and beliefs by examining the evidence for and against them
    - substituting the negative thinking with more realistic thinking.

Homework. The therapist will often set 'homework', e.g. graded task assignments, so the client can continue the modification outside of the therapy session.

Unhelpful thinking patterns are modified by techniques such as examining the evidence for the thoughts and identifying the underlying beliefs.

Addressing avoidance. Avoidance of particular activities and situations is a key feature of many problems, including anxiety and depression, which in turn contributes to unhelpful thinking patterns. Avoidance can be addressed by structured graded activities.

Other CBT strategies and techniques may include relaxation and distraction techniques.

A common misconception about CBT is that it is just 'positive thinking'. This is not the case; the aim of CBT is not to teach the client to think positively but to teach the client to think realistically.

DIALECTICAL BEHAVIOURAL THERAPY

Dialectical behaviour therapy (DBT) is a psychosocial treatment developed by clinical psychologist Marsha Linehan following her unsuccessful attempts to apply CBT to a group of young women who all fitted the criteria for diagnosis of borderline personality disorder. DBT aims specifically to create a practical way of helping people with borderline personality disorder. It is a hybrid approach created out of a variety of disparate elements. It makes use of self-monitoring, there is also an emphasis on the here and now and much of the therapeutic technique is borrowed from CBT, including the style of open and explicit collaboration between client and therapist. The 'dialectical' in DBT refers to the way in which it uses a broad way of thinking that emphasises the limitations of linear ideas about causation. For further details see Linehan (1993a, 1993b).

HUMANISTIC THERAPY

Humanistic therapy derives from humanistic psychology and is based on the work of Abraham Maslow, Carl Rogers and others. Person–centred therapy (PCT), also known as non-directive psychotherapy or client-centred therapy, was developed by Carl Rogers. PCT is concerned with the quality of life — how people grow, develop and become who they are. Rogers (1951, 1961) believed that people are essentially social, creative beings and have an inherent tendency to become fully functioning individuals able to express more and more of their potential. Psychological disorders arise from blocks to the person's attempts to reach their potential. PCT is best used to treat clients with relationship problems, anxiety or depression.

In PCT personality theory is known as a self-theory of personality and is concerned with the person's conceptual construction of himself and how s/he then behaves in the world in accordance with that self-concept. The self-concept can be understood in terms of the way we describe ourselves. Similar to Freud, Rogers believed that childhood events are significant in shaping our adult personalities, i.e. children need to feel *unconditionally* loved and valued by people who are significant to them. Rogers (1961) described *conditions of worth*, which refers to the ways in which our self-concepts are shaped by the judgements (love) of others in early childhood, which can be *conditional* or *unconditional*. If love is offered *unconditionally* then children are able to be naturally expressive and accepting of all their feeling. However if love is *conditional*, i.e. given only to the child if s/he behaves in a certain way, then the child begins to think of him/herself in terms of the evaluations of others (*external locus of evaluation*). Hence people with a self-concept that comprises many negative conditions of worth are likely to have low self-esteem and are unlikely to place much trust in their own experience or feelings (*internal locus of evaluation*). For example, if a person has internalised evaluations of poor self-worth then s/he is likely to behave in a way that fulfils this part of their self-concept, which can become self-destructive and unhealthy (Merry 1995).

Principles of PCT in Practice

PCT places much of the responsibility for the treatment process on the client, with the therapist taking a non-directive role. According to Rogers, the client knows best and the client, not techniques and methods, is at the centre of the process.

The therapist encourages the client to express his/her feelings and does not suggest how the person may wish to change, but by listening and then mirroring back (paraphrasing) what the client reveals, helps the client to explore and understand their feelings for themselves and to reach a state of realisation that they can help themselves (Mearns and Thorne 2003).

Core conditions. Rogers (1951, 1961) identified three core conditions as essential to creating a therapeutic relationship: unconditional positive regard; empathetic understanding; and congruence.

- Unconditional positive regard or acceptance means that the therapist accepts the client as a person rather than judging the person by his/her behaviour, thoughts or feelings. This does not mean that the therapist does not make assessments or condones destructive behaviour, rather it means separating the individual from his/her behaviour.

- Empathetic understanding means demonstrating to clients a deep empathetic understanding of the client's 'inner world', i.e. feeling *with* the client (empathy) as opposed to feeling *for* the client (sympathy).
- Congruence means that the therapist remains genuine, real or authentic in his/her relationships with clients.

Two primary goals of PCT are increased self-esteem and greater openness to experience positive condition of worth. The therapist initiates mutual decision making, identifying the client's problems and needs. Goals are achieved through problem-solving ability, promoting stages of change towards self-actualisation.

UNDERSTANDING HUMAN SYSTEMS — FAMILY THERAPY

Systemic approaches draw on general systems theory as well as family therapy to understand communication within families as well as looking at the wider social context. Family therapy, also referred to as family systems therapy, is a branch of psychotherapy that works with families and couples to nurture change and development (Nichols and Schwartz 2007). It emphasises family relationships as an important factor in psychological health. Systems therapy differs from other theoretical orientations in that there is no underlying theory of personality or motivation and change is viewed as a change in the functional properties of the system rather than the individual characteristics of any member of the system (Bor *et al.* 1996).

Whereas most theoretical orientations focus on the individual as the unit of analysis (e.g. psychodynamic therapy), the basic assumption underpinning all versions of family therapy is that the distress or maladjusted behaviour of individual family members is best understood as a manifestation of something going wrong at a systemic level, for example through ineffective communication between family members (Becvar and Becvar 2005). Family therapists view the family as a system of interacting members and are interested in what goes on *between* people (interpsychic) rather than what goes on *in* people (intrapsychic). Family therapy has been used effectively in cases where individuals in families suffer from:

- serious psychological disorders (e.g. schizophrenia, eating disorders and addictions)
- interactional and transitional crises in a family's life cycle (e.g. divorce).

It can also be used to support other psychotherapies and medications.

The Principles of Family Therapy Practice

A family therapist usually meets several members of the family at the same time in the therapy sessions. This allows for patterns of interactions to be observed by the therapist and family and any changes to be shared. The systemically orientated therapist is primarily interested in the system within which the person lives and how this system works. Therapy interventions are aimed at properties of the system rather than aspects of the experiences of individuals. The therapist is not so much concerned with *why* people behave the way they do (cause), but *how* they behave (process) and with what consequences (Bor *et al.* 1996). The goal of the systemic therapist therefore is to facilitate change at a systemic level, for example by rewriting the implicit rules, shifting the balance between different parts of the system or improving the effectiveness of how communication/feedback is transmitted.

Sessions

Systemic approaches are characterised by teamwork, with some workers in the room with the family and others acting as observers to reinforce neutrality. This approach normally entails using a one-way screen that separates the therapist and the family from the rest of the team. The team (behind the screen) can offer feedback of their observations and impressions to the therapist and/or the family. Working this way also enables the team to detect subtle interaction patterns that occur in the complex dynamic of a family's way of being together. The family are aware that that there are people watching from behind the screen. Usually the family attend a limited number of high-impact sessions rather than an extended number of 'gentler' or more supportive sessions.

Hypothesis-forming

The fundamental process in assessment is creating a hypothesis about the presenting problem. A hypothesis directs the therapist to think about the problem in a particular way and to seek particular types of information from the family.

Neutrality

Neutrality is the ability to avoid forming an alliance with particular family members or sub-groups. The therapist adopts a detached, neutral stance to prevent any bias and to be able to hear multiple perspectives within the family. Maintaining neutrality is important as it is the system, and not any one individual, that is the target of change.

Circular Questioning

Circular questioning is a potent assessment tool and intervention that increases the amount and quality of information that comes out of the interview (Becvar and Becvar 2005). Circular questioning links the family members together, as one person's answers to a question can be used to generate a question to another family member: for example, rather than asking a family member what he feels about something that has happened in the family, the therapist could ask the family member how he feels about what his brother thinks about it, thus introducing both an awareness of the links between the different perspectives and raising the possibility of generating multiple descriptions of the same event. Hence circular questioning may prove a useful tool for elaborating the nature of the problem and getting the family to develop a representation of its own dynamics.

Genograms

A genogram is a pictorial display constructed by the therapist. It goes beyond a traditional family tree by allowing the user to visualise hereditary patterns, repetitive patters of behaviour and hereditary tendencies. Some family therapists use genograms to explain family dynamics to the client/family.

GROUP THERAPY

Group therapy is a form of psychotherapy in which one or more therapists facilitate a small group of clients together as a group. A group comprises a number of people who share some common interest or concern and who stay together long enough for the development of a network of relationships which involves all members of the group. The theoretical approach underpinning group therapy may include humanistic psychology, cognitive behavioural approach, psychoanalytical theory and other schools of counselling and psychotherapy. Groups can be used for many mental health problems concerning interpersonal relationships.

The focus of group therapy is on the individual's way of relating within a group. The members of the group interact with one another in such a manner that each person influences and is influenced by each other person. This situation allows the group members to understand and learn about being in a relationship and how relating to others influences getting their needs met (Gilbert and Shmukler 1996). The term 'group dynamics' is used to describe the general study of the behaviour of people in groups and more specifically to refer to the theories of group behaviour. Group dynamic material is an analysis of the observations by the facilitator(s) of what they see happening in the group, e.g. the roles of group members, patterns of communication. In group therapy the activity of the whole and the activity of the parts must both be studied.

Each group is unique in its particular constellation (membership) and climate, yet common themes emerge across groups that appear to reflect shared human concerns, e.g. the need to belong, the need to be accepted. Hence 'both the uniqueness and the universality contribute to the learning potential of a group as these reflect the nature of our psychological make-up and the world in which we live' (Gilbert and Shmukler 1996:444). While group therapy primarily consists of a 'talking therapy' it may also include other therapeutic modes, e.g. psychodrama, play therapy. Groups have advantages in that they can provide multiple sources of feedback and are often time- and cost-effective. As a therapeutic approach, there is evidence that group therapy leads to successful outcomes for people living with mental health problems including depression, anorexia nervosa, schizophrenia and alcohol dependency, and for suicidal adolescents (Roth and Fonagy 2005).

Stages in the Life of a Group
There are a number of different views of group development and while they may focus on different aspects of group life and use different ways to describe the various stages, they share many ideas.

Figure 9.2 Stages in the life of a group

Bion (1961) — Three types of basic assumption	Tuckman (1965)	Yalom (1970) — Three stages
Dependency	Forming	Orientation
Pairing	Storming	Conflict
Fight/flight	Norming	Cohesiveness
	Performing	

Types of Groups used in Mental Health
In clinical practice, groups are formed for a variety of reasons and a group is constructed along very specific lines for a particular purpose. The conductor (facilitator) of the group may be a user of mental health services, a nurse, a carer, etc. Some self-help groups may function without the role of a facilitator.

Groups may be large or small, open or closed; they may use different approaches (e.g. psychodynamic, CBT, humanistic); and they may have different tasks (e.g. supportive, educational).

Figure 9.3 Factors to consider in forming and facilitating a group

Forming a Group	Facilitating a Group
Selecting members; number in group; inclusion/exclusion criteria	Facilitation skills/role: • ensuring adherence to ground rules • encouraging and enabling members' participation • fostering atmosphere of open discussion • challenging people who may be acting in a manner harmful to the group
Agreeing ground rules (boundaries), e.g. • time, length, frequency of meetings • location • start and end dates • open/closed • addition of new members • attendance	Level of trust: people are more likely to participate in a group if they trust the group and feel safe in sharing information with others in the group

Forming a Group	Facilitating a Group
Task of group: goals	Cohesion: a group is cohesive when all members share a common therapeutic goal
Confidentiality	Group roles: in groups the roles and functions may be allocated or adopted by group members, e.g. the peacemaker, joker, aggressor, information-giver, helper, etc.
Role of group facilitator and participants	Power and influence: the process whereby group members influence, or are influenced by others, through the exercise of power
Theoretical approach, e.g. CBT, humanistic	Bringing the group to a close in a manner that does not leave unresolved tensions, and applying consistency in starting and ending on time

Strengths and Challenges of Group Therapy
Group therapy presents both strengths and challenges as a therapeutic approach for both the facilitator and members of the group. These include the following (Wright 1989).
Strengths:
- group acts as a social microcosm of society
- group acts as a container
- universality
- offers feedback
- intimacy/belonging
- learning to develop tolerance of others
- cost effective
- group can act as a role model.

Challenges:
- threatening
- increases defences
- less intimate
- less individual time
- power/powerlessness
- rivalry within group
- splitting — the process of turning one against another in the group
- group members forming into small cliques
- scapegoating — the role of the scapegoat is to act as a recipient for all the hostile and guilty feelings the group has.

CONCLUSION

Psychotherapeutic approaches are an important component of treatment for helping individuals, families or groups with mental health problems. Each psychotherapeutic approach seeks to provide a model of human behaviour as well as a focus for the level to which an intervention is addressed within the therapeutic relationship. However, each theoretical orientation wrestles with the dilemma of trying to provide evidence to support its efficacy, particularly given the increasing demand on resources in mental health care. Nevertheless, there is evidence to support the use of different psychotherapeutic approaches to assist people who experience problems and who are often incapacitated by these problems. This being the case, it is important that nurses have an understanding of their use in mental health nursing.

Reflective Questions
1. If you were to seek psychotherapy what would be your treatment of choice in psychological therapies (counselling) and for what reasons?
2. What psychotherapeutic approach would you like to know more about and how might this assist you in your clinical practice?
3. What psychotherapeutic approaches have you been exposed to in your clinical placements and how have they benefited (or not) individuals, families or groups?
4. What are the key commonalities and differences between psychodynamic therapy, cognitive behaviour therapy, humanistic therapy, family therapy and group therapy?

References
Asay, T. P. and Lambert, M. J. (1999) 'The empirical case for the common factors in therapy', in M. A. Hubble, B. L. Duncan and S. D. Miller (eds), *The Heart and Soul of Change: What Works in Therapy?* Washington, DC: American Psychological Association.
Beck, A. (1976) *Cognitive Therapy and the Emotional Disorders.* New York: New American Library.
Becvar, D. S. and Becvar, R. J. (2005) *Family Therapy: A Systemic Integration* (6th edn). Boston: Allyn and Bacon.
Bion, W. R. (1961) *Experiences in Groups.* London: Tavistock.
Bor, R., Legg, C. and Scher, I. (1996) 'The systems paradigm' in R. Woolfe and W. Dryden (eds), *Handbook of Counselling Psychology.* London: Sage.
Department of Health (UK) (2001) *Treatment Choice in Psychological Therapies and Counselling.* London: Department of Health.
Ellis, A. (1962) *Reason and Emotion in Psychotherapy,* New Jersey: Lyle Stuart.
Ellis, A. (1977) 'The basic clinical theory of rational-emotive therapy' in A. Ellis and R. Grieger (eds), *Handbook of Rational Emotive Therapy.* New York: Springer.

Gilbert, M. and Shmukler, D. (1996) 'Counselling psychology in groups' in R. Woolfe and W. Dryden (eds) *Handbook of Counselling Psychology*. London: Sage.

Jacobs, M. (1994), *Psychodynamic Counselling in Action*. London: Sage.

Jacobs, M. (2006) *The Presenting Past: The Core of Psychodynamic Counselling and Therapy* (3rd edn). Buckingham: Open University Press.

Kelly, G. (1955) *The Psychology of Personal Constructs* (vols 1 and 2). New York: Norton.

Linehan, M. (1993a) *Cognitive Behavioural Therapy for Borderline Personality Disorder*. New York: Guilford Press.

Linehan, M. (1993b) *Skills Training Manual for Treating Borderline Personality Disorder*. New York: Guilford Press.

McLeod, J. (1998) *An Introduction to Counselling* (2nd edn). Buckingham: Open University Press.

Mearns, D. and Thorne, B. (2003) *Person–Centred Therapy Today: New Frontiers in Theory and Practice*. London: Sage.

Meichenbaum, D. (1985) *Stress Inoculation Training*. New York: Pergamon Press.

Merry, T. A. (1995) *Invitation to Person Centred Psychology*. London: Whurr Publishers.

Nichols, M. P. and Schwartz, R. C. (2007) *The Essentials of Family Therapy*. Boston, Mass: Pearson/Allyn and Bacon.

O'Kelly, G. (1998) 'Countertransference in the nurse–patient relationship', *Journal of Advanced Nursing*, 28 (2), 391–7.

Patterson, C. H. (1986) *Theories of Counselling and Psychotherapy* (4th edn). New York: Harper Collins.

Rogers, C. (1951) *Client Centred Therapy: Its Current Practice, Implications and Theory*. Boston: Houghton Mifflin.

Rogers, C. (1961) *On Becoming a Person*. London: Constable.

Roth, A. and Fonagy, P. (2005) *What Works for Whom? A Critical Review of Psychotherapy Research* (2nd edn). New York: Guildford Press.

Sandler, J., Holder, A., Dare, C. and Dreher, A. (1997) *Freud's Models of the Mind*. London: Karnac Books.

Stark, M. (1994) *A Primer on Working with Resistance*. NJ: Aronson.

Strupp, H. H. (1978) 'Psychotherapy research and practice — an overview' in A. E. Bergin and S. L. Garfield (eds), *Handbook of Psychotherapy and Behaviour Change* (1994) (2nd edn). New York: Wiley.

Trower, P., Casey, A. and Dryden (1994) *Cognitive Behavioural Counselling in Action*. London: Sage.

Tuckman, B. W. (1965) 'Developmental sequences in small groups'. *Psychological Bulletin*, 63: 384–99.

Westbrook, D., Kennerley, H. and Kirk, J. (2007) *An Introduction to Cognitive Behaviour Therapy: Skills and Applications*. London: Sage.

Wilkins, P. (1997) 'Congruence and countertransference: similarities and differences'. *Counselling*, 8, (1) 36–40.

Wright, H. (1989) *Groupwork: Perspectives and Practice*. Middlesex: Scutari Press.

Yalom, I. D. (1970) *The Theory and Practice of Group Psychotherapy*. New York: Basic Books.

10
Psychosocial Interventions
Mark Monahan, Louise Doyle and Brian Keogh

Since the 1950s pharmacological interventions have been the mainstay in treatment approaches to serious mental illness. However, despite the usefulness of pharmacological treatments, it is now generally acknowledged that optimum outcomes for severe mental illness cannot be achieved by medication alone. The limited response of some individuals to pharmacological treatment and a high incidence of adverse effects, in conjunction with limitations in concordance with medication regimes, has led to a quest for choice and a range of treatment options with reduced reliance on medication (Mental Health Commission 2005). Recently a range of interventions for severe mental illness has evolved both as adjuncts to pharmacological treatments and as interventions in their own right. These approaches are broadly classified as psychosocial interventions (PSI). This chapter provides an introduction to some of the common principles and approaches included in psychosocial interventions.

WHAT ARE PSYCHOSOCIAL INTERVENTIONS?

Psychosocial interventions are a range of activities designed to enhance an individual's social and psychological functioning. Interventions focus primarily on working with people with psychosis, their families and caregivers through developing social skills, interpersonal relationships, and communication. Definitions are underpinned by a vision of recovery and encompass models of service delivery such as case management and assertive outreach. The concept has grown to represent both an ideological standpoint in contemporary mental health and a political movement within healthcare. The success of a psychosocial interventions approach is contingent on the delivery of care in a holistic and integrated manner.

TERMINOLOGIES IN PSYCHOSOCIAL INTERVENTIONS

A varied terminology has developed to discuss psychosocial interventions in the management of psychosis or schizophrenia. Tension exists between the medical model's perception of illness and those who seek an alternative to this perspective. The use of terms such as hallucination, delusion and negative symptoms is seen to contribute to the development of labelling and stigmatisation associated with the diagnosis. A counter perspective, presented by groups such as the Hearing Voices Network, is that the features associated with the diagnosis of schizophrenia are responses to an inability to cope with phenomena experienced by a significant proportion of the population, and this inability to cope manifests in 'illness'. The terms 'voice hearing' and 'strange thoughts' have now entered mental health vocabulary. Accordingly, the language of psychosocial intervention, while not completely decrying the perception of illness, has attempted to represent both perspectives in developing interventions and, in many instances, the terms have become interchangeable.

STRESS AND VULNERABILITY AS APPLIED TO PSYCHOSIS

The Stress Vulnerability Model has become a major premise for the use of psychosocial interventions. Zubin and Spring (1977) presented an alternative perspective to severe mental illness with the proposal of the Stress Vulnerability Model for schizophrenia (see Chapter 2). It views the well-being of an individual as a complex interaction between a wide range of factors, both intrinsic and extrinsic. Nuechterlein and Dawson's (1984) development of the model explains this as a series of complex interactions between personal vulnerability factors, personal protectors, environmental protectors, potentiators and stressors. These factors govern and influence the individual's interaction with life. Simply put, the consequence of stressors that exceed the individual's capacity to cope (vulnerability) result in signs and symptoms that are typically interpreted as the diagnosis of schizophrenia.

BENEFITS OF PSYCHOSOCIAL INTERVENTION

Psychosocial interventions aim to decrease a person's vulnerability to illness through improving coping skills and reducing the impact of stressful events and situations. The approach emphasises improvement in social functioning and communication. The objective is to decrease distress and disability and ultimately improve the quality of life for individuals. Interventions do not decrease the incidence of symptoms, but assist in the management of persisting psychotic symptoms and in the development of understanding and insight. Interventions enhance the effectiveness of pharmacological interventions, improve depressive symptoms, and prevent relapse. Figure 10.1 presents an overview of the different approaches to psychosocial interventions.

Figure 10.1 Approaches to psychosocial interventions

Psychological	Social
• Cognitive Behaviour Therapy	• Employment/education
— Normalisation	• Social skills training
— Focusing	• Life skills training
— Influencing beliefs	• Social inclusion
— Coping strategy enhancement	• Functional improvement
• Symptom reduction	• Well-being and quality of life
• Stress reduction	

Family interventions	Educative
• Psycho-education	• Relapse prevention
• Communication training	• Medication management/concordance
• Problem solving	• Health promotion

Currently no studies clearly show that psychosocial interventions are effective without the concurrent use of pharmacological interventions and they should not be considered as a direct alternative. The combination of these approaches is considered to be the most effective treatment. The growth in the popularity of PSI may be attributable to the challenge it presents to existing thinking on severe mental illness, and how it prioritises the needs of the severe mentally ill, as this group was previously perceived as disadvantaged by stigma and neglected as a population. In this regard, PSIs provide opportunities to enhance services by tailoring interventions to meet the needs of individual users and their families.

Despite growing evidence of effectiveness, many of these approaches are still not widely available in clinical environments. It is argued that some techniques, such as Cognitive Behaviour Therapy (CBT), should not be used without specialist education or clinical supervision (Siddle and Everitt 2002). However, the application of the principles involved is increasingly perceived as valuable in the potential that they can add to nurses' interventions in everyday clinical situations (Keen 2003) and educational programmes now seek to build upon these principles. For example, the Thorn Programme has now become synonymous with working with severe mental illness using evidence-based psychosocial interventions and is now open to all groups working in the mental health field.

ENGAGING CLIENTS WITH SEVERE MENTAL HEALTH PROBLEMS

The success of a PSI approach may be attributable not merely to improving psychological or social functioning but also to its role in strengthening and developing the therapeutic relationship (Goering and Stylianos 1988). Engagement is a prerequisite for embarking on a psychosocial intervention approach. Historically, engaging clients with severe mental health problems was an area embarked upon with some trepidation. It was considered that people with a diagnosis of schizophrenia were unable to collaborate in a working relationship because of their impaired mental state (Wolpe 1958). This idea prevailed into the 1980s, when it was still regarded as pointless and possibly damaging to discuss symptoms such as hallucinations and delusions with clients (Hamilton 1980). Current thinking considers that ignoring hallucinations and delusions, a primary cause of distress for many clients, creates a significant obstacle to the development of a meaningful therapeutic relationship (Repper 2002). Addressing concerns about the client's illness may lead to more satisfactory outcomes and improve their engagement with the health services. However, today professionals rarely ask 'what do the voices say?', with a result that there remains tension and difficulty in interactions (McCabe et al. 2002).

When working with clients a 'naive' approach can offer a potential avenue in the development of the relationship (Mills 2006). Rather than entering the equation as an expert, this approach allows for open engagement on the client's terms and permits the development of new insight. This requires treatment as an equal, with discussion rather than interrogation being most effective. When engaging, it is essential that the needs identified by the individual must take priority. Practicality dictates that if factors such as financial or social concerns require attention, these will need to be resolved before the person will be willing to engage. A synopsis of research on clients' perceptions of their needs is detailed in Figure 10.2.

Figure 10.2 Research on clients' analysis of needs

Social
- Self-organisation
- Self-help
- Social networks
- Reducing stigma
- Advocacy
- Equal opportunity

Financial
- Meaningful employment
- Adequate income, finance and resources
- Assistance with housing

Services
- Choice
- Accessibility

Relationship
- Warmth
- Understanding
- Respectful
- Empathy
- Intimacy
- Privacy
- A satisfying sex life
- A satisfying social life
- Happiness
- Help to come to terms with problems
- Physical health

Sources: Estroff 1981; Shepherd et al. 1995; Read 1996; Mental Health Commission 2005

Simple practical interventions often offer the best basis for establishing the relationship, in particular interventions that focus on skill development or social competency. With psychosocial intervention, patience is required and it must be accepted that trust will take time to develop. In this instance, informal, frequent contact, with flexibility and willingness to engage with the individual across a range of different environments may offer the best route. Ultimately, engagement can only occur if the interventions being considered are acceptable to the client (Repper 2002).

ASSESSMENT OF CLIENTS

Psychosocial assessment requires a detailed evaluation of clients that focuses on the identification of goals and outcome-orientated interventions. Assessment in serious mental illness is acknowledged as difficult and there is concern that existing assessment approaches do not translate into effective interventions in practice (Gamble and Brennan 2006). A wide range of structured assessment tools now exists, which are applicable to severe mental illness. It is important to emphasise that assessment should be co-ordinated and involve the entire multi-disciplinary team. The isolated use of assessments can lead to inappropriate outcomes and create barriers to team functioning. Figure 10.3 identifies the key aspects of psychosocial assessment.

Figure 10.3 Key aspects of psychosocial assessment

Risk
- Suicide
- Violence

Social
- Need and Functioning
- Financial
- Accommodation
- Employment

Symptoms
- Hallucinations
- Delusions
- Negative symptoms
- Depression

Medication
- Use and effect

Relapse prevention
- Early warning signs
- Coping strategies

Supports
- Carer involvement
- Carer needs

Quality of Life

Health needs
- Health promotion

WORKING WITH VOICES AND STRANGE THOUGHTS

From the stress/vulnerability perspective, the presence of hallucinations or voices can be interpreted as an extreme form of normal experience and in theory, everybody may be susceptible. Kingdon and Turkington (1994) identify the probability that it is a naturally occurring phenomenon, with research recording a two to three per cent incidence in the general population (Tien 1991). Significantly, the presence of auditory hallucinations, although occurring in only 30 per cent of schizophrenia diagnoses, manifests in an 84 per cent likelihood of receiving the diagnosis (Lewinsohn 1968). Romme and Escher (1996) report that 28 per cent of all psychiatric patients have heard voices at some time, with auditory hallucinations occurring across a range of conditions such as bipolar disorder, affective disorder, personality disorder and anxiety states. Most voice hearers experience both positive and negative voices. However, negative voices predominate for those who present as clients and the ability to cope with the voice is a factor which may differentiate the need for psychiatric care (Honig *et al.* 1998). These people report being more afraid of the voices, finding them upsetting, and disrupting their daily life. Romme and Escher (2000) identify that the ability of voice hearers to express their experiences freely is intensely liberating. The ability to acknowledge voices openly can allow voice hearers to make a choice about how to react, allowing a degree of control and the alleviation of powerlessness and dependency.

Figure 10.4 Stages in developing coping strategies for voices and strange thoughts

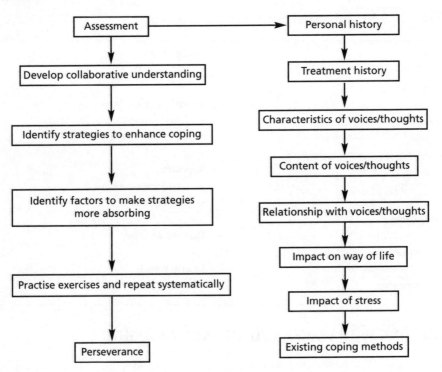

The foundation for interventions for voice hearers begins with the development of an understanding of the client's experience with voice hearing. Often this is a difficult process, owing to clients' fear in talking openly about the experience or fear of being punished by the voice. It should also be expected that the voices may be active and comment on the process during the assessment, thereby limiting engagement (Mills 2006). The stages in developing coping strategies for voices and strange thoughts and the factors in assessment are outlined in Figure 10.4. The timescale for the assessment process and interventions should not be hurried and an assessment can take several sessions to complete.

According to the Stress Vulnerability Model, voices and strange thoughts may be exacerbated by stressful life events as the individual struggles to cope. Thus, interventions targeted at meeting physical and social needs, frequently a source of stress, may protect against the incidence of the phenomenon. Interventions generally fall into two categories: simple techniques that can be used to assist the individual gain control over voices; and longer-term methods that focus on assisting the individual to develop an understanding of the experience. Common strategies for coping with voices and strange thoughts are illustrated in figure 10.5.

Figure 10.5 Strategies for coping with voices and strange thoughts

Physical

Relaxation techniques
- Breathing exercises
- Having a bath

Activity
- Playing a musical instrument
- Singing

Exercise
- Walking
- Workout

Using earplugs

Medication use/increase

Social/Behavioural

Distraction
- Listening to music
- Reading aloud
- Counting backwards
- Describing an object in detail
- Watching TV

Peer support
- Talking to family member or friend
- Self-help group
- Phone helpline

Avoidance of trigger situations/people

Use of satisfying experience

Cognitive

Interaction with the voices
- Telling voices to stop
- Replying to the voices (using mobile phone in company)
- Designating a time and duration
- Dismissing voices
- Postponing orders from the voices

Writing down what the voices say and want

Testing/checking whether voice content is true

Creating boundaries on content

Anticipating the voices

Substituting different orders for commands

Source: Romme and Escher 2000; Mills 2006

Initial short-term interventions must be monitored for effectiveness as inappropriate interventions may generate more emotional distress or in some cases be detrimental to physical health or involve physical harm. Inappropriate coping mechanisms may also lower confidence and self-esteem or trigger negative responses in other people.

COGNITIVE BEHAVIOUR THERAPY IN PSYCHOSIS

Evidence is emerging of the effectiveness of cognitive behaviour therapy in psychosis. Initial work in this field was done with persistent delusions and hallucinations where it was shown to reduce symptom severity and decrease the duration of hospital stays. Four of the most popular approaches — normalisation, focusing, influencing beliefs and coping strategy enhancement — are outlined below.

Normalisation (Kingdon and Turkington 1991)
Normalisation is an education-based intervention also known as 'de-catastrophisation'. This approach suggests that hearing voices is not purely related to the illness, it contextualises the voice hearer's experiences with those of others who experience the phenomenon, drawing on the research into sleep deprivation, sensory deprivation, hostage situations and those relating to sexual abuse as illustrations. The outcomes of this approach show that it is effective in decreasing anxiety and powerlessness associated with the experience.

Focusing (Bentall et al. 1994)
The initial development of this approach was with long-term voice hearers who were resistant to neuroleptic medication. The intervention is structured on a sessional basis and requires the person to examine the characteristics of the voice, what is said by the voice, the thoughts the individual has related to the experience, and the meanings the voices generate. It is done in a gradual four-stage approach, akin to systematic desensitisation. Progress is made at the pace of the individual and depends on the level of anxiety created when working through the process. The results of the approach when compared with distraction techniques show the same levels of symptom reduction but the level of the individual's self-esteem is increased.

Influencing Beliefs (Chadwick et al. 1996)
This approach is based on the premise that there is a point between an individual's perception of voices and their subsequent behaviour. This intermediate point, and ultimately the person's ability to cope (coping response), are governed by their beliefs about their voices. Whether voices are benevolent or malevolent heavily influences their behaviour. In this approach, the therapeutic relationship focuses on interventions that challenge the person's beliefs as to the nature and intent of the voices, thereby increasing the individual's ability to cope with the phenomenon.

Coping Strategy Enhancement (Yusupoff and Tarrier 1996)

The emphasis in this approach is on developing a clear understanding of what happens when the voice is heard. It tries to establish what the individual does in the interval before they experience the voice again and what their pattern of response is. With this understanding the therapist seeks to build upon the effectiveness of the person's existing coping strategies and seeks to develop these further. It comprises a three- phase process: assessment; establishing the individual's motivation and desire to gain control over voices; and the development of suitable intervention or training programme tailored to the individual.

The use of cognitive behaviour therapy in psychosis is considered effective when it is expertly applied, in particular in its benefits to both positive and negative symptom reduction (Tarrier *et al.* 1998; Kinderman and Cooke 2000). Current indications are that it can be effective in the medium term however long-term effects are not sustained, and may not provide additional benefits over standard treatments or supports (Jones *et al.* 2004).

MEDICATION MANAGEMENT

The use of psychotropic medications remains one of the mainstays of psychiatric treatment, however there is considerable evidence to suggest that many people do not take their medication as prescribed. It has been established that continuing on regular medication can significantly reduce relapse rates. Consequently there has been an effort to target 'non-compliance' among those who are prescribed these medications. In addition, there has been recognition that the term 'compliance' is value-laden and suggests an authoritative relationship between the client and the prescriber/carer (Marland and Sharkey 1999). Accordingly, the terminology has moved from 'compliance' through 'adherence' to 'concordance', which suggests a more collaborative and partnership approach to care.

The factors contributing to a client's decision not to take their medication as prescribed are numerous and diverse. They include:

- Side-effect profile of prescribed medications.
- Lack of insight into the illness: individuals may believe that they are not ill and therefore have no need to take medication.
- Clinical features of illness, e.g. paranoia.
- Secondary gain from illness, e.g. people who are manic may enjoy the feeling of elevation.
- Lack of symptoms, particularly in prophylactic use.
- Refusal to accept diagnosis.
- Beliefs about treatment: many people believe that medications should not have a primary role in treating mental health problems.
- Fear of drug addiction.
- Quality of relationship with the prescriber – paternalistic or collaborative?
- Treatment setting: home versus hospital.

- Dual diagnosis: co-morbidity of a mental health problem and a substance abuse problem increases the rate of non-concordance.
- Poor knowledge and understanding of medication.
- Polypharmacy/complex regimes leading to inability to understand medications.

Non-adherence with psychotropic medications regimens can have a range of effects including an increase in relapse rate leading to an increased number of hospitalisations. This in turn may cause a loss of occupational/recreational opportunities and may lead to a decrease in social functioning. Non-adherence may also increase the burden on carers and mental health services. It is therefore essential that interventions aimed at improving adherence rates are developed and implemented. A medication management approach must highlight the importance of interactions that encourage client involvement, choice and independence. It must also aim to address the reasons behind non-adherence. The following are common interventions in a medication management approach:

- Assessment of mental state: an initial assessment of the client's illness is important both prior to commencement of psychotropic medications and also during treatment to assess the medication efficacy. A baseline measurement of symptoms prior to administration of medications is also important to distinguish symptoms from side effects. A scale such as the KGV symptom scale can be utilised (Krawiecka *et al.* 1977).
- Assessment of side effects: assessment of the severity of side effects of medication is an important aspect of medication management. They may go undetected as clients may not report them and nurses may not ask about them (Bennett *et al.* 1995). A side effect rating scale such as the LUNSERS (Day *et al.* 1995) can help to provide an accurate picture of the extent of side effects and how they impinge on clients' lives.
- Management of side effects: many side effects can be managed medically by downward titration of dosage, switching to other pharmacological therapies or introducing other medications to alleviate side effects. Side effects can also be managed symptomatically by including interventions to alleviate common side effects such as constipation, dry mouth, weight gain etc.
- Compliance therapy (Kemp *et al.* 1997): this is a cognitive-behavioural intervention that has adapted techniques from motivational interviewing and psycho-education. The aims of the therapy are to develop an open dialogue about medication and to encourage discussion about the pros and cons of pharmacological treatment. It promotes a partnership approach between the client and the mental health professional to aid 'negotiating medication'. Compliance therapy involves working with clients to address their beliefs and perceptions about medication, their ambivalence about change and their expectations about treatment outcomes. Education is also a key component and aims to provide information to clients about their illness and their medication. However, while education is useful in improving people's knowledge about their medication, when used *in isolation* from the other

components of compliance therapy, it does not increase concordance (Gray *et al.* 2002). Finally, compliance therapy also involves a behavioural component, which is concerned with incorporating the medication regime into the everyday routine of the client.

'Mental health nurses play a central role in helping patients manage their medication more effectively' (Gray *et al.* 2002:283). Understanding the factors that affect a person's decision to take their medication and working collaboratively with them in addressing these factors is crucial if clients are to benefit from the positive effects of medication while minimising adverse effects.

PREVENTING RELAPSE

According to Birchwood and Spencer (2001:1212) 'Relapse in psychosis is conventionally defined as the re-emergence or exacerbation of the frank psychotic symptoms.' Research internationally has reported on the effects of medication and psychosocial interventions in relation to the recurrence of mental health problems with a decrease in number of relapses being the measure of positive outcome (van Meijel *et al.* 2004). This section describes interventions aimed at preventing relapse involving recognition of early warning signs, the use of relapse signatures and the implementation of an action plan.

The Process of Relapse

Much of what is written about the process of relapse concentrates on illnesses such as schizophrenia, bipolar affective disorder or problems associated with substance misuse. It should be noted that relapse varies among individuals and can occur over a short or extended timeframe. Birchwood and Spencer (2001) offer a three-stage model of psychotic relapse, which is described in Figure 10.6.

Figure 10.6 Psychological aspects of early relapse (Birchwood and Spencer 2001)

Stage	Process
1. First stage of relapse	Symptoms such as reduced attention span, derealisation or racing thoughts occur.
2. Dysphoria	Decreased interest, low mood, changes in self-care, preoccupation with mental life.
3. Pre-psychotic or psychotic phase	Hears voices, may appear suspicious, have ideas of reference.

Van Meijel *et al.* (2003) describe an intervention protocol that helps nurses, and people vulnerable to relapse, to develop a relapse prevention plan. Although originally intended for people with schizophrenia and schizoaffective disorder, the four basic steps can be easily applied to different people with different mental health problems. Figure 10.7 presents a diagram of this intervention protocol.

Figure 10.7 The intervention protocol (van Meijel *et al.* 2003)

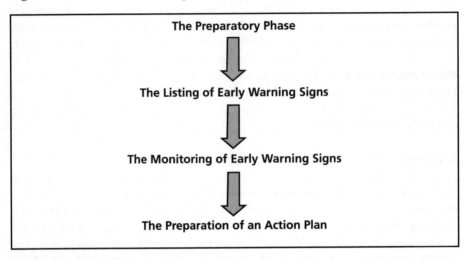

The Preparatory Phase
This phase of the intervention protocol sets the scene for working collaboratively with the client and other significant people such as the client's family or other members of the client's support network. This creates 'a basis for collaboration ... to make concrete agreements about the involvement of various people in the preparation of the plan' (van Meijel *et al.* 2003:167).

Early Warning Signs
Early warning signs of impending psychosis can be described as subtle or explicit symptoms that occur in the preceding days or weeks before the client is said to have relapsed. They are sometimes referred to as prodromal symptoms and are often similar to the symptoms of the particular illness. They can be divided into two types (Figure 10.8).

Figure 10.8 Early warning signs

Early Warning Symptoms	Idiosyncratic Behaviours
• Dysphoria • Increased anxiety • Sleep disturbances • Appetite disturbances • Auditory hallucinations • Feelings of uneasiness (Sutton 2004)	These refer to those subtle behaviours or symptoms that may appear and are exclusive to that particular person e.g. the person starts to spend long periods alone or there is a change in dress or make-up patterns. (van Meijel *et al.* 2004)

The recognition of early warning signs forms the basis for most interventions targeting relapse prevention and are imperative to the development of a relapse signature, which is described by Birchwood *et al.* (2000:95) as 'a set of general and idiosyncratic symptoms, occurring in a specific order, over a particular time period, that serve as early warning signs of impending psychotic relapse'. They identify a number of strategies, which are useful in helping the client and nurse to identify these subtle early symptoms or stressors/events that may have precipitated their relapse.

Monitoring Early Warning Symptoms
During this phase the nurse, with the client and significant members of the social network, reviews the client for any early signs of impending relapse. This stage is crucial in implementing the action plan (van Meijel *et al.* 2003).

The Action Plan
During the action plan phase, the client, the social network and the nurse develop an extensive and inclusive plan. Central to the aims of the plan is the recovery of the client and interventions are designed to meet the individual needs of the client and their unique experiences. The plan uses a range of interventions including stress management strategies, medication, information giving, and utilisation of the client's support network including professional assistance (van Meijel *et al.* 2003).

WORKING WITH FAMILIES AND FRIENDS

In serious mental illness the attitudes of families and friends towards the person, and how they understand and react to the person's experiences, can influence recovery. A good family environment, avoiding excessive emotion and stress in family relationships, can be a major factor in improving stabilisation and in preventing relapse. Accordingly, the role of working with families is recognised as effective in influencing outcomes in serious mental illness (Penn and Mueser 1996). A co-operative approach is identified as working best with families. These approaches usually involve both individual and group sessions. Sessions are based on education and the development of practical problem-solving strategies. The objectives of family intervention are outlined in Figure 10.9.

Figure 10.9 Objectives of educational interventions with families

- Communicate up-to-date information
- Provide support
- Reduce feelings of guilt
- Decrease feelings of blame
- Increase understanding of condition
- Provide information on treatment/rationale
- Provide realistic expectations regarding outcomes
- Provide practical advice about managing the condition
- Enable families to become participants in care
- Feel positive about treatment and relationships
- Reinforce notion of recovery

The shift to community-based care has placed a significant burden on families in this regard, as they too attempt to cope. Parents and carers express the need to be empowered as partners in the caring equation, receiving appropriate information and advice. Families, parents and carers need to experience understanding, empathy and respect when they engage with services. Families now play a key role in support for the client and in maintaining adherence to medication regimes. Accordingly, effective family support services need to be in place to reflect the important role parents, families and carers play in a person's healing.

The term 'expressed emotion' (EE) evolved to describe a situation in which clients living with relations who were critical or over-involved in their care were more prone to relapse (Kuipers *et al.* 2002). The phenomenon is characterised by behaviours such as yelling, shouting, fighting, and repeated critical or hostile comments, which are attributable to an increase in stress for the client. It is now regarded as an established factor in short-term relapse in schizophrenia (Kavanagh 1992; Bebbington and Kuipers 1994; Butzlaff and Hooley 1998) and therapies aimed at lowering high EE are now considered as a long-term preventative approach (Marom *et al.* 2005). Three primary factors are identified in the concept: critical comments; hostility; and emotional over-involvement.

Reader (2002) highlights that these responses are indicative of the families' attempts to cope with the problems that confront them and to do what they think is best for the client in the absence of support and information. For optimum outcomes addressing EE, programmes should target these key areas including psycho-education in this approach. However, the availability of family interventions through public services, with constraints around therapists' availability outside conventional working hours, coupled with the ability of family members to engage in programmes, has limited the provision and uptake of services.

CONCLUSION

The growing evidence base as to the effectiveness of psychosocial interventions in severe mental illness, combined with improvements in pharmacological interventions, offer a renewed hope for recovery to clients. The more widespread use of psychosocial interventions requires changes in education programmes for all mental health professionals and the development of a co-ordinated multidisciplinary approach.

Reflective Questions
1. Discuss strategies you might use with a client experiencing auditory hallucinations.
2. How might mental heath nurses help families better understand severe and enduring mental illness?
3. Think about how you might help a client design an action plan to prevent relapse.
4. Consider the role a mental health nurse can play in helping clients manage their medications.

References

Bebbington, P. and Kuipers, E. (1994) 'The predictive utility of expressed emotion in schizophrenia'. *Psychological Medicine*, 24, 707–18.

Bennett, J., Done, J. and Hunt, B. (1995). 'Assessing the side-effects of antipsychotic drugs: a survey of CPN practice'. *Journal of Psychiatric and Mental Health Nursing*, 2 (3), 315–30.

Bentall, R. P., Haddock, G. and Slade, P. D. (1994) 'Cognitive behavior therapy for persistent auditory hallucinations: from theory to therapy: innovations in cognitive-behavioral approaches to schizophrenia'. *Behavior Therapy*, 25(1), 51–66.

Birchwood, M. and Spencer, E. (2001) 'Early intervention in psychotic relapse', *Clinical Psychology Review*, 21(8), 1211–26.

Birchwood, M., Spencer, E. and McGovern, D. (2000) 'Schizophrenia: early warning signs', *Advances in Psychiatric Treatment*, 6, 93–101.

Butzlaff, R. and Hooley, J. (1998) 'Expressed emotion and psychiatric relapse: a meta-analysis'. *Archives of General Psychiatry*, 55, 547–52.

Chadwick, P., Birchwood, M. and Trower, P. (1996) *Cognitive Therapy for Delusions, Voices and Paranoia*. Chichester: Wiley.

Day, J. C., Wood, G., Dewey, M. and Bentallo, R. P. (1995) 'A self-rating scale for measuring neuroleptic side-effects. Validation in a group of schizophrenic patients'. *British Journal of Psychiatry*, 166, 650–3.

Estroff, S. (1981) *Making It Crazy: Ethnography of Psychiatric Clients in an American Community*, Berkeley: University of California Press.

Gamble, C. and Brennan, G. (2006) *Working with Serious Mental Illness*. London: Harcourt.

Goering, P. and Stylianos, S. (1988) 'Exploring the helping relationship between schizophrenic client and rehabilitation therapist'. *American Journal of Orthopsychiatry*, 58(2), 271–80.

Gray, R., Wykes, T. and Gournay, K. (2002) 'From compliance to concordance: a review of the literature on interventions to enhance compliance with antipsychotic medication'. *Journal of Psychiatric and Mental Health Nursing*, 9, 277–84.

Hamilton, M. (1980) *Fish's Schizophrenia*, London: Wright PSG.

Honig, A., Romme, M. A., Ensink, B. J., Escher, S., Pennings, M. H. and Devries, M. W. (1998) 'Auditory hallucinations: a comparison between patients and nonpatients'. *Journal of Nervous and Mental Disease*, 186(10), 646–51.

Jones, C., Cormac, I., Mota, J. and Campbell, C. (2004) 'Cognitive behaviour therapy for schizophrenia'. *Cochrane Database of Systematic Reviews* (Issue 4), Art. No.: CD000524.pub2. DOI: 10.1002/14651858.CD000524.pub2.

Keen, T. M. (2003) 'Post-psychiatry: paradigm shift or wishful thinking? A speculative review of future possibles for psychiatry'. *Journal of Psychiatric and Mental Health Nursing*, 10(1), 29–37.

Kemp, R., Hayward, P. and David, A. (1997) *Compliance Therapy Manual*. London: Bethlem and Maudsley NHS Trust.

Kinderman, P. and Cooke, A. (2000) *Understanding Mental Illness*. London: British Psychological Society.

Kingdon, D. G. and Turkinston, D. (1991) 'The use of cognitive behavior therapy with a normalizing rationale in schizophrenia. Preliminary report'. *Journal of Nervous and Mental Disorder*, 179(4), 207–11.

Kingdon, D. G. and Turkington, D. (1994) *Cognitive-behavioral Therapy of Schizophrenia*, London: Psychology Press.

Krawiecka, M., Goldberg, D. and Vaughn, M. (1977) 'A standardised psychiatric assessment scale for rating chronic psychotic patients'. *Acta Psychiatrica Scandinavica* 55, 299–308.

Kuipers, L., Leff, J. and Lam, D. (2002) *Family work for schizophrenia. A practical guide*, London: Gaskel.

Lewinsohn, P. M. (1968) 'Characteristics of patients with hallucinations'. *Journal of Clinical Psychology*, 24 (4), 423.

McCabe, R., Heath, C., Burns, T. and Priebe, S. (2002) 'Engagement of patients with psychosis in the consultation: conversation analytic study'. *British Medical Journal*, 326, 549.

Marland, G. R. and Sharkey, V. (1999) 'Depot neuroleptics, schizophrenia and the role of the nurse: is practice evidence based? A review of the literature'. *Journal of Advanced Nursing*, 30(6), 1255–62.

Marom, S., Munitz, H., Jones, P. B., Weizman, A. and Hermesh, H. (2005) 'Expressed emotion: relevance to rehospitalization in schizophrenia over seven years'. *Schizophrenia Bulletin*, 31 (3), 751.

Mental Health Commission (2005) *Quality in Mental Health – Your Views*. Dublin: Mental Health Commission.

Mills, J. (2006) 'Dealing with voices and strange thoughts' in C. Gamble and G. Brennan (eds) *Working With Serious Mental Illness: A Manual for Clinical Practice*. London: Elsevier.

Nuechterlein, K. and Dawson, M. (1984) 'A heuristic vulnerability/stress model of schizophrenic episodes'. *Schizophrenia Bulletin,* 10, 300–12.

Penn, D. and Mueser, K. (1996) 'Research update on the psychosocial treatment of schizophrenia'. *American Journal of Psychiatry*, 153: 606–17.

Read, J. (1996) 'What we want from mental health services' in J. Read and J. Reynolds (eds) *Speaking Our Minds*. Basingstoke: Macmillan Press.

Reader, D. (2002) 'Working with families' in N. Harris, S. Williams, S. and T. Bradshaw (eds) *Psychosocial Interventions for People with Schizophrenia: A Practical Guide for Mental Health Workers*. Basingstoke: Palgrave Macmillian.

Repper, J. (2002) 'The helping relationship' in N. Harris, S. Williams, S. and T. Bradshaw (eds) *Psychosocial Interventions for People with Schizophrenia: A Practical Guide for Mental Health Workers*. Basingstoke: Palgrave Macmillian.

Romme, M. and Escher, S. (1996) *Understanding Voices. Coping with Auditory Hallucinations and Confusing Realities*. Maastricht: University of Maastricht.

Romme, M. and Escher, S. (2000) *Making Sense of Voices: A Guide for Mental Health Professionals Working with Voice-Hearers*. London: Mind Publications.

Shepherd, G., Murray, A. and Muijen, M. (1995) 'Perspectives on schizophrenia: A survey of user, family carer and professional views regarding effective care'. *Journal of Mental Health*, 4, 403–22.

Siddle, R. and Everitt, J. (2002) 'Assessment and therapeutic interventions with positive psychotic symptoms' in N. Harris, S. Williams, S. and T. Bradshaw (eds) *Psychosocial Interventions for People with Schizophrenia: A Practical Guide for Mental Health Workers*. Basingstoke: Palgrave Macmillian.

Sutton, D. L. (2004) 'Relapse signatures and insight: implications for CPNs'. *Journal of Psychiatric and Mental Health Nursing*, 11, 569–74.

Tarrier, N., Yusupoff, L., Kinney, C., McCarthy, E., Gledhill, A., Haddock, G. and Morris, J. (1998) 'Randomised controlled trial of intensive cognitive behaviour therapy for patients with chronic schizophrenia'. *British Medical Journal*, 317 (7154), 303–7.

Tien, A. Y. (1991) 'Distribution of hallucinations in the population'. *Social Psychiatry and Psychiatric Epidemiology*, 26(6), 287–92.

van Meijel, B., van der Gaag, M., Kahn, S. R. and Grypdonck, M. (2003) 'Relapse prevention in patients with schizophrenia: the application of an intervention protocol in nursing practice'. *Archives of Psychiatric Nursing*, 17(4), 165–72.

van Meijel, B., van der Gaag, M., Kahn, S. R. and Grypdonck, M. (2004) 'Recognition of early warning signs in patients with schizophrenia: A review of the literature'. *International Journal of Mental Health Nursing*, 13, 107–16.

Wolpe, J. (1958) *Psychotherapy by Reciprocal Inhibition*. Stanford CA: Stanford University Press.

Yusupoff, L. and Tarrier, N. (1996). 'Coping strategy enhancement for persistent hallucinations and delusions' in G. Haddock and P. D. Slade (eds), *Cognitive-behavioural Interventions with Psychotic Disorders*. London: Routledge.

Zubin, J. and Spring, B. (1977) 'Vulnerability: a new view of schizophrenia'. *Journal of Abnormal Psychology*, 86(2), 103–26.

11
Treatment Modalities in Psychiatric Nursing Practice

Declan Patton

Mental health care has historically been based on the medical model. The philosophical underpinning of this medical model of psychiatry was that mental illness was something that required diagnosis, treatment and cure through medical intervention. This medical approach for the treatment of mental illness primarily involved the use of pharmacological interventions and other medical interventions, for example electroconvulsive therapy (ECT). It was with the advent of psychotherapeutic approaches that mental healthcare moved towards more person-centred or non-medical treatment approaches. Although the debate continues over which approach is best in the treatment of mental illness, contemporary mental healthcare involves the use of an array of medical and non-medical approaches, many of which are used in tandem. From a medical perspective, the prevailing approach to the treatment of a majority of mental disorders is pharmacological intervention, through the use of medications generally known as psychotropic medications/drugs, while the other main medical intervention used in the treatment of some mental disorders is ECT.

The aim of this chapter is twofold. First, drugs used in the treatment of schizophrenia, depression, mania, anxiety and addictions will be described. Examples of common medications used in the treatment of each illness will be given as well as an overview of their indications, actions and possible side effects. The role of the nurse in medication administration will also be described. Second, the use of ECT in mental healthcare will be examined as well as the role of the nurse in preparing someone for ECT and in caring for him/her after the procedure. The overriding aim of this chapter is to provide mental health/psychiatric nursing students with an understanding of the medical treatments that they will generally encounter in their clinical practice. In doing this, the chapter will remain practice-focused.

PHARMACOLOGICAL PRINCIPLES OF PHARMACOKINETICS AND PHARMACODYNAMICS

Pharmacokinetic and pharmacodynamic principles are pertinent to all medications and are issues with which the administering nurse must be familiar. Principles underpinning pharmacodynamics and pharmacokinetics can be found in more detail in Keltner and Folks (2005). According to Greenstein and Gould (2004) pharmacokinetics is best summed up by posing the question, 'what factors determine the formation and maintenance of a therapeutic level of a drug in the bloodstream?' More specifically, pharmacokinetics may be summarised as the way in which the administered drug moves from its administered site to the bloodstream, which is called absorption. How the administered drug moves from the bloodstream to the rest of the body (and more specifically the receptor site at which the drug will have an effect) is known as distribution. Ideally, enough of the drug should reach the receptor site to have a therapeutic effect as opposed to causing a toxic reaction. In order for any psychotropic drug to attach itself to a receptor site, it must first cross the blood/brain barrier. The blood/brain barrier regulates the amount of substances that enter the brain and the speed at which they enter. Drug metabolism refers to the way in which the body alters the shape of a drug. Removal of the drug from the body is known as elimination. Drugs are eliminated from the body primarily in urine and to a lesser extent in bile, breast milk, perspiration and expiration of air.

Pharmacodynamics is the name given to the action and effects of a drug, i.e. how drugs bring about their therapeutic effect and side effects. Two terms most common in examining the issue of pharmacodynamics are 'site of action', which refers to the actual receptor site on which a drug works, and 'mode of action', which refers to the effects on the body that that drug has through attaching itself to a particular receptor site. For example, it is thought that antipsychotic drugs (particularly typical antipsychotics) bind themselves to the D2 receptor site with the result that the person experiencing psychosis becomes less preoccupied with the perceptual or thought disorder that they are experiencing. Although the role of the psychiatric nurse in administering medication will be discussed later in the chapter, it is clear at this early stage that any practising nurse administering medication must be aware of issues relating to the action of medications.

ANTIPSYCHOTIC DRUGS

Antipsychotic medications are classified as being typical or atypical and are used to treat a wide variety of psychiatric signs and symptoms, not just psychosis. While psychotic, the person generally cannot distinguish between distorted thoughts and perceptions that are stimulated internally and the reality of the external environment.

Antipsychotic drugs are used to treat people experiencing psychosis, although their effects are palliative as opposed to curative. Antipsychotic drugs may also be called neuroleptic medication or, more traditionally, major tranquillisers (as the effect of these drugs was largely sedative). Until comparatively recently people requiring treatment with antipsychotic drugs were prescribed, on a more or less wholesale basis, drugs that are now known as traditional or typical antipsychotics, e.g. Haloperidol (Serenace) and Chlorpromazine (Largactil). These types of antipsychotic drugs were particularly effective in treating the positive effects of psychosis, e.g. delusions and hallucinations. However, according to Keltner and Feldman (cited in Keltner and Folks 2005) these traditional antipsychotic drugs continue to be prescribed as their general effectiveness is widely recognised and they are cheaper than atypical antipsychotics.

Figure 11.1 Common antipsychotic drugs (typical and atypical)

Typical antipsychotics	
Generic drug name	Drug trade name
Chlorpromazine	Largactil
Flupenthixol	Depixol
Zuclopenthixol	Clopixol
Trifluperazine	Stelazine
Haloperidol	Haldol/Serenace

Atypical antipsychotics	
Generic drug name	Drug trade name
Clozapine	Clozaril
Risperidone	Risperdal
Olanzapine	Zyprexa
Quetiapine	Seroquel
Amisulpride	Solian
Zotepine	Zoleptil

Those antipsychotic drugs that have been marketed since 1990 are known as atypical antipsychotics. The outstanding difference between typical and atypical antipsychotics is that atypical antipsychotics can help minimise the negative symptoms associated with schizophrenia, as well as the positive symptoms. Negative symptoms manifest through such features as apathy, demotivation and poor level of social skills, etc. In summarising the distinct differences between typical and atypical antipsychotic drugs the following observations may be made:

- Atypical antipsychotics have a reduced risk for the occurrence for extra pyramidal side effects. These are side effects closely associated with the use of typical antipsychotic drugs.
- Atypical antipsychotic drugs block serotonin receptors, which inhibit dopamine release. This action causes an increase in dopamine activity in the mesocortical dopamine pathway. This may reduce the risk of side effects associated with typical antipsychotics.
- Atypical antipsychotics are effective in treating the positive and negative symptoms of psychosis. As one can imagine, this makes them immediately more appealing to service users and providers.
- Atypical antipsychotics reduce the risk of tardive dyskinesia and neuroleptic

malignant syndrome (NMS) (Keltner and Maus Feldman cited in Keltner and Folks 2005). Tardive dyskinesia is an extra pyramidal side effect whose onset usually occurs after a period of prolonged antipsychotic drug use.

The effects of antipsychotic drugs are usually seen within the first two weeks (Richards *et al.* 1999), although some antipsychotics can have a sedative effect within the first hour. The phenomenon known as the 'dopamine hypothesis' may be used to illustrate the action of antipsychotic drugs. According to this hypothesis, the psychotic symptoms associated with schizophrenia are caused by an elevated level of dopamine in the brain. Antipsychotic drugs work by decreasing the amount of dopamine, subsequently lessening the psychotic symptoms. They generally cause a feeling of indifference in the person experiencing psychosis (Healy 2005). For example, if a person is experiencing auditory hallucinations, after receiving antipsychotic medication the person will talk of how they are now not that bothered by the voices with which they were previously preoccupied. On a more critical note it could be said that antipsychotics do not cure the core symptoms of a psychotic episode (e.g. a hallucination or delusion); rather, they ensure that the patient is less preoccupied by the hallucination or delusion. Considering this, it is essential that patients continue with their antipsychotic drug regime even after symptoms have subsided. If patients fail to take their medication, the symptoms that previously disturbed them will often re-emerge (Parker *et al.* 1998).

For patients who have difficulty complying with their antipsychotic medication, the prescription and administration of depot antipsychotic medication may be considered as an alternative (Marland and Sharkey 1999). This means that instead of the patient receiving an oral daily dosage of an antipsychotic drug they will receive an antipsychotic drug via intramuscular injection at periods of two to four weeks, depending on the medication type and dosage prescribed. Common depot antipsychotic drugs can be seen in Figure 11.2. These longer-acting maintenance depots are to be differentiated from clopixol acuphase, which is a short-acting preparation, generally given intramuscularly and used in the management of acute agitation and aggression.

Figure 11.2 Common antipsychotic depot drugs

Generic drug name	Drug trade name
Flupenthixol	Depixol
Zuclopenthixol	Clopixol
Fluphenazine	Modecate
Haloperidol	Haldol
Risperidone	Risperdal consta

The most common peripheral nervous system side effects of antipsychotic drugs may be summarised as:

- dry mouth
- constipation
- blurred vision
- lowered blood pressure upon standing (orthostatic hypotension)
- urinary retention
- weight gain
- sedation.

Central nervous system side effects usually affect the extra pyramidal system and are known as extra pyramidal side effects (EPSEs). These are summarised below:

- *Akathesia*, an altered emotional state that leads to the patient becoming restless,occasionally engaging in impulsive aggressive behaviour.
- *Dystonia* occurs when a muscle goes into spasm. This event may be called a dystonic reaction, e.g. oculogyric crisis, locked jaw.
- *Dyskinesia* relates to abnormal movements, of which one of the most common is the pin rolling finger movement.
- *Late onset dyskinesia*, or *tardive dyskinesia* as it is more commonly known, is common in long-term usage of typical antipsychotics.

Central nervous system side effects may be deemed more serious than peripheral nervous system side effects and are often treated by prescribing alternative antipsychotic drugs or other medical drugs. A further major adverse reaction to using antipsychotic drugs is neuroleptic malignant syndrome, which is caused by the person being in a hypodopaminergic state due to excess dopamine blockade (Keltner and Maus Feldman cited in Keltner and Folks 2005). It is described in more detail in Chapter 22. Anticholinergic drugs are often used to combat the motor side effects of antipsychotics. These medications antagonise the action of acetylcholine in the brain. What this means is that the patient will experience inhibitory side effects, which may include constipation, dry mouth, dizziness and blurred vision. Indeed, many of these anticholinergic side effects mirror peripheral nervous system side effects. Commonly used anticholinergic drugs are listed in Figure 11.3.

Figure 11.3 Commonly used anticholinergic drugs

Generic drug name	Drug trade name
Orphenadrine	Disipal
Procyclidine	Kemadrin
Bisperiden	Akineton
Benzhexol	Artane
Benzatropine	Cogentin (available in injection only)

DRUGS USED IN THE TREATMENT OF DEPRESSION

According to Lilja *et al.* (2006) drug treatment is usually the first line of treatment used for depression. More specifically, antidepressants are the drug of choice in treating depression. As well as assisting in the treatment of an acute episode of depression, long-term antidepressant treatment usually continues for at least four to six months after recovery from an acute episode. Although antidepressants are very much the first-line treatment for depression, electroconvulsive therapy is another option, though this is usually viewed as a last option for some physicians.

According to Healy (2005), there are four groups of antidepressant medication. Tricyclic, selective serotonin reuptake inhibitors (SSRI) and monoamine oxidase inhibitor (MAOI) antidepressants make up the first three groups. The final group are classified as 'other antidepressants' as their modes of actions or indications do not readily match those in the other classes. Antidepressants do not have the immediate effects that antipsychotic drugs have, often taking between two and four weeks before patients start to feel better. The depressed person will usually feel more energised after taking antidepressants for a number of weeks. With this increase in energy the person will become more interested in life and experience fewer feelings of sadness and hopelessness; however, therapeutic effects on mood can take longer.

Tricyclic antidepressants are usually given orally and act in a way that reduces the reuptake of certain neurotransmitters, e.g. serotonin and noradrenaline, from post-synaptic receptor sites. Inhibiting reuptake of these neurotransmitters ensures that increased levels of the neurotransmitters are available at post-synaptic receptor sites. Similar to antipsychotic drugs, antidepressants may bring about peripheral and central nervous system side effects. One of the major drawbacks to using tricyclic antidepressants is that even though they have a low risk for abuse they may be fatal in overdose due to their cardiotoxic nature. Considering this, the use of these antidepressants could be questioned, as suicidal thoughts and intent are often a symptom of depression, and people who want to engage in self-harm may be at greater danger if prescribed these drugs. Examples of tricyclic antidepressants are shown in Figure 11.4.

Figure 11.4 Tricyclic antidepressants

Generic drug name	Drug trade name
Clomipramine	Anafranil
Dothiepen	Prothiaden
Lofepramine	Gaminil
Doxepin	Sinequan
Trimipramine	Surmontil
Amitryptiline	Tryptizol

Selective serotonin reuptake inhibitors (SSRIs) are another group of antidepressants whose use has grown in recent times, mainly because they are not as cardiotoxic as tricyclics. SSRIs are so called as they are thought to specifically block the reuptake of serotonin. However, Healy (2005) questions the blanket use of SSRIs given the paucity of evidence relating to dysfunctional serotonin systems in people with depression, claiming that SSRIs may have more anxiolytic properties than anything else. As stated already, SSRIs have a relatively low lethality rate in overdose (Keltner and Folks 2005). The side effects most closely associated with SSRIs are:

- gastrointestinal tract complaints
- headache
- dizziness
- anxiety
- agitation
- insomnia
- sexual dysfunction.

Further to this, SSRIs may produce a state named 'serotonin syndrome' (Healy 2005) (see Chapter 22). Examples of commonly used SSRIs can be found in Figure 11.5.

Figure 11.5 Selective serotonin reuptake inhibitors (SSRIs)

Generic drug name	Drug trade name
Citalopram	Cipramil
Fluoxetine	Prozac
Paroxetine	Seroxat
Sertraline	Lustral
Fluvoxamine	Faverin

Monoamine oxidase inhibitors (MAOIs) are usually prescribed to be dispensed orally as a third-line pharmaceutical agent after other antidepressants have been tried. This would seem to be because of the potential that MAOIs have of causing adverse reactions. These adverse reactions are made more likely because patients taking MAOIs have to avoid food containing tyramine while taking the medication. People who do not adhere to a specific MAOI diet are at risk of developing high blood pressure, which may result in a hypertensive crisis. Monoamine oxidase inhibitor drugs block monoamine oxidase, a major enzyme involved in the inactivation of norepinephrine, serotonin and dopamine. The consequence of this is an increased number of these neurotransmitters. The action of MAOIs contrasts with how tricyclics and SSRIs work, which is by preventing the reuptake of neurotransmitters from post-synaptic neurons. Commonly used MAOIs can be found in Figure 11.6. The use of these drugs has decreased in recent years.

Figure 11.6 Monoamine oxidase inhibitors (MAOIs)

Generic drug name	Drug trade name
Moclobemide	Manerix
Phenelzine	Nardil
Tranylcypromine	Parnate
Isocarboxazid	Isocarboxazid

OTHER ANTIDEPRESSANTS

Other antidepressants are also available and are classified because their mode of action does not readily fit into the other classes or, in the case of Tryptophan, are licensed only for prescription in treatment-resistant depressions and only dispensed under specialist supervision (BNF 2007).

Figure 11.7 Other antidepressant drugs

Generic drug name	Drug trade name
Flupenthixol	Fluanxol
Mirtazepine	Zispin
Nefazedone	Dutonin
Reboxitine	Edronax
Tryptophan	Optimax
Venlafaxine	Efexor

DRUGS USED IN THE TREATMENT OF MANIA

Although antipsychotic drugs can be used in the treatment of an acute episode of mania and antidepressants can be used if the person fluctuates between mania and depression, in this section two medication types used in the treatment of mania will be discussed – lithium and anticonvulsant drugs. Although the exact action of lithium is unknown, it is used in the treatment of acute mania and as a mood stabiliser in people with bipolar affective disorder (BPAD). It can also be said that by being a mood stabiliser, lithium acts in a prophylactic way in that it decreases the chances of the person relapsing into mania or depression (Schou 1999; Tondo et al. 2001).

People who are prescribed lithium require a physical examination beforehand, including electrocardiogram, thyroid, hepatic and renal function tests, to rule out any abnormalities prior to the commencement of treatment. Serum-lithium measurements are also taken during the time they are taking the drug. The serum-lithium measurements are required because a therapeutic serum level of lithium is not much lower than a toxic level. Lithium serum levels greater than 1.5mEq/L usually result in toxic effects (see Chapter 22). Common side effects of lithium include (Healy 2005):

- passing greater volumes of urine. This is because lithium inhibits the action of the antidiuretic hormone (ADH)
- kidney damage (in cases of exposure to toxic levels of lithium)
- rashes and acne are common
- weight gain
- tremor
- if discontinuation of lithium is deemed to be prudent, then slow discontinuation is more desirable than rapid discontinuation as affective morbidity is associated with the latter (Baldessarini *et al.* 1999).

Anticonvulsant drugs such as carbamazepine (tegretol) and sodium valproate (epilim) have been used in the treatment of mania. Carbamazepine is used to treat acute episodes of mania in those who are resistive to lithium therapy. It has also proved useful in the treatment of rapid cycling BPAD. Sodium valproate has a more rapid onset and is used to treat acute episodes of mania, and it can also be used as a mood stabiliser. The side effects of carbamazepine include:

- dizziness
- drowsiness
- nausea
- confusion.

Common side effects of sodium valproate include:

- stomach cramps
- lethargy
- ataxia
- slurred speech.

DRUGS USED TO TREAT ANXIETY

Benzodiazepines is the drug group most commonly used in the treatment of anxiety, although it has been stated that these drugs, while alleviating anxiety, do not address the issue of helping the individual become more aware of their stressors. Therefore, as a general rule, benzodiazepines should be used only in the short term. As a drug group benzodiazepines have a rapid onset and are effective in the treatment of many anxiety disorders. They are known as a receptor agonist as they increase the action of gamma aminobutyric acid (GABA), an inhibitory neurotransmitter. On a more critical note, benzodiazepines can cause sedation and may be addictive, especially with alcohol. Tolerance can develop over a relatively short period, with patients experiencing withdrawal symptoms if sudden discontinuation occurs (Keltner and Folks 2005). Benzodiazepines are usually administered orally but may be administered by intramuscular injection. Commonly encountered side effects of Benzodiazepines include:

- sedation
- decreased mental acuity
- people taking benzodiazepines should be warned against using machinery or driving
- ortostatic hypotension.

Figure 11.8 Common benzodiazepines

Generic drug name	Drug trade name
Diazepam	Valium
Chlordiazepoxide	Librium
Lorazepam	Ativan
Alprazolam	Xanax
Prazepam	Centrax

Beta blockers (e.g. propranolol) can also be used to treat anxiety. These drug types are used mainly in the treatment of hypertension, angina and cardiac arrhythmias. In treating anxiety these drugs inhibit the peripheral symptoms of anxiety, e.g. hand tremors. By inhibiting these symptoms the person with anxiety may become less preoccupied with these 'anxiety symptoms'. Possible side effects of beta blockers are (Healy 2005):

- shortness of breath
- decreased blood supply to the peripheries
- sleeping difficulties.

HYPNOTICS

Drugs used in the treatment of insomnia are generally known as hypnotics. Some of the benzodiazepines drugs have been manufactured specifically to treat insomnia (e.g. Nitrazepam, Fluazepam) although any benzodiazipine given at night should promote sleep. The use of these drugs has decreased over the past number of years due to their potential for tolerance and dependence. Other hypnotics such as Zolpidem (Stilnoct), Zopiclone (Zimovane) and Zaleplon (Sonata) are not classed as benzodiazipines but act on the same receptors (BNF 2007). Another hypnotic, chloral hydrate, is also available but its use is not widespread. Clomethiazole (Hemineverin) is indicated for insomnia in elderly patients due to its decreased potential for a 'hangover' effect following use (BNF 2007). The hypnotic drugs have several possible side effects:

- tolerance after two to four weeks; prolonged use should be avoided
- it is possible that upon completion of a course of hypnotics the person will experience sleep difficulties (rebound insomnia)
- broken sleep pattern
- hangover effect
- dependence.

DRUGS USED TO TREAT ADDICTIONS

Substance misuse co-exists with many mental illnesses, for example drug-induced psychosis. In terms of alcohol abuse and subsequent withdrawal, the effects of withdrawal on the person depends on how much they had been drinking and if they had a co-existing mental illness or a history of a co-existing mental illness. A benzodiazepine such as chlordiazepoxide (Librium) may be used to manage withdrawal symptoms and to offset the occurrence of delirium tremens, a syndrome associated with acute alcohol withdrawal and within which psychosis may develop. When Librium is prescribed it is usually done so in a way that ensures the patient commences on a high dose that is gradually reduced. If delirium tremens does develop and the person becomes psychotic then an antipsychotic drug may be prescribed. As a deterrent against using alcohol, a person may be prescribed disulfiram (Antabuse). This will usually be prescribed once the person has withdrawn from alcohol. Disulfiram will cause extreme physical sickness in the person if it is combined with alcohol. Acamprosate calcium (Campral EC) is also available and can be used to maintain abstinence in patients with alcohol dependence syndrome by reducing cravings. It can be used even if the patient relapses, but if the patient continues to consume alcohol it should be discontinued (BNF 2007).

Opioid addiction is when someone continues to use opiates in the face of ever-increasing opioid use problems. Symptoms of opioid withdrawal include anxiety, restlessness, runny nose, tearing, nausea and vomiting. Methadone hydrochloride is a highly effective agent in reducing the signs and symptoms of opioid withdrawal. Methadone is administered orally and is usually taken as a substitute for heroin. The patient prescribed methadone must be stabilised on a daily dose of methadone. Once stabilised, the drug can be slowly tapered.

ELECTROCONVULSIVE THERAPY (ECT)

In ECT, a seizure is induced artificially by an electrical current being passed through the brain. This happens through electrodes being placed on one temple (unilateral ECT) or both temples (bilateral ECT), or through two electrodes being placed on the forehead (bi-frontal ECT). Usually ECT is indicated in the treatment of depression that is unresponsive to antidepressant drugs. Times do occur when ECT is a first-line treatment, for example if the patient prefers ECT, there is a history of non-compliance with medication, there are greater risks involved with taking medication or a rapid response is required. Usually, no more than 12 applications of ECT should be administered over a three- to four-week period. The action of ECT upon the brain is not exactly known and side effects relate mainly to short-term memory loss and headaches after the procedure, with bone fractures being rare (Nott and Watts 1999).

The nurse has a vital role to play in caring for someone undergoing ECT (Gass 1998), particularly before and after the procedure. Initially the patient may feel anxious and frightened about what ECT entails. The patient may be considering ECT as a treatment option or have consented to receiving the treatment. The nurse should talk to the patient, explaining what the procedure entails and what it will mean in terms of helping the patient recover from his/her illness. As with talking to a patient about medication, this information should be imparted in a manner that the patient understands. In order to ensure the patient knows what the nurse is saying the nurse should stop at intervals to ask the patient if he/she understands and if they have any questions.

Of course, it is possible that the patient will be quite depressed and perhaps not receptive to what the nurse has to say. This does not mean that such a patient should be ignored. All patients have a right to know what treatment and care they will be receiving and afforded an opportunity to ask questions about elements of treatment and care. In the days prior to treatment commencing, the patient will undergo a full medical assessment including an electrocardiograph and a chest X-ray. As a general anaesthetic is administered, the patient is usually fasted for ten to twelve hours prior to the procedure. On the morning of the procedure pre-treatment care consists of the following:

- Check and record the patient's vital signs; report abnormalities to the patient's responsible medical officer.
- Ensure the patient removes false teeth, prostheses and jewellery, as well as nail varnish from the toenails and fingernails.
- Encourage the patient to wear comfortable clothes and to use the toilet prior to receiving the treatment.
- Escort the patient to the treatment suite, taking medical notes or the patient's case file (if an integrated care system exists) and signed consent form.
- On entering the treatment suite introduce the patient to each member of the treatment team.
- Assist the patient onto a bed and ask him/her to remove their socks.

After the patient has received the treatment and has had a grand mal seizure the following nursing care should be undertaken:

- Remove the patient (remaining on the bed where they received ECT) to a recovery area where they will immediately be placed upon humidified oxygen therapy.
- Observe the patient's cardiac rhythm, blood pressure, oxygen saturation rate and pulse.
- Wait for the patient to regain consciousness and allow him/her to remove their oxygen mask.
- Re-orientate the patient if confused.
- Return the patient to the unit, in a wheelchair if required.
- Reassure the patient by explaining the treatment that they have just had and any ill effects they may be experiencing, e.g. a headache.
- On return to the unit the patient may request food or may want to rest.
- It is also good practice to measure the patient's vital signs in the first three to

four hours after treatment. This should happen every 15 minutes. Any abnormalities should be reported immediately.
• Document in the nursing or integrated care notes the care given to the patient throughout the day.

Medications administered during ECT are as follows:
• Atropine, a prototypical anticholinergic, is occasionally administered intravenously. When used in ECT, atropine inhibits salivation and respiratory tract secretions.
• A short-acting anaesthetic, e.g. methohexital (Brevital), is administered intravenously.
• A muscle relaxant, e.g. succinlycholine (Anectine), is administered to inhibit the motor response that may come with the patient receiving ECT.
• Throughout this initial medical preparation, oxygen is provided to the patient by the anaesthetist.
• A benzodiazepine may have to be administered post-ECT if the patient awakens in an agitated state.

ROLE OF THE PSYCHIATRIC NURSE IN ADMINISTERING MEDICATION

The role of the psychiatric nurse in medication administration may be summarised as follows:
• While assessing the patient the nurse ascertains what the patient's target symptoms are. These symptoms are then, in association with the wider medical team, addressed through prescribed medication.
• Medication administration should be included in the patient's care plan. Ideally, the patient is included in the construction of his/her care plan (Harris et al. 2002).
• The nurse will administer the prescribed medication. It is imperative that, prior to administering any drug via any route to a patient, the nurse ensures that the correct patient, dose, route and drug are identified. Double-checking medication is not mandatory but is good practice when administering intramuscular injections.
• In evaluating a patient's care, the nurse will evaluate the effects of prescribed medication on his or her mental state. This can be noted by observing the patient or talking to them or their family (when appropriate) about how the medication they are taking is helping them think or behave differently.
• Assessing and monitoring side effects.
• The nurse has a central role in ensuring and/or increasing patient concordance with medication (Marland and Sharkey 1999).

Patient and family education about treatment, and in this case medication treatment, is of paramount importance (Usher and Arthur 1997). There are a number of reasons for this:

- It is every patient's right to be informed of the treatment they are receiving.
- There is an onus on the nurse to ensure that the patient complies with prescribed medications to help prevent a relapse. At the core of this duty is removing knowledge deficits that the patient or family may have about the medication that has been prescribed. It could be said that there are, and always will be, risks involved in informing patients about their medications; however, it is the professional duty of the nurse to impart knowledge about any treatment the patient is receiving.

More specifically, areas of education should include the following:
- Side effects: the nurse should talk about side effects that may inhibit a patient's willingness to take medications, such as decreased sexual arousal. The nurse should always ask the patient about how they are responding to a drug.
- Safety: the nurse should ask questions such as, Is the person taking his/her medication? Do the patient and family know what to do if symptoms of the illness arise? Can the drug be abused? Can the drug be discontinued abruptly?
- Attitudes towards medication should be explored by the nurse, who should ascertain whether the patient and family view the use of medication as something to be avoided.
- The patient and family should be educated about how the medications they have been prescribed interact with other substances, such as alcohol.
- The nurse will have to be aware of the information required by special groups, e.g. adolescents, older persons and pregnant women.

CONCLUSION

This chapter began by giving a brief overview of the use of psychotropic drugs, placing their relevance within the medical model of psychiatry, but also recognising that psychotropic drugs may achieve their best results when combined with other treatment approaches from other paradigms of psychiatry. Issues relating to pharmacokinetics and pharmacodynamics were then outlined. Broadly, pharmacodynamics and pharmacokinetics are concerned with a drugs metabolism, action and therapeutic effect. Psychotropic drugs used in the treatment of psychosis, depression, mania, anxiety and addiction were then described. It was the purpose of the author to provide a working clinical understanding of these drugs for undergraduate student nurses. Specific issues relating to drugs used in treating the aforementioned illnesses can be found in one of the many pharmacological textbooks relating to psychiatry or indeed general medicine. What is apparent is that there is a variety of drugs that can be used to treat any named mental illness and, indeed, there is, in some cases, potential for drugs to be used in association with each other. The role of the nurse in ECT and the drugs used in this treatment were described. Again, a practice focus was maintained throughout, highlighting the imperative of the nurse in ensuring that patients are prepared prior to ECT and that they are cared for afterwards. Finally, patient compliance with medication was addressed through the lens of the nurse's role in administering medication and in ensuring that the patient and his/her family are informed about what medications have been prescribed. Fulfilling this fundamental duty may well increase the rate with which patients comply with their medication regimens with the knock-on effect that a decreasing number of relapses are experienced. Considering that re-admission rates to Irish psychiatric hospitals accrue annually at approximately seventy per cent there is an obvious need for nurses to ensure that they play their part in helping patients understand the medication treatment they are receiving.

Reflective Questions

1. What are the benefits of patients being prescribed psychotropic drugs for a diagnosed mental illness?
2. What is the nurse's role in preparing a patient to receive ECT for the first time?
3. What factors should the nurse take into consideration when planning education sessions about the medications that a patient has been prescribed?
4. How may the nurse promote concordance with prescribed medication?

References

Baldessarini R. J., Tondo, L., and Viguera, A. C. (1999) 'Discontinuing lithium maintenance treatment in bipolar disorders: risks and implications'. *Bipolar Disorders*, 1, 17–24.

British National Formulary (BNF) (2007), www.bnf.org.

Gass, J. P. (1998) 'The knowledge and attitudes of mental health nurses to electro-convulsive therapy'. *Journal of Advanced Nursing*, 27, 83–90.

Greenstein, B. and Gould, D. (2004) *Trounce's Clinical Pharmacology for Nurses*. London: Churchill Livingstone.

Harris, N. R., Lovell, K. and Day, J. C. (2002) 'Consent and long-term neuroleptic treatment'. *Journal of Psychiatric and Mental Health Nursing*, 9, 475–82.

Healy, D. (2005) *Psychiatric Drugs Explained* (4th edn). London: Elsevier Churchill Livingstone.

Jarventausta, K. and Leinonen, E. (2000) 'Neuroleptic malignant syndrome during olanzepine and levomepromazine treatment'. *Acta Psychiatrica Scandanavia*, 102, 231–3.

Keck, P. E., Pope, H. G., Cohen, B. M., McElroy, S. L. and Nierenberg, A. A. (1989) 'Risk factors for neuroleptic malignant syndrome: a case–control study'. *Archives of General Psychiatry*, 46, 914–18.

Keltner, N. L. and Folks, D. G. (2005) *Psychotropic Drugs* (4th edn). St Louis: Elsevier Mosby.

Lilja, L., Hellzen, M., Lind, I. and Hellzen, O. (2006) 'The meaning of depression: Swedish nurses' perceptions of depressed inpatients'. *Journal of Psychiatric and Mental Health Nursing*, 13, 269–78.

Marland, G. R. and Sharkey, V. (1999) 'Depot neuroleptics, schizophrenia and the role of the nurse: is practice evidence based? A review of the literature'. *Journal of Advanced Nursing*, 30(6), 1255–62.

Nielsen, J. and Bruhn, A. M. (2005) 'Atypical neuroleptic malignant syndrome caused by olanzapine'. *Acta Psychiatrica Scandanavia*, 112, 238–40.

Nott, M. R. and Watts, J. S. (1999) 'A fractured hip during electro-convulsive therapy', *European Journal of Anaesthesiology*, 16, 265–7.

Parker, G., Lambert, T., McGrath, J., McGorry, P. and Tiller, K. (1998) 'Neuroleptic management of schizophrenia: a survey and commentary on Australian psychiatric practice'. *Australian and New Zealand Journal of Psychiatry*, 32, 50–8.

Richards, S. S., Musser, W. S. and Gershon, S. (1999) *Maintenance Pharmacotherapies for Neuropsychiatric Disorders*. Philadelphia: Brunner/Mazel.

Schou, M. (1999) 'The early European lithium studies'. *Australian and New Zealand Journal of Psychiatry*, 33, S39–S47.

Tondo, L., Hennen, J. and Baldessarini, R. J. (2001) 'Lower suicide risk with long-term lithium treatment in major affective illness: a meta analysis'. *Acta Psychiatrica Scandanavia*, 104, 163–72.

Usher, K. J. and Arthur, D. (1997) 'Nurses and neuroleptic medication: applying theory to a working relationship with clients and their families'. *Journal of Psychiatric and Mental Health Nursing*, 4, 117–23.

SECTION 3

Clinical Application to Practice

12

Care of the Person with a Mood Disorder

Louise Doyle and Catherine Delaney

The mood disorders of depression and elation have been referred to in the Old Testament and in the writings of Homer and Hippocrates, and are probably the oldest recorded mental illnesses (McKeon 1995). Mood disorders, or affective disorders, can be defined as disorders in which the predominant feature is the disturbance or alteration of a person's mood/affect, and is exhibited through the person's emotions and behaviours. There is a range of mood disorders, which include depression and mania to varying degrees of severity and also a combination of both – bipolar disorder. This chapter sets out to discuss the aetiology and presenting features of mood disorders and identifies the appropriate assessment and nursing care principles for a client experiencing such a disorder. The range of treatments available for depression and mania are also briefly outlined.

Depression has been a growing phenomenon both nationally and internationally over the past number of years. The World Health Organisation have projected that by the year 2020 depression will be the second leading cause of disability worldwide and the leading cause of disability in developing regions (Murray and Lopez 1997). In Ireland, mood disorders account for the largest number of admissions to psychiatric hospitals. In their annual report of admissions to psychiatric units and hospitals Daly *et al.* (2006) identified that depressive disorders accounted for almost one third (31 per cent) of admissions to psychiatric units and hospitals in 2005 and were the most frequent cause of admission. Similarly, episodes of mania accounted for 13 per cent of admissions.

AETIOLOGY OF MOOD DISORDERS

Estimates of depression range from ten to twenty-five per cent for women over their lifespan and five to twelve per cent for men, a ratio of approximately two to one. For bipolar disorder, the prevalence rate is approximately one to two per cent of the population, with no significant difference between women and men. As with most mental health problems, there is rarely one single causative factor for mood disorders, rather there is a combination of predisposing and precipitating factors that when combined increase one's likelihood of being affected by a mood disorder. The factors contributing to a diagnosis of mood disorder can be classified as genetic, biological, environmental/social and psychological. These will be only briefly outlined: there is a more exhaustive account of the aetiology of mental health problems in Chapter 2.

Genetic Factors

As with most mental health problems, genetics play a role in the aetiology of mood disorders. Twin studies have identified a concordance rate of twenty per cent in dizygotic twins and a rate of sixty to seventy per cent in monozygotic twins for bipolar disorder (Bertelsen *et al.* 1977). For unipolar depression, concordance rates of twenty-five per cent in dizygotic twins and forty to fifty per cent in monozygotic twins have been found (Price 1968; McGuffin *et al.* 1991). Furthermore, adoption studies, which examined the incidence of mood disorders in those children born to parents with a mood disorder but adopted out at birth, have found that those children also had an increased rate of mood disorder (Mendlewicz and Rainer 1977).

Biological Factors

As with most mental health problems, there are theories about an imbalance of certain neurotransmitters in the aetiology of mood disorders. In particular, a reduction in the neurotransmitters serotonin and noradrenaline appears to play a role in the causation of depression (Cleare 2000).

Social Factors

The results of the influential study by Brown and Harris (1978) suggest a relationship between social stressors and depression. In this study carried out on two samples of depressed women, several factors were found to increase the risk of developing depression and included: the lack of a confiding relationship; unemployment; three or more children under the age of 14 at home; and the loss of mother before the age of 11. Social isolation is also a powerful predisposing factor for depression (Cleare 2000).

Psychological Factors

Various psychological theories have been developed in an attempt to explain the mood disorders. Psychoanalytic theory views depression as a turning inward of anger and hostility while mania is described as a defence against depression. Cognitive theories focus on distorted patterns of thinking and memory, which not only cause depressive feelings but also play a role in the persistence of the disorder.

CLASSIFICATION OF MOOD DISORDERS

Mood disorders are classified by both the *Diagnostic and Statistical Manual of Mental Disorder* (DSM-IV-TR) (APA 2000) and by the *International Classification of Diseases and Related Health Problems* (ICD-10) (WHO 1992). Figure 12.1 provides an outline of the most commonly diagnosed mood disorders according to both diagnostic classifications. (For a full classification and description of mood disorders, refer to the DSM-IV-TR and the ICD-10.)

Figure 12.1 Commonly diagnosed mood disorders

DSM-IV-TR	ICD-10
Mood Episodes	*Mood Affective Disorders*
Major Depressive Episode	Manic episode
Hypomanic Episode	Hypomania
Manic Episode	Mania without psychotic symptoms
Mixed Episode	Mania with psychotic symptoms
Depressive Disorders	*Bipolar affective disorder*
Dysthymic Disorder	Current episode hypomanic
Major Depressive Disorder: Single Episode	Current episode manic without psychotic symptoms
Major Depressive Disorder: Recurrent	Current episode manic with psychotic symptoms
Depressive Disorder not otherwise specified	Current episode mild or moderate depression
	Current episode severe depression without psychotic symptoms
Bipolar Disorders	Current episode severe depression with psychotic symptoms
Bipolar I Disorder	Current episode mixed
Bipolar II Disorder	
Cyclothymic Disorder	
Bipolar Disorder not otherwise specified	*Depressive episode*
	Mild depressive episode
	Moderate episode
	Severe depressive episode without psychotic symptoms
	Severe depressive episode with psychotic symptoms
	Recurrent depressive disorder
	Current episode mild
	Current episode moderate
	Current episode severe without psychotic symptoms
	Current episode severe with psychotic symptoms
	Persistent mood affective disorders
	Cyclothymia
	Dysthymia

As is evident, there are a number of different diagnoses within the spectrum of mood disorders. The most common of these diagnoses is depression, which can range from mild to severe and presents as a low mood that is more intense and persistent than normal unhappiness. Mania, the polar opposite of depression, can also occur on its own but is more likely to occur as part of bipolar disorder (BPD). Bipolar disorder is a cyclical disorder that consists of the occurrence of manic episodes in addition to depressive episodes. The diagnosis of BPD usually involves the occurrence of two major mood episodes (usually one depression and one mania). BPD can be rapid cycling (i.e. four or more episodes have occurred during the previous twelve months). Manic episodes usually begin abruptly whereas depression most often has a gradual onset. Similarly, the duration of a manic episode tends to be shorter than that of a depressive episode.

Below are some of the most common symptoms listed for depression and mania. These symptoms may occur with differing degrees of severity ranging from mild to severe, and it is important to note that individuals will usually not experience all of these symptoms. Just as the contributing factors to mood disorders can be divided into psychological, biological and social factors, so too can the features of depression and mania.

FEATURES OF DEPRESSION

Psychological features:
- depressed mood for at least two weeks
- anhedonia (inability to take pleasure in activities)
- apathy
- avolition (lack of motivation)
- feelings of worthlessness
- a sense of hopelessness and bleak outlook for the future, guilt, despair
- profound sadness for others
- inability to think, concentrate and make decisions
- decreased self-esteem
- over-reaction to minor mistakes
- excessive reassurance seeking
- suicidal thoughts/suicidal behaviour
- in severe cases, psychotic features such as delusions (e.g. nihilistic delusions, delusions of poverty).

Physical features:
- change in appetite (usually lack of appetite leading to weight loss, but in some cases over-eating may occur)
- sleep disturbance (may take the form of difficulty getting to sleep at night, early morning wakening or in some cases hypersomnia)
- tiredness
- decreased energy

- decreased activity level
- psychomotor retardation (slowed motor activity, e.g. slower movements, less gesticulating when talking, etc.)
- slower speech (monosyllabic and monotone)
- decreased bowel activity
- decreased libido and decreased sexual activity
- loss of interest in physical appearance (e.g. unkempt)
- possible agitation (e.g. hand wringing, picking at clothes).

Social features:
- social withdrawal/isolation and avoidance of others
- difficulty in communicating
- dysfunctional interpersonal skills
- loss of interest in college/job leading to possible expulsion from college or loss of employment
- difficulty with existing relationships with family/friends.

FEATURES OF MANIA

Psychological features:
- elevated mood for a persistent period of time (elevating towards euphoria)
- flight of ideas (abrupt change of topic in conversation)
- pressure of speech (increase in pressure and volume of speech)
- changes in speech content (e.g. overuse of alliteration, rhyming slang, word association, etc.)
- inflated self-esteem
- lack of judgement
- poor concentration and attention span
- distractability
- irritability (mood can quickly change from elation to irritability/aggression)
- labile mood (e.g. can become suddenly tearful)
- over-optimism
- perceptual disorders (appreciation of colours as especially vivid)
- in some cases, psychotic features (particularly delusions of grandeur).

Physical features:
- increased energy
- hyperactivity
- undertaking too many activities (but not completing any)
- hypersexuality
- decreased need for food and drink
- decreased need for sleep
- lack of attention to personal hygiene
- inappropriate clothing (e.g. summer clothes in winter)
- wearing very bright/garish clothing and make-up.

Social features:
- interfering behaviour (individual may involve themselves in other clients' personal business)
- social and sexual disinhibition
- overfamiliarity
- extravagant spending (may spend beyond their means, run up large debts, etc.)
- marked impairment of social functioning (which can affect employment/college performance, etc.).

It is apparent that depression and mania are in many respects polar opposites of each other, although some common areas are evident. While it is important for the mental health nurse to be able to recognise the symptoms of a mood disorder, it is even more important that they can recognise the impact that these symptoms have on the client and on their ability to live their lives and interact with those around them. The next section of this chapter outlines the nursing assessment of a client presenting with both depression and mania and identifies appropriate nursing interventions for both mood disorders. See Chapter 5 for a more detailed discussion on undertaking a nursing assessment.

ASSESSMENT OF A CLIENT WITH DEPRESSION

Assessing a client's needs should be a collaborative project between the nurse and client and, where appropriate, their family. However, on initial presentation, the severity of depressive symptoms may preclude the client taking an active role in this assessment. It is important to remember, however, that assessment is not a static one-off occurrence but rather a continuous process that aims to identify the client's changing needs. Central to this process is the establishment and development of the therapeutic relationship between nurse and client. Establishing such a relationship allows for a partnership approach to care, where the client has an active role to play in identifying their own needs and developing appropriate interventions to meet those needs. A good nurse/client relationship allows for a fuller disclosure from the client as they have more confidence and trust in the nurse and are more willing to let them enter their personal world. The assessment of a person who presents with depression requires a holistic approach, encompassing the physical, psychological and social impact of depression on the individual.

Physical Assessment
Important points to assess are in particular diet/hydration, sleep, psychomotor retardation and sexual activity. As previously identified, both diet and sleep are affected by depression and continued poor dietary intake and poor sleep pattern will not positively contribute towards a successful recovery. A disturbed sleep pattern is particularly problematic for a person who is feeling depressed as feelings of hopelessness, guilt and other negative feelings are often magnified during

periods of insomnia. Diet/hydration are also particularly important as it is common for a person who is feeling depressed to significantly reduce their dietary intake and, even more crucially, their fluid intake, which could lead to dehydration and therefore further problems.

The presence of psychomotor retardation should also be noted. This would be obvious in noting a reduction and slowing down of movement. The combination of psychomotor retardation and a poor dietary intake may also contribute to constipation. Sexual activity is another area which also requires attention but is often overlooked by nurses, either through embarrassment or because they believe it is not an important area to focus on (Higgins *et al.* 2005). However, a reduction in sexual activity can have a severe impact on a client's self-esteem and on the quality of their relationship with their partner. It is therefore important that mental health nurses ask about changes in sexual activity in a sensitive manner, while recognising that it is an important aspect of human life. Finally, due to the apathy and general lack of motivation that often accompanies depression, attention to personal hygiene can be compromised. Individuals who take great care about their appearance when well may, when depressed, lose all interest in meeting their self-care needs. This is another area that mental health nurses should be cognisant of.

Psychological Assessment

Psychologically, the main areas to assess are mood, communication and the presence of suicidal ideation. Many tools have been developed to help accurately assess the extent of depressive feelings and to identify a change in severity of these feelings. One such commonly used tool is Beck's Depression Inventory (Beck 1961, Beck *et al.* 1996). Using this self-report inventory, individuals respond to 21 items on a scale from zero to three to assess the intensity of depressive symptoms. The use of such a tool by nurses can, *in collaboration* with a nursing assessment, help to identify the extent to which depressive symptoms are affecting the person's life.

In most cases, depression is accompanied by low mood, which is subjectively reported by the individual concerned and can be objectively assessed by mental health professionals. However, in a minority of cases, individuals may not report low mood but may instead identify vague physical symptoms such as generalised aches and pains, abdominal pain and/or excessive tiredness. This masked depression can be difficult to assess and there is a need for mental health nurses to be aware of the different ways in which depression may present. Assessing how an individual communicates with other people, e.g. nurses, family members, other clients, can give an insight into the extent of the depressive symptoms.

In severe depression, the individual may be completely uncommunicative and may avoid opportunities to interact with others or when spoken to may reply in a monosyllabic and monotone manner. For those with moderate depression, communication with others may identify negative views about themselves. They may be self-accusative and may attribute negative meanings to everyday events. Assessing the nature of the client's communication can provide the mental health nurse with valuable information about how they feel about themselves. This is particularly relevant if individuals do not willingly disclose these feelings when asked during the nursing assessment.

Assessing the risk of suicide or self-harm is also particularly important for a person with depression. A more detailed account of the assessment and interventions for a client engaging in suicidal behaviour will be provided in Chapter 15, but an overview of the salient points to mood disorders will be provided here. Suicidal behaviour, especially completed suicide, is strongly associated with both diagnosed and undiagnosed mental health problems, depression in particular. The mental health nurse should be alert to the risk of suicide when caring for a depressed person. Observation is important because of the high risk of self-harm and suicidal feelings that are associated with depression. The person may feel despair and also feel unable to improve their situation. The feelings of worthlessness and hopelessness that indicate that their lives are not worth living and that they have nothing to look forward to in the future could be strong risk factors for suicide. The person could have specific plans regarding how they will end their life (Chioqueta and Stiles 2003) and it is therefore important that this is sensitively but skilfully assessed by the nurse. A particularly high-risk time for suicide is when the individual is beginning to recover, usually during the first weeks of treatment with antidepressant medications. It is during this period that psychomotor retardation improves and energy levels rise, but mood remains low. In this case, the person now has the energy and motivation to carry out a suicidal act, which they may not have been able to do before. The nurse should conduct a risk assessment of the person in an attempt to identify the risk of suicidal behaviour (see Chapter 15).

Social Assessment

It is important to identify the effect depression has had on the person's ability to function socially, occupationally and interpersonally. Most people who experience moderate to severe depression experience an inability to go about their normal daily routines due to a lack of motivation and a lack of energy. This obviously has an impact on the person's ability to hold down a job or attend and perform at school/college. Similarly, social withdrawal and uncommunicativeness may mean that family and friends of the individual are frustrated at the person's apparent 'laziness', not understanding the inherent difficulties in daily functioning that are common with depression. This may cause disharmony within these relationships. When assessing this area, the mental health nurse again must be cognisant of the person's previous social functioning.

NURSING INTERVENTIONS FOR A CLIENT WITH DEPRESSION

Physical Interventions

Physical interventions should focus initially on improving diet and hydration. As previously outlined, it is important to establish the individual's normal dietary intake and to develop interventions aimed at returning normal nutrition for the individual concerned. Some basic but important principles in this area focus on providing small but nutritious meals for the person and establishing their likes and dislikes. It can be very off-putting for a person who has lost their appetite if large meals consisting of food they don't normally eat are constantly placed before them. Rather, where possible, small portions of food which the client normally eats should be provided. While this may prove difficult in some in-patient environments, every effort should be made to facilitate this. Similarly, increasing fluid intake is also important particularly if the person is severely depressed and does not spontaneously eat or drink.

Attention needs also to be paid to improving sleep for the client. Basic measures such as avoiding caffeine and promoting a restful environment are important here. It is also important to establish the individual's normal sleep patterns as it is both unreasonable and unrealistic to expect someone to sleep for eight hours every night if they normally function quite well on less.

In the initial stages of moderate/severe depression, the individual may also need some gentle coaxing regarding attending to personal hygiene needs. Taking a bath can have a relaxing and soothing effect on a person and this simple task may provide an opportunity for therapeutic interactions between the nurse and the client.

Dealing with issues around a decrease in sexual activity is also important. While this may not be an immediate priority for someone experiencing severe depression, as the depression begins to lift this aspect will again become important and can have an important role to play in improving self-esteem. It may be useful to help the client (and where appropriate, their partner) to recognise a decrease in libido as a symptom of depression rather than as a personal failing (which it may be interpreted as). Informing the client that sexual activity will improve as the depression lifts can give optimism to the person experiencing this often distressing symptom.

Psychological Interventions

Psychological interventions with a client who is experiencing depression should focus on improving mood and improving negative self-esteem. A depressed person may have negative and unreasonable feelings about themselves and the nurse can discuss these with the person (Schwecke 2003). While these pervasive negative feelings may require a formal programme of intervention with trained therapists such as cognitive behavioural therapy (CBT), Parsons (2004) suggests that nurses may draw on CBT techniques such as challenging negative attributions and cognitions and teaching the client to replace negative thoughts with more realistic and constructive thoughts.

The qualities of a good therapeutic relationship are again important here, for example by demonstrating empathy to indicate that the person's feelings are understood. Similarly, being available and accessible to the client when they want to talk is also important. However, some clients, particularly in the initial stages of a severe depression, may not wish to actively communicate with nurses and may prefer to spend time alone. This does not mean, though, that this vulnerable group should be forgotten about. Sitting silently with a person for intervals throughout the day can be comforting to someone who is severely depressed by reminding them that they are not alone. These periods of silence can be built on and can move to periods when an effort is made to engage the person in conversation as their mood begins to lift.

If a client has indicated that they are experiencing suicidal ideation or feelings, more specific interventions will be required. These are presented in more detail in Chapter 15, but measures such as reducing the opportunities for the client to harm themselves and knowing the whereabouts of the client in an in-patient unit are essential. A 'special' nurse undertaking one-to-one observation may be required. During this period the nurse can play an important role by being supportive and acknowledging the feelings that the person is experiencing.

Social Interventions

Social interventions should aim to increase social and occupational functioning. In an in-patient unit, this may begin by encouraging the client to become involved in the ward routine and activities. During the initial stages of a depressive episode, the client may not have the motivation or energy to engage in any activities. However, as the person's mood begins to lift, they should be encouraged to become involved in activities they previously enjoyed. This can range from simple things like reading the newspaper to more formal occupational therapy. The nurse should, however, be aware that the concentration levels of a person who is depressed may be impaired and this may have an impact on the activities they choose to engage in. Furthermore, there should be a gentle emphasis on encouraging activities involving other people, which can help to counteract social withdrawal. As previously highlighted, relationships between family and friends can become strained when a person is experiencing a mood disorder. In these instances it may be appropriate for the mental health nurse to become involved by helping educate the client and their family on various aspects of the illness, including how to recognise and manage symptoms, how to manage the side effects of prescribed medication and how to maximise wellness and prevent relapse. It may be helpful to the client and their family to advise them of self-help groups that provide support and advice on how to strive towards and maintain a successful recovery. Such groups in Ireland include GROW and AWARE.

ASSESSMENT OF A CLIENT WITH MANIA

As with a client who is experiencing severe depression, a person who is manic on initial presentation may be too unwell to play a meaningful role in their initial assessment. However, every effort should be made to involve the client in the assessment of their needs and the planning of interventions to meet these needs once their mood has stabilised sufficiently.

Physical Assessment

The physical assessment of a person presenting during a manic episode will take much the same format as a client with depression. Important areas to assess include diet/hydration, sleep pattern, expressing sexuality and self-care deficits. When a person is manic, they are often simply too busy to be distracted with such mundane activities as eating and drinking. As a result, an individual may go for the whole day or even several days with minimal dietary intake. Adequate intake of fluids is particularly important. As the person is usually very active, extra fluid intake may be required to prevent dehydration.

Similarly, a person's sleep pattern is often negatively affected as a person who is manic may be too overactive to sleep. Restlessness, an abundance of energy and an overactive mind can all prevent sufficient sleep. It is very important to monitor the client's sleeping pattern and to ensure that they are getting enough rest because they may become completely exhausted.

The expression of sexuality for a client who is manic is usually different from when their mood is normal. When manic, hypersexuality may be present and there is often a lack of judgement with regard to sexual behaviour. In many cases, this may not pose a significant problem for the client, but it can in some cases. This is particularly the case if their sexual behaviour becomes aggressive or insulting to other people or if their behaviour is so out of character that it may cause them extreme embarrassment when their mood returns to normal (see Clinical Vignette, below, for an example). Furthermore, the risk of sexually transmitted infections and unwanted pregnancies is increased as lack of judgement may lead to a failure to use contraception.

Finally, attention to self-care needs to be assessed. Personal hygiene needs often increase if someone is overactive, but in many cases the client is too preoccupied to shower/bathe. It may also be the case that the client is wearing inappropriate clothes for the weather (e.g. shorts in winter) or very garish/loud clothing. Wearing very colourful clothing is obviously not a problem in itself, but it can become a problem if this is completely out of character. This may have an impact on the person's dignity when their mood returns to normal.

Psychological Assessment

The main areas to assess here are mood, self-image and communication. In a client who is manic their mood is elevated. The important point to assess is how this elevated mood manifests itself in terms of the effect on self-image and its effect on the nature and content of communication with other people. Heightened mood can often turn quickly to irritability and anger, and observation and assessment of this is important. A person experiencing a euphoric mood tends also to have an elevated self-esteem, bordering on grandiosity. They may believe themselves to be particularly beautiful or particularly intelligent.

Along with an elevated mood, a person may have flight of ideas, with many thoughts continually rushing through their mind. This in turn leads to pressure of speech: the client is trying to articulate their thoughts, but this occurs in a pressurised, disjointed manner. This makes meaningful communication with others difficult, frustrating and even exhausting for the client. Social and sexual disinhibition may also cause problems for the individual as their communication with other people may be inappropriate. It may be difficult for the client experiencing a manic episode to understand why other individuals are not responding to them or feeling the same way they do.

Social Assessment

Social assessment involves examining how the client is interacting with other people and how their manic episode is affecting their social and occupational functioning. Any mental health problem can put pressure on the family of the individual affected, but mania can cause a particular problem. Extreme overactive behaviour is very difficult to manage in the home environment and this, coupled with the sometimes inappropriate nature of communication (rude, insulting, etc.), and possible overspending and running up debts, can all serve to cause a significant strain in the interactions between the client and their family. It is therefore important that the mental health nurse assess the nature of interaction between the client and their family. Families are one of the main providers of support and this support needs to be encouraged and protected. Occupational functioning is also likely to have been adversely affected by the client's manic behaviour. While some people who have experienced mania report higher productivity during this period, for most people being manic and the associated effect on concentration means that the ability to perform adequately in work/college/school is compromised.

NURSING INTERVENTIONS FOR A CLIENT WITH MANIA

Physical Interventions

During a manic phase, the person's distractibility is so pronounced that to encourage them to sit down and eat a full meal may be unrealistic. In this case, in order to ensure that the person is receiving adequate nutrition, snacks such as sandwiches, fruit, etc. should be regularly provided to the person. In particular it is important that fluid intake is maintained, so drinks should be regularly given to the client.

Encouraging sleep and rest is very important for a person who is expending a large amount of energy daily. Clients often report that they do not feel tired, or that they feel refreshed after only a couple of hours' sleep. It is important when encouraging rest for these clients that they have a restful and quiet environment that is free from distractions. In a ward environment, it is also important to be aware of other clients' need for sleep and rest. For this reason and to minimise distraction it may be better for the client experiencing mania to have a room of their own where appropriate. If sleepless nights continue the short-term use of a hypnotic may be required to prevent physical and mental exhaustion.

In terms of self-care deficits, the client may not want to 'waste time' having long baths, so encouraging regular showers may be more appropriate.

If a client is expressing hypersexuality that is adversely affecting other people or has the potential to adversely affect the client's own dignity when their mood returns to normal, this needs to be addressed. In this case, setting firm limits to behaviour, not reinforcing inappropriate behaviour, and close supervision are all required. It is important to remember that the mental health nurse is not trying to discourage sexual feelings or acting on these feelings, it is the *inappropriate* reaction to the feelings, which may offend others, and later upset the client, that is discouraged.

Psychological Interventions

Psychological interventions for a client experiencing mania focus initially on aiming to minimise the adverse effects of mania, including racing thoughts and pressure of speech, which can affect the person's ability to communicate effectively. While the concomitant use of medication can help to alleviate these symptoms, the mental health nurse can use distraction techniques in an attempt to concentrate the person's mind on less stressful experiences. This can include encouraging the person to engage in light activities with a nurse, which also helps to expend some of the excessive energy the client might experience. The mental health nurse must, however, be cognisant of the client's poor concentration and should introduce activities in which this will not be a major problem.

Similarly, one-to-one activities may be the best choice initially as involving a client in group activities may provide too much stimulation to an already over-active mind. Elevated mood can turn easily to agitation and the client's heightened self-esteem and sometimes offending behaviour may annoy other clients on a unit. In this situation, it is important to be aware of the effect the client is having on other clients and vice versa, and in some situations they may need to be removed if the risk of an altercation arises. The key to providing nursing interventions to a client experiencing a manic episode is to do so in a calm, reassuring and consistent manner so that the client and other people on the unit feel safe.

Finally, being aware of the effect of the client's manic behaviour on their self-esteem and dignity is important when their mood begins to return to normal. As identified, clients may act in a way that is out of character and socially embarrassing to them. It is important that the client and their family are reminded that these actions are a feature of the mania and not a feature of the person's actual personality. It is particularly important, though, to be aware of the person's mood level. In some cases, an individual's mood may continue to lower to the extent that they become depressed, and this depression may be compounded by the affront to their dignity and their family's reaction to their manic behaviours.

Social Interventions

As previously identified, the reaction of a person's family and friends is critical in their recovery from their mood disorder. Families may find it difficult to understand that behaviour such as overspending, and a rude and aggressive attitude, is actually a feature of the illness and in many cases cannot be prevented.

It is important for the mental health nurse, where appropriate, to educate the client and the family about how to manage these symptoms with minimal adverse effects. Practical issues such as keeping a low credit allowance on credit cards and having only minimal funds available on short notice may help to minimise the stress and financial difficulty associated with overspending.

Clients and their family should also be educated regarding how to manage the side effects of medications they may be taking and how to manage and respond to signs of relapse. Support groups may be beneficial in promoting understanding and fostering recovery.

Outlined above are the main points to consider when assessing and developing nursing interventions for a client experiencing depression and a client experiencing mania. In order to maximise successful outcomes, a partnership approach to both the assessment and the development of interventions must be utilised as soon as the client can actively engage in the process. It is also crucial to remember that individual clients present with very individual needs and individual contexts and these must be recognised when assessing needs and developing interventions to meet those needs.

TREATMENT OF MOOD DISORDERS

The contemporary treatment of mental health problems is discussed in Chapter 11 and for this reason only a very brief outline of the *main* treatments commonly used to treat mood disorders will be provided here.

Pharmacotherapy

Pharmacological treatment of mood disorders remains the most common form of treatment. (For a full description of the medications used for mood disorders and for further information on dosage, side effects, etc. consult the British National Formulary.) In depression, the selective serotonin re-uptake inhibitors (SSRIs) are the most commonly used pharmacological treatment. They have fewer adverse effects than older antidepressant medications and do not have a sedative effect, which greatly benefits those who work or attend college/school. However, some of these medications can have a negative impact on sexual activity (see Chapter 24) and this in turn can adversely affect self-esteem and relationship with partners. As a result, clients should be educated about what to potentially expect when taking these medications and, where possible, how to manage side effects. Some SSRI medications have the added bonus of having anxiolytic properties, which can be beneficial for those who have an anxiety component to their depression.

For most clients experiencing mania or bipolar disorder a mood stabiliser will be required. The most common mood stabiliser used is lithium, which is effective in regulating mood but does have a range of adverse effects and can become toxic. For this reason, nurses must be aware of the blood lithium levels of clients on this medication and should also be familiar with the regular side effects and the signs of toxicity. As a physical work-up is required before commencing lithium and it can take several days to have a therapeutic effect, an antipsychotic agent may be prescribed in the first days of acute mania to help calm the client and reduce psychotic symptoms if present. Other drugs which can be used as mood stabilisers include carbamazepine (which is particularly useful for rapid cycling bipolar disorder) and sodium valproate.

Psychotherapeutic Interventions

Psychotherapeutic interventions such as cognitive behavioural therapy can be particularly effective when used by a trained therapist with a client experiencing depression. The basic aim of this approach is to help the individual to identify and modify negative thoughts and attributions. Individual psychotherapy, group therapy and family therapy are all interventions that may facilitate a client's recovery from a mood disorder. These interventions are considered in more detail in Chapter 9.

Electroconvulsive Therapy (ECT)

Electroconvulsive therapy is a controversial form of treatment but one which is still used in psychiatric practice in Ireland today. It is particularly beneficial for clients with severe depression and is normally used in combination with pharmacotherapy. For a further discussion of ECT, see Chapter 11.

Complementary Treatments

Non-traditional interventions such as the use of herbal medications, relaxation therapy, homoeopathy and acupuncture are becoming more popular with individuals who are reluctant to rely solely on medical treatment of their mental health problem. While these interventions may not actively treat the symptoms of mood disorder, they can in many cases help clients to cope with their symptoms a little better. Similarly, there has also been a renewed consideration of the benefits of a healthy diet and exercise in managing symptoms and preventing relapse.

As there are many causes of mood disorders the available treatment regimes should reflect this. Relying solely on medication to alleviate emotional and mental distress often results in a less than optimum experience for clients who may benefit from psychotherapeutic interventions to help explore some of their feelings and values. Complementary therapies may aid relaxation and help to cope with the often distressing effects of an illness, including the adverse effects of medication. Ideally, most treatment options need not and should not be used in isolation; rather a combination of suitable therapies can help a person to a meaningful and lasting recovery.

Clinical Vignette

Joan is a 58-year-old woman who was admitted to an in-patient psychiatric unit during an acute manic episode. Joan has a long history of bipolar disorder, and has had frequent hospitalisations for both depressive and manic states. She is a nun and lives within a supportive community in a convent. Joan's current admission was precipitated by her decision to stop taking her medication as she believed that it was keeping her mood too low.

During her admission, Joan's mood was very elevated. She was very talkative but conversation was difficult as her thought content and speech pattern was very disjointed. She acted in a very sexual way, taking off her clothes in the open unit, and the content of her speech was very sexual. This was not a feature of Joan's character when her mood was normal. As Joan's manic episode resolved, other clients on the unit began to tell her of her overtly sexualised behaviour when she was manic. This was deeply distressing to Joan and had a negative impact on her self-esteem.

Reflective Questions

1. How would you identify that a person is experiencing a depressive episode rather than a period of unhappiness?
2. How would you initiate, develop and maintain a therapeutic relationship with a client who is severely depressed?
3. With reference to the clinical vignette above, how might you have intervened to help manage the sexual behaviour exhibited by Joan on an in-patient unit?
4. Again with reference to the vignette, how might you work with Joan to help alleviate the distress she feels as a result of her manic behaviour?

References

American Psychiatric Association (APA)(2000) *Diagnostic and Statistical Manual of Mental Disorders* (DSM-IV-TR) (4th edn: text revision). Washington DC: APA.

Beck, A. T. (1961) 'An inventory of measuring depression'. *Archives of General Psychiatry*, 4, 561–71.

Beck, A. T., Steer, R. A. and Brown, G. K. (1996) *BDI—II Manual*. San Antonio: The Psychological Corporation.

Bertelsen, A., Harvald, B. and Hauge, M. (1977) 'A Danish twin study of manic-depressive disorders'. *British Journal of Psychiatry*, 130, 330–51.

Brown, G. W. and Harris, T. O. (1978) *Social Origins of Depression: A Study of Psychiatric Disorder in Women*. London: Tavistock.

Chioqueta, A. P., and Stiles, T. C. (2003) 'Suicide risk in outpatients with specific mood and anxiety disorders. *Crisis: The Journal of Crisis Intervention and Suicide Prevention*, 24(3), 105–112.

Cleare, A. (2000) 'Affective disorders', in P. Wright, J. Stern and M. Phelan (eds), *Core Psychiatry*. London: WB Saunders.

Daly, A., Walsh, D., Ward, M., and Moran, R. (2006) *Activities of Irish Psychiatric Units and Hospitals 2005*. Dublin: Health Research Board.

Higgins, A., Barker, P and Beglet, C. M. (2005) Neuroleptic medication and sexuality: the forgotten aspect of education and care. *Journal of Psychiatric and Mental Health Nursing*, 12(4), 439–46.

McGuffin, P., Katz, R. and Rutherford, J. (1991) 'Nature, nurture and depression: a twin study'. *Psychological Medicine*, 21, 329–35.

McKeon, P. (1995) *Coping with Depression and Elation*. London: Sheldon Press.

Mendlewicz, J. and Rainer, J. D. (1977) Adoption study supporting genetic transmission in manic-depressive illness. *Nature*, 268, 327–9.

Murray, C. G. L. and Lopez, A. D. (1997) 'Alternative projections of mortality and disability by cause 1990–2020: global burden of disease study'. *Lancet*, 349, 1458–504.

Parsons, S. (2004) 'The person with a mood disorder', in I. Norman and I. Ryrie (eds), *The Art and Science of Mental Health Nursing. A Textbook of Principles and Practices*. Berkshire: Open University Press.

Price, J. (1968) 'The genetics of depressive behaviour', in A. Coppen and S. Walk (eds.), *Recent Developments in Affective Disorders. British Journal of Psychiatry* Special Publications no. 2.

Schwecke, L. H. (2003) 'Models for working with psychiatric patients', in N. L. Keltner, L. H. Schwecke and C. E. Bostrom (eds), *Psychiatric Nursing* (4th edn). St Louis: Mosby.

World Health Organisation (WHO) (1992) *The ICD-10 Classification of Mental and Behavioural Disorders. Clinical Descriptions and Diagnostic Guidelines*. Geneva: WHO.

13

Care of the Person with a Perceptual Disorder

Gerry Maguire and John McDonald

The aim of this chapter is to identify and discuss the primary perceptual disorders relating to mental health and their implication for psychiatric nursing practice in Ireland. Perception, by definition, involves identification and initial interpretation of a stimulus based on information received through the five senses of sight, hearing, taste, touch and smell (Stuart and Laraia 2005). The primary perceptual disorder discussed in this chapter is schizophrenia, though schizophreniform disorder, schizo-affective disorder, delusional disorder, brief psychotic disorder, along with other less common perceptual disorders, will also be considered. Various nursing interventions for clients with schizophrenia will be discussed, together with an outline of the aetiology, classification, symptomatology and illness trajectory of schizophrenia.

UNDERSTANDING SCHIZOPHRENIA

Schizophrenia is a complex psychiatric diagnosis encompassing a range of symptoms including disorder of thought, perception, volition and behaviour. The disorder is described as a 'psychotic' illness, meaning that the person may have no insight into their illness or behaviour and/or may be perceived as being out of touch with reality.

Schizophrenia is often misunderstood and misinterpreted. Psychiatrist Emil Kraepelin (1893) was the first person to draw a distinction between what he termed dementia praecox ('premature dementia') and other psychotic illnesses. Eugen Bleuler, a Swiss psychiatrist, introduced the term 'schizophrenia' (1911), having found Kraepelin's term misleading. The word schizophrenia derives from the Greek *schizo* meaning 'split' and *phrenia* meaning 'mind'. Bleuler wanted to describe the split between what is perceived, what is believed and what is objectively real. It is important that the nurse understands that this does not mean that the person with schizophrenia is suffering from a 'split personality', a rare hysterical condition with which schizophrenia is often confused in society.

It is generally accepted that schizophrenia affects approximately one in every one hundred people worldwide (Barker 2003) while approximately three per cent of the general population suffer from the range of psychotic disorders. Daly *et al.* (2006) reported that in Ireland, schizophrenia accounted for twenty per cent of all psychiatric in-patient admissions to psychiatric units during 2005. Furthermore, they found that while schizophrenia is often viewed as an extremely debilitating illness, 18 per cent of those with the diagnosis who were admitted to Irish psychiatric units were discharged within one week and 86 per cent were discharged within three months. Schizophrenia is a serious mental illness which often requires periods of hospitalisation or community care. Therefore the nurse is in a prime position to develop and maintain a programme of interventions, in collaboration with the client, to promote recovery.

AETIOLOGY OF SCHIZOPHRENIA

Commonly, the illness is first diagnosed in adolescence or early adulthood, usually from the age of 15 to 30 years, although it may also be diagnosed in later life. There is evidence to suggest that schizophrenia rates are slightly increased in males whereas the rate for schizo-affective disorder is somewhat higher for females (Baldwin *et al.* 2005). There is an increased rate of schizophrenia in single, separated and divorced people, as it appears that being in a relationship acts as a buffer against this condition. While no single cause is attributable to the diagnosis, it seems clear that genetic, biological and psychological factors, together with environmental and social influences, may contribute to the development of schizophrenia.

Genetic Factors
It is suggested that genetic vulnerability coupled with environmental stressors can act to cause schizophrenia (Harrison and Owen 2003). There is considerable evidence to support the view that schizophrenia has an inherited or genetic component, with some estimates as high as eighty per cent. Also, Stuart and Laraia (2005) claim that there is compelling evidence to support the genetic basis, evidenced by identical twin studies which confirm an increased incidence. Adoption studies further confirm that the incidence of developing schizophrenia resembles that for the birth parents rather than for the adoptive parents (Harrison and Owen 2003).

Biological Factors
One of the most debated aetiological theories of schizophrenia is the dopamine hypothesis. This hypothesis suggests that symptoms of schizophrenia are caused by an overactivity of the neurotransmitter dopamine in the brain. Evidence supporting this theory includes the fact that drugs such as amphetamines and cocaine, which are known to increase dopamine levels, also produce psychotic symptoms. Furthermore, typical antipsychotic drugs, e.g. haloperidol, which block dopamine at the D2 receptor reduce the positive symptoms of psychosis. The dopamine hypothesis is the basis for the pharmacological interventions in schizophrenia. However, for now the dopamine hypothesis remains a hypothesis, yet to be conclusively proven.

There is increasing evidence that cannabis use can trigger an acute psychotic episode and worsen the outcome in those already known to suffer a perceptual disorder. Cannabis is the commonest illegal drug in Europe and approximately one in six of 15–64-year-olds have used the drug (McCarney 2006). A review of the evidence has suggested that cannabis doubles the risk of developing schizophrenia on the individual level, and may be responsible for up to eight per cent of cases (Arseneault et al. 2004). The drug appears to hold a particularly strong affinity for dopamine receptors which as previously identified are implicated in schizophrenia.

Research in early neurodevelopment suggests there is increasing evidence that prenatal exposure to infections increases the risk for developing schizophrenia later in life (Brown 2006). It is also proposed that exposure to environmental influences during childhood may interact with neurobiological risk factors to influence the possibility of later onset of schizophrenia. Positive or negative effects of a child's environment may interact with genetics and the processes of neurodevelopment, with long-term consequences for brain function.

Current research focuses on the differences in structure or function in certain parts of the brain in those with a diagnosis of schizophrenia. Early evidence for differences in the neural structure in the brain originated from the discovery of ventricular enlargement in clients with a schizophrenia diagnosis, for whom negative symptoms were most evident (Flashman and Green 2004). Other research, using magnetic resonance imaging (MRI) techniques, claims that there is reduced grey matter density as well as decreased pituitary volume, which is most evident in the frontal lobes and the hippocampus.

Environmental and Social Factors

Factors such as poverty, homelessness and discrimination appear to be involved in an increased risk of schizophrenia or relapse, due to the high levels of stress they engender. Research has consistently demonstrated the association between living in an urban environment and the risk of developing schizophrenia; even after factors such as drug use, ethnicity and social class have been taken into account (Van Os 2004). A Swedish study found a 68–77 per cent increased risk of psychosis for people living in the most urbanised environments, a significant proportion of which is likely to be accounted for by schizophrenia (Sundquist et al. 2004).

Psychological Factors

Childhood experiences of abuse or trauma have also been recognised as risk factors for a diagnosis of schizophrenia later in life (Janssen et al. 2004; Schenkel et al. 2005). Negative attitudes towards individuals with schizophrenia (or who are at risk of developing the illness) can have a significant adverse effect on the person. Issues such as critical comments, hostility and intrusive or controlling attitudes (termed 'high expressed emotion') from family members correlate with a higher risk of relapse in schizophrenia.

The stress-vulnerability model has also been used to explain the aetiology of schizophrenia (Zubin and Spring 1977). This model purports that every person has a different level of vulnerability to the development of a psychotic illness. Individuals are more or less vulnerable as a result of biological factors (e.g. genetics) and/or psychological factors (e.g. resilience to stress). According to the stress-vulnerability model, it is only when environmental stresses are present that vulnerability will result in the development of problems. When vulnerability is great, relatively low levels of stress may be enough to cause problems. Conversely, when the person is more resilient (when vulnerability is low), problems will develop only when higher levels of environmental stress are experienced.

SYMPTOMS OF SCHIZOPHRENIA

Symptoms of schizophrenia are commonly divided into positive and negative symptoms.

Positive Symptoms
Hallucinations
A hallucination is a sensory distortion of reality in the absence of an external stimulus. While the most common hallucination is hearing voices, a hallucination may also involve seeing (visual), tasting (gustatory), smelling (olfactory) or feeling (tactile) something that is not real.

- An auditory hallucination involves hearing sounds, most commonly one or more voices talking to the patient or to each other.
- A visual hallucination may take the form of a flash of light, a vision or the appearance of some object or person. This should be differentiated from an illusion where reality is misinterpreted but in the presence of external stimuli.
- An olfactory or gustatory hallucination typically involves the perception of distinct foul smells or tastes, such as faeces or urine.
- A tactile hallucination may cause the person to experience pain or discomfort without an external stimulus.

Delusions
A delusion is a strongly held belief in something which is untrue and outside the person's cultural beliefs. Examples include grandiose, paranoid, religious, nihilistic and somatic delusions.

- Grandiose delusion: a delusion of grandeur may take the form of the person believing they are someone famous.
- Paranoid delusion means the person may believe they are being watched by others or that someone is going to do them harm.
- Religious delusional ideation tends to relate to the person having unusual or obsessive religious beliefs.
- Nihilistic delusions involve thoughts of hopelessness and the person believes they do not exist despite evidence of those around them.
- In somatic delusions the person may believe that they are seriously ill while displaying symptoms of much less severity.

Thought Disorder

This describes the condition in which thinking patterns become disorganised. It includes:

- Thought withdrawal, which involves the belief that one's thoughts are being removed from their conscience.
- Thought broadcasting means the person believes their thoughts are being shared with others or that others can pick up their thoughts (e.g. by transmitters in hair, teeth, etc.).
- Thought insertion is a 'made' thought — the thought is not the person's own.

Negative Symptoms

- **Flattening or blunting of affect** is a reduction or lack of emotional expression, including monotonous voice, lack of eye contact, and restricted facial expression.
- **Avolition** describes a lack of motivation or desire to do anything.
- **Anhedonia** is the inability to experience pleasure from normally pleasurable life events.
- **Catatonic behaviour** is characterised by an apparent unawareness of the environment, decreased motor activity or excess and aimless motions, bizarre postures and lack of self-care.
- **Alogia**: poverty of speech. The person displays difficulty with speech, inability to carry on a conversation, short and sometimes disconnected replies to questions and a lessening of fluency in their conversation.

CLASSIFICATION AND DIAGNOSIS OF PERCEPTUAL DISORDERS

Schizophrenia and other perceptual disorders are classified by both the *Diagnostic and Statistical Manual of Mental Disorders* (DSM-IV-TR) (APA 2000) and by the *ICD-10 Classification of Mental and Behavioural Disorders* (WHO 1992). Figure 13.1 provides an outline of both classifications.

Figure 13.1 Classification of perceptual disorders DSM-IV-TR and ICD 10

DSM-IV-TR	ICD 10
Contains five sub-classifications of schizophrenia:	A conventional classification system encompassing:
1. *Catatonic type:* marked absences or peculiarities of movement are present	1. *Paranoid type:* the principle symptom is of paranoid delusions
2. *Disorganised type:* thought disorder and flattened affect are present together	2. *Hebephrenic type:* affective changes are prominent, delusions and hallucinations fleeting and fragmentary, behaviour irresponsible and unpredictable
3. *Paranoid type:* delusions and vivid, often horrifying, hallucinations are present but thought disorder, disorganised behaviour, and affective flattening are absent	3. *Catatonic type:* dominated by prominent psychomotor disturbances

DSM-IV-TR

4. *Residual type:* positive symptoms are present at a low intensity only
5. *Undifferentiated type:* psychotic symptoms are present but the criteria for paranoid, disorganised or catatonic types have not been met

Other disorders of perception identified by the DSM-IV-TR include:

Schizophreniform disorder — the essential features are the same as for schizophrenia except:
- the total duration of the illness is at least one month but less than six months
- impaired social/occupational functioning is not a requirement

Schizoaffective disorder — schizophrenic and depressive symptoms are both prominent in the same episode of illness

Delusional disorder — the presence of one or more non-bizarre delusions that persist for at least one month

Brief psychotic disorder — essential feature is the presence of delusions, hallucinations, disorganised speech or grossly disorganised or catatonic behaviour for at least one day but less than one month

Shared psychotic disorder — the essential feature is a delusion that develops in an individual who is involved in a close relationship with another person who already has a psychotic disorder with prominent delusions (folie a deux)

ICD 10

4. *Simple schizophrenia:* an insidious but progressive development of oddities of conduct and an inability to meet the demands of society

Other disorders of perception identified by the ICD-10 include:

Undifferentiated schizophrenia – psychotic conditions meeting the general diagnostic criteria for schizophrenia but not conforming to any of the sub-types above

Residual schizophrenia — characterised by long-term presence of negative symptoms

Post-schizophrenic depression — refers to an episode of depression in the aftermath of a schizophrenic illness

Schizotypal disorder — characterised by eccentric behaviour and anomalies of thinking that resemble schizophrenia

Persistent delusional disorder — long-standing delusions constitute the only, or most conspicuous, clinical manifestation

Delusional disorder — characterised by the development of a single delusion or a set of related delusions which may be persistent and sometimes lifelong

Acute and transient psychotic disorders — a heterogenous group of disorders characterised by the acute onset of psychotic symptoms such as delusions and hallucinations, and by the severe disruption of ordinary behaviour

Diagnosing Schizophrenia

Schizophrenia often involves deterioration from a previous high level of functioning to a lower level, often in such areas as personal care, interpersonal relationships, academic achievement and work. The sub-clinical or prodromal phase of the illness may appear as if the client were suffering from an affective disorder such as depression. The duration of untreated psychosis (DUP), which is the time lapse between the first clinical symptom and initiation of treatment, for a first episode of schizophrenia is suggested at between 72 and 104 weeks. A lengthy DUP is associated with increased risk of relapse, more hospitalisations, less likelihood of returning to work, worse course and 'short-term' outcome, increased suicidality as well as increased costs (Scully *et al.* 2000).

When diagnosing a disorder of perception, such as schizophrenia, the mental health professional will first examine the self-reported experiences of the patient and/or those close to him/her. There is currently no recognised biological test for schizophrenia. However, the completion of a medical history, nursing assessment, physical examination, mental state examination (MSE) and risk assessment should confirm the diagnosis. Other tests that may be undertaken include a magnetic resonance imaging (MRI) scan, computerised tomography (CT) scan and standard blood tests. These tests should lead to the exclusion of any other medical condition that might explain such a bizarre presentation, e.g. organic brain disease, substance abuse, and other conditions such as vitamin deficiency or hormonal imbalances. The nurse should be aware of the need to conduct a differential diagnosis, i.e. excluding the presence of a psychiatric condition other than schizophrenia (dementia, mood disorder, acute psychotic episode).

Early recognition and intervention at the first sign of psychosis is important, though it should be recognised that the diagnosis usually takes a long time. However, the nurse or other mental health professional may be reluctant to inform the client of the diagnosis, even when it is certain, for fear of labelling and the social stigma the illness may bring.

The nurse must take into account their own cultural and social background when assessing the symptoms of schizophrenia in clients from differing socio-economic or cultural situations. Ideas that may appear to be delusional in one culture (e.g. witchcraft) may be commonly held in another. In some cultures, visual or auditory hallucinations with a religious content (e.g. apparitions) may be a normal part of religious experience. The mental health professional should consult either the DSM-IV-TR or the ICD-10 classifications in order to ascertain the essential features required for a diagnosis of schizophrenia or other perceptual disorder.

CONTEMPORARY APPROACHES TO CARE AND TREATMENT

The feasibility of providing care to people with a perceptual disorder depends on adequate resourcing of community-based multi-disciplinary mental health teams. It is essential that team members are sufficiently educated and trained in the provision of current best evidence-based practice in response to individual client needs (Mental Health Commission 2006). The treatment for a client experiencing a perceptual disorder will revolve around the bio-psycho-social approach. The goals of treatment are to eliminate symptoms, reduce the risk of relapse and the severity of the illness while also improving the level of social functioning and relationships. Treatment for schizophrenia is in general lifelong and includes medications, professional counselling, and support from family or community services.

Assessment
It is important that the nurse is aware that many clients with symptoms relating to a perceptual disorder will present first at primary care level, perhaps visiting their GP. Following an initial assessment, the client may continue to be cared for at primary care level or referred to the specialist psychiatric services. The primary indicator for a referral to the psychiatric services is the risk to self or others. A comprehensive review of the literature identified that the risk for suicide is much greater for those with a diagnosis of schizophrenia (Hawton *et al.* 2005). The client must be comprehensively assessed, normally with one or more of the following tools, as part of the overall assessment:
- global assessment of function (GAF score)
- structured clinical interview for DSM-IV-TR (SCID)
- positive and negative symptom scale (PANSS)
- Beiser scale (to assess for onset of psychosis)
- local nursing assessment matrix.

This assessment will examine the client's quality of life, neurological state, co-morbid drug abuse, previous psychiatric history, specific symptomatology and understanding about their beliefs and illness. In general, the nurse will assess for the presence of hallucinations, delusions, thought disorder, self-care deficits, family dynamic, poor interpersonal functioning, disordered affect, altered volition, and disturbed behaviour. Also, medication management and the promotion of concordance should be addressed.

Planning
The overall goal of nursing care is to help the client to recognise the psychosis and to assist them to develop strategies to manage the symptoms. One of the first care-related decisions is whether to care for the client in hospital or in the community. With the advent of improved community multi-disciplinary team care it may not always be necessary to admit the client to in-patient care (see Chapter 7). However, in some cases and dependent upon the findings of the initial assessment, the decision may be taken to admit the client to an approved acute in-patient unit (DoHC 2001).

Early intervention and a flexible approach in the management of care are essential for the client. The client must be involved in decision making at all stages of their care in order that they will continue with the programme in the long term. In order to achieve this, good communication skills, involving the establishment of a therapeutic relationship fostered on mutual trust and respect (Stuart and Laraia 2005), are paramount.

There should be a focus on the recovery (Mental Health Commission 2005) of the client from this debilitating condition, which includes a return to normal work, social and family life. Client and family psycho-education must be a priority throughout the process. It is vital that the nurse and all the members of the multidisciplinary team are aware of the stigma and social isolation associated with schizophrenia and become involved in preventive strategies in order to ameliorate these effects on the person.

Implementation
Hallucinations
When the client expresses hallucinatory phenomena, the nurse should remain calm: attempts at reasoning may lead to arguments and even anger. It will be necessary to observe for behaviour that suggests the presence of a hallucination, particularly if the client is not forthcoming. An assessment of both the nature and content of the hallucination is essential. It is important to monitor for any precipitating stressors relating to the illness or hallucination. The client needs to feel reassured that the nurse is listening and that she/he understands that these experiences may be very frightening. The nurse must never imply a belief in the voices. You might say that while you do not hear them, you would like to know about the client's experience of the voices in order to gain a greater understanding and be more specific with proposed nursing and medical interventions. Using distraction may also assist the patient to focus on other activities of their choosing, e.g. listening to music, or becoming involved in organised activities in the unit or in the community (see Chapter 10).

Delusions
The nurse should be mindful not to attempt to reason with the client in relation to their delusional beliefs, as this may prove useless and frustrating. It is important that the meaning of the delusions for the person is investigated. The nurse should acknowledge the plausible elements of the delusion, but if the client asks 'Do you believe?', respect that this is their experience and state that you do not share their belief, while exploring the underlying feelings the client attaches to the delusion. It is important that the nurse is empathic and should not whisper or laugh in the vicinity of a person experiencing delusions as this may exacerbate the delusional state.

Thought Disorder
The client with schizophrenia, due to thought disorder, may experience difficulties in concentration and making decisions. Supportive psychotherapy will always be a treatment option for this client. Cognitive behaviour therapy (CBT) is the most common of these 'talk therapies'. CBT aims to promote an understanding of the client's experience and to reduce distress caused by symptoms, promote adaptive coping responses, address self-esteem issues, reduce occupational and social disability, and lower the risk of relapse. In order to maintain client engagement it

is important to ensure that there are shared goals and ownership at all stages of treatment. It may be necessary to review and summarise learning tasks so as to clarify the person's knowledge and awareness. Interventions should be paced and experiences normalised so as to facilitate understanding.

Self-care Deficits

The client with schizophrenia can experience a general deterioration in their personal care and general appearance. The nurse should employ tactful prompting to improve this aspect of care in order to maintain the client's dignity and sense of self-worth. A normal well-balanced diet is encouraged, sometimes involving the support of the dietician. It is important to ensure that the patient is enjoying a regular sleep pattern. In order to promote health and well-being, smoking and excessive alcohol intake should be discouraged. The client may also benefit from social skills training or advice on re-training in order to advance their lives.

Previous History, Insight and Judgement

The experienced nurse, due to the often inherent chronicity of this condition, will develop knowledge of the client over time. Due to the nature of the illness, there can be potential for aggressive behaviour. De-escalation techniques can help to prevent aggressive outbursts (see Chapter 20). Supportive psychotherapy, in the context of the therapeutic nurse–client relationship, can facilitate the development of insight into the illness and their behaviour. This can also reduce the risk of harm to self or others.

Commonly, issues of adherence with treatment arise in the care of the client with schizophrenia, primarily due to their lack of insight into their illness. Non-adherence with the nursing care plan can range from any deviation from the programme of care including non-adherence to written client contracts, attendance at outpatient appointments or failure to follow professional advice. The relationship with the nurse is one of the most important predictors of compliance. This therapeutic alliance should be utilised to: explore clients' beliefs about their illness; address their concerns about medications; educate them about the effects and benefits of concordance with their medications; and encourage questions in an open and honest manner.

Volition and Affect

Clients with schizophrenia may experience lack of motivation. The nurse should encourage meaningful interactions and personal responsibility. Social inclusion should be encouraged through the use of reality orientation, creative group activities and other therapeutic interactions. It is important to be aware of changes in the client's mood and to address this as necessary.

Interpersonal Relationships

It is important that there is excellent communication between the various members of the multi-disciplinary team (MDT). The client must be at the centre of all planned interventions. Family members, and/or a significant other, may be involved as collaborators by sharing their observations of the client's experiences with the nurse or key worker. The mental health professional should be able to assess their ability to cope with the burden of care based on their own health needs, other responsibilities or stressors, or other financial or social burdens.

If the client is in regular contact with their family, it is feasible to engage them in the care process.

Schizophrenia can be a bewildering and destructive force in the lives of family members and friends of the person affected by the disorder. If there are relationship difficulties within the family, particularly if these are impinging on the well-being of the client, family support and education can be very helpful. Generally, family members are the first to notice something is wrong, whether it is social withdrawal and isolation, obsessive-type behaviour, paranoia, or a lack of logic and common sense in conversation. Family members often feel great frustration, confusion and resentment about a loved one's strange behaviour. They may become tired of making allowances for the person's behaviour, angry about the distrustful or paranoid behaviour and embarrassed because the person is acting so strangely. Additionally, it can be difficult to seek treatment because the affected individual, believing their visions, voices and delusions to be real, may insist that nothing is wrong and object to seeing a doctor. Support and information for family and friends is vital and they should be given written information as well as being advised about support groups that are available. Treatment options for schizophrenia are good, and a supportive network is crucial to helping a person succeed in the long term.

Pharmacotherapy

Pharmacological interventions may form part of the first line of treatment for the client with schizophrenia. Specifically the use of anti-psychotic medications can provide relief from the positive and in some cases the negative symptoms of schizophrenia. Current practice suggests that atypical antipsychotic medications (e.g. risperidone, olanzapine) are commonly prescribed before the typical anti-psychotic medications (e.g. chlorpromazine, haloperidol). Atypical antipsychotic medications have shown improved efficacy in treating negative symptoms (Healy 2005). However, all antipsychotic medications are known to cause a range of distressing side effects. In response to this, Solutions for Wellness, a programme devised by a pharmaceutical company, was developed to support clients in remaining active and enjoying a healthy well-balanced diet.

Evidence over the past twenty years suggests that discontinuing treatment may lead to a rapid relapse. Any decision to reduce or stop antipsychotic medication must be taken between the individual client and their mental health team. The current consensus is that this decision should not be taken until at least two years after the initial episode (Healy 2005). Even so, up to eighty per cent of individuals relapse within one year of stopping their antipsychotic medication. However, new evidence shows improved long-term outcomes for atypical antipsychotics, with

34 per cent of clients relapsing over two years on risperidone compared to 60 per cent on haloperidol (Healy 2005). For further information on antipsychotic medications, see Chapter 11.

Non-adherence with medication regimes may include any deviation from a doctor/health care professional's advice and includes partial adherence, taking sub-therapeutic dosage and complete cessation of medication. This is more common with typical than atypical drugs, perhaps because of the lower side-effect profile of typical drugs. All attempts to ensure or improve adherence must be based on a collaborative rather than authoritarian relationship with the client.

Electroconvulsive Therapy (ECT)

ECT may be used in conjunction with, or to augment pharmacotherapy, but it is no longer considered a first-line treatment (see Chapter 11). It may be particularly beneficial in the presence of affective symptoms or in catatonic schizophrenia. Psychosurgery is an extremely rare procedure and is not a recommended treatment for schizophrenia in Ireland.

Evaluation

The ultimate goal of therapeutic interventions is to reintegrate the client into society and to support them into the future. It must be recognised that the risk of relapse is high for this illness. Potential causes of relapse include sudden reduction in medication, non-adherence issues, previous psychiatric history, male gender, being single, the presence of negative symptoms, a lengthy first episode and an insidious onset.

Ongoing support for the client with schizophrenia is extremely important. Support services may include drop-in centres, day centres, visits from the community psychiatric nurse, and patient-led support groups such as the Irish Advocacy Network. Indeed in recent years the importance of service-user-led recovery-based movements has grown substantially throughout Europe and America. Groups such as the Hearing Voices Network and, more recently, the Paranoia Network, have developed a self-help approach that aims to provide support and assistance outside the traditional medical model adopted by mainstream psychiatry. By avoiding framing personal experience in terms of criteria for mental illness or mental health, they aim to destigmatise the experience and encourage individual responsibility and a positive self-image.

Schizophrenia Ireland, which was founded in 1975, is recognised as being the primary national organisation concerned with promoting the interests and articulating the needs of those affected by schizophrenia. The organisation comprises clients, family members, concerned friends and mental health professionals. They advocate on behalf of service users on three levels: that clients have the same rights, entitlements and opportunities as those available to other members of society; that relatives and families should be supported and fully recognised by the statutory services for the important role they provide; that those with a diagnosis of schizophrenia should not suffer stigmatisation or prejudice in their daily lives.

Mental Health Ireland is another locally based national organisation involved in advocating for all those affected by mental health problems within their community.

In keeping with the national framework document, *A Vision for Change* (DoHC 2006) it is imperative that there is a renewed emphasis on prevention of schizophrenia, education of communities and early detection and treatment for those who require it in order to promote a meaningful recovery.

Clinical Vignette

Paul is a 20-year-old single man who lives at home with his parents. He has been expressing paranoid thoughts towards his parents despite their best intentions. He has been hearing voices, which are familiar, but confusing and frightening to him. He says that the voices are telling him he is a bad person and that he must be punished. He is suggesting that the radio is talking about him and therefore cannot bear to have it on. He has become increasingly isolated because of his views and spends most of his time alone in his room. Although Paul has always taken pride in his appearance, recently self-care has deteriorated. In response to their concerns, his parents have brought him for a psychiatric assessment.

Reflective Questions

1. What are the primary aetiological factors associated with schizophrenia?
2. What are the principle treatment options that may be utilised in the care and treatment of the client in this vignette?
3. What is the role of voluntary organisations and statutory agencies and how might they assist the client in the process of recovery?
4. What is the role of the family in relation to a community-based model of care and how might they be supported in their role?

References

American Psychiatric Association (APA) (2000) *Diagnostic and Statistical Manual of Mental Disorders* (DSM-IV-TR) (4th edn: text revision). Washington DC: APA.

Arseneault L., Cannon, M., Witton, J. and Murray, R. M. (2004) 'Causal association between cannabis and psychosis: examination of the evidence'. *British Journal of Psychiatry*, 184, 110–17.

Baldwin, P., Browne, D., Scully, P. J., Quinn, J., Morgan, M., Kinsella, A., Owens, J., Russell, V., O'Callaghan, E. and Waddington, J. (2005) 'Epidemiology of first-episode psychosis: illustrating the challenges across diagnostic boundaries through the Cavan–Monaghan study at 8 years'. *Schizophrenia Bulletin* 31(3): 624–38.

Barker, P. (2003) *Psychiatric and Mental Health Nursing: The Craft of Caring*. London: Arnold.

Brown, A. S. (2006) 'Prenatal infection as a risk factor for schizophrenia'. *Schizophrenia Bulletin*, 32 (2), 200–2.

Daly, A., Walsh, D., Ward, M. and Moran, R. (2006) *Activities of Irish Psychiatric Units and Hospitals 2005*. Dublin: Health Research Board.

Department of Health and Children (2001) *The Mental Health Act* Dublin: Government Publications.

Department of Health and Children (2006) *A Vision for Change*. Dublin: Stationery Office.

Flashman, L. A. and Green, M. F. (2004) 'Review of cognition and brain structure in schizophrenia: profiles, longitudinal course, and effects of treatment'. *Psychiatric Clinics of North America*, 27 (1), 1–18, vii.

Harrison, P. J. and Owen, M. J. (2003) 'Genes for schizophrenia? Recent findings and their pathophysiological implications'. *Lancet*, 361 (9355), 417–9.

Hawton, K., Sutton, L., Haw, C., Sinclair, J. and Deeks, J. (2005) 'Schizophrenia and suicide: systematic review of risk factors'. *British Journal of Psychiatry* 187: 9–20.

Healy, D. (2005) *Psychiatric Drugs Explained* (4th edn). Edinburgh: Elsevier.

Janssen, L., Krabbendam, L., Bak, M., Hanssen, M., Vollebergh, W., De Graaf, R. and Van Os, J. (2004) 'Childhood abuse as a risk factor for psychotic experiences'. *Acta Psychiatrica Scandinavica*, 109, 38–45.

McCarney, G. (2006) 'Cannabis Use and Psychosis'. Conference paper delivered at the ACAMH/Lucena Clinic Services conference, Dublin: 21 June 2006.

Mental Health Commission (2005) *A Vision for a Recovery Model in Irish Mental Health Services — Discussion Paper*. Dublin: Mental Health Commission.

Mental Health Commission (2006) *Multidisciplinary Team Working: From Theory to Practice — Discussion Paper*. Dublin: Mental Health Commission.

Schenkel, L. S., Spaulding, W. D., Dilillo, D. and Silverstein, S. M. (2005) 'Histories of childhood maltreatment in schizophrenia: relationships with premorbid functioning, symptomatology and cognitive deficits'. *Schizophrenia Research*.

Scully, P. J., Coakley, G., Kinsella, A. and Waddington, J. L. (2000) 'Psychopathology, executive (frontal) and general cognitive impairment in relation to duration of untreated psychosis', in *Psychological Medicine*: Cambridge University Press.

Stuart, G. W. and Laraia, M. T. (2005) *Principles and Practice of Psychiatric Nursing* (8th edn). St Louis: Elsevier Mosby.

Sundquist, K., Frank, G. and Sundquist, J. (2004) 'Urbanisation and incidence of psychosis and depression: follow-up study of 4.4 million women and men in Sweden'. *British Journal of Psychiatry*, 184(4): 293–8.

Van Os, J. (2004) 'Does the urban environment cause psychosis?' *British Journal of Psychiatry*, 184(4): 287–8.

World Health Organisation (WHO) (1992) *The ICD-10 Classification of Mental and Behavioural Disorders. Clinical Descriptions and Diagnostic Guidelines*. Geneva: WHO.

Zubin, J. and Spring, B. (1977) 'Vulnerability — a new view of schizophrenia'. *Journal of Abnormal Psychology* 86(2), 103–26.

14

Explaining and Treating Anxiety Disorders

Agnes Tully

Anxiety disorders are among the most common mental health disorders and are reported to affect as much as ten to fifteen per cent of the western world population. They are illnesses often related to our biological structure and/or personal experiences and have a propensity to run in families (Barlow 2002). Today it is unlikely for people with anxiety as a primary diagnosis to require in-patient care. Anxiety thus falls essentially within the remit of the primary care arena. This chapter will examine the origins and meaning of anxiety. It will also outline the causes and effects of anxiety on the individual, and will discuss the following anxiety disorders: generalised anxiety disorder, panic disorder, post-traumatic stress disorder, obsessional compulsive disorder, and phobic disorders. Treatment modalities for anxiety disorders will also be outlined and discussed.

THE CONCEPT OF ANXIETY

Anxiety has been defined as 'a state wherein a person feels a strong sense of dread' (Frisch and Frisch 2006:191) This feeling of dread and impending doom gives rise to a number of unpleasant or upsetting symptoms, which include physical, behavioural, cognitive and attentive responses (Beck *et al.* 1985). Physical, psychological and behavioural symptoms of anxiety are listed in Figure 14.1.

All of us are familiar with the concept of anxiety as a short-term feeling associated with events or thoughts that make us feel anxious. For example, the night before an important exam or thinking about a particularly unpleasant event. Generally these feelings pass and we are able to recognise the source of the anxiety. When feelings of anxiety are present for long periods of time and impact on our day-to-day life we may be described as having an anxiety disorder. The term 'anxiety disorder' is used as an umbrella term to include a number of anxiety-related conditions. A central aspect of anxiety, which differentiates it from other mental health disorders, is that it is based primarily on anticipation of future problems and this leads to avoidance of situations that are perceived as being anxiety-provoking. People with a panic disorder, for example, avoid situations or places that might trigger a panic attack. This avoidance of feelings of anxiety generally forms the basis of the disorders, and interventions target this aspect of the person's behaviour among other problems.

Figure 14.1 Physical, psychological and behavioural symptoms of anxiety

Physical Symptoms	Psychological Symptoms	Behavioural Symptoms
• Muscle tension	• Tension	• 'Flight' from situations
• Headaches	• Worry, dread,	• Avoidance of fear-
• Neck pain/tension	apprehensiveness	evoking situations or
• Restlessness	• Poor concentration	places
• Startled reactions	• Irritability	• Restlessness
• Chest pains	• Poor memory	• Speech difficulties
• Breathlessness	• Confusion	• Hyperventilation
• Hyperventilation	• Fearfulness (of losing	• Inhibition
• Lump in the throat	control, of losing one's	
• Sweating/feeling	mind)	
clammy	• Feeling panicky	
• Nausea	• Early insomnia	
• Exhaustion	• Perceptual disturbances,	
• Palpitations	e.g. depersonalisation	
	and derealisation	

Source: Saunders and Wills 2003; Varcolis 2002; Turner 2003

PREVALENCE OF ANXIETY DISORDERS

Between one third and one quarter of people attending primary care services have some form of psychological problem. Anxiety disorders and depression are the most common disorders (Rogers *et al.* 2004; Saunders and Wills 2003; Brown and Barlow 1992). While there are many theories about the stress and pressure of modern-day living, there is no evidence suggesting that anxiety disorders are any more prevalent than they used to be (Saunders and Wills 2003). However, anxiety as a condition is better recognised and many new terms are being used to describe it, such as 'stressed out' or 'burnt out' (Saunders and Wills 2003; Turner 2003).

CLASSIFICATION OF ANXIETY DISORDERS

The anxiety disorders as classified by the DSM-IV-TR (APA 2000) are listed below. Given the scope of this chapter only the more common of these will be described in further detail.
• generalised anxiety disorder
• panic disorder with agoraphobia
• panic disorder without agoraphobia
• agoraphobia without history of panic disorder
• obsessive compulsive disorder

- post-traumatic stress disorder
- social phobia
- specific phobia
- acute stress disorder
- anxiety disorder not otherwise specified
- anxiety due to a general medical condition
- substance-induced anxiety disorder.

AETIOLOGY OF ANXIETY

No single factor has been identified as the cause of anxiety or any of its related disorders. People get anxious for many reasons. Disease, drugs and hospitalisation can cause a general sense of unease. Waiting for a painful procedure or anticipating test results of an important diagnostic nature will make many of us nervous; some people get anxious when they have to make a presentation at work or cover for their boss; many of us feel anxious when we feel someone significant disproves of us.

Theoretical explanations of the nature and causes of anxiety vary widely. Personality theorists support the notion that individual differences in disposition lead people to respond differently to stressful experiences. Such approaches are known as the 'trait theories', meaning that traits or characteristics or personality influence responses (Rogers et al. 2004).

Genetic studies have shown that up to a third of first-degree relations of anxious clients have a similar condition. Thus anxiety does tend to run in families (APA 2000). Twin studies have demonstrated a genetic component in both panic disorder and obsessive compulsive disorder (APA 2000). Phobias were also shown to be genetically predisposed in up to forty per cent of cases (Kendler et al. 1992). First-degree relations of people with social phobia were found to be more at risk of developing this disorder than the general population (APA 2000; Turner 2003).

Brain imaging and neurochemistry can help to identify areas of the brain responsible for our reactions to anxiety. Biological theorists assert that anatomical pathways in the limbic system facilitate the transmission of anxiety-related responses back and forth (Varcolis 2002; Yates 2005). There is also the gamma aminobutyric acid (GABA) benzodiazepine theory, which suggests that the calming effect of GABA, which is inhibited in anxiety disorder, may be facilitated or disinhibited with the administration of benzodiazepines (Saunders and Wills 2003; Varcolis 2002).

Barlow (2002) draws the conclusion that being 'highly strung', 'nervous' or 'emotional' has a genetic component in that it runs in families. This conclusion is supported in the works of a number of authors (Eysenck 1967; Gray and McNaughton 1996). There is indeed strong evidence of an inherited personality dimension of emotionality or neuroticism or anxiousness (Clarke et al. 1994; Barlow 2002). However, what seems to be inherited is a 'vulnerability' or a 'predisposition' to developing an anxiety disorder (Kendler et al. 1995).

Cognitive behaviourists believe that faulty patterns of thought and learned behaviour may be responsible for the development of anxiety disorders. For example, people who experience the physical symptoms of anxiety such as shortness of breath or palpitations do not associate these symptoms with anxiety. Consequently they may believe that these symptoms are more serious than they are. When the person experiences palpitations they believe that they are having a heart attack, making the symptoms worse and heightening other physical and psychological symptoms of anxiety. The person becomes finely attuned to any physical inconsistencies, reinforcing the idea that something terrible is going to happen and creating a vicious circle of anxiety.

CO-MORBID CONDITIONS WITH ANXIETY

Some people have a single anxiety disorder (e.g. specific phobia) and nothing else. However, it is very common for an anxiety disorder to co-exist with another mental disorder. Research has shown that anxiety disorders and depression occur together quite frequently (Lang and Stein 2001). In fact Kessler (1999) reported that 58 per cent of patients with major depression were found also to suffer from anxiety, and 93 per cent of patients diagnosed with bipolar disorder were also found to have an anxiety disorder. When co-morbidity occurs the illness tends to be more severe and more chronic in nature (Varcolis 2002). Other disorders commonly diagnosed concurrent with an anxiety disorder include substance abuse, somatisation and other anxiety disorders (Sartorius *et al.* 1996).

DEFENCES AGAINST ANXIETY

Defence mechanisms are psychological processes that guard persons from anxiety. According to Freud these are tactics which the ego develops to help deal with the id and the super ego. In distorting reality, there is a change in perception which allows for a lessening of anxiety, with a corresponding reduction in felt tension. Common defence mechanisms associated with reducing anxiety include:
- Denial — unpleasant feelings or realities are escaped from by ignoring their existence.
- Displacement — emotions are redirected to a substitute target.
- Repression — this involves pushing uncomfortable thoughts into the unconscious.
- Somatisation — the conversion of anxiety symptoms into physical symptoms.

GENERALISED ANXIETY DISORDER

Generalised anxiety disorder (GAD) is much more than the normal experience of day-to-day worrying. With GAD every aspect of worry — its intensity, duration and frequency — is exaggerated. Even when people know they are worrying far more than situations necessitate, they cannot seem to extricate themselves from the rut of worry because of this ongoing tension, and daily functioning is interfered with. People with GAD can be irritable and often have trouble sleeping, concentrating or working effectively.

Features of generalised anxiety disorders include tension, worry, apprehension, restlessness, fatigue and poor concentration (APA 2000; Saunders and Wills 2003). The DSM-IV-TR (APA 2000) definition of GAD requires an individual's worry and anxiousness to be accompanied by three or more of the following symptoms on most days for six months.

- restlessness, edginess, tension
- being easily exhausted
- poor concentration
- irritability
- muscle tension
- disturbance in sleep pattern.

Those suffering from GAD worry incessantly about personal adequacy, personal relationships, health, finance, etc. Much time is also spent anticipating future problems (e.g. 'Will I be ok'? or 'What if I feel anxious?').

PANIC DISORDERS

Panic attacks are an integral feature in a number of anxiety disorders. However, if the panic attacks are the central cause for concern a diagnosis of panic disorder is likely (Barlow 2002). The DSM-IV-TR (APA 2000) describes panic disorder as recurrent episodes of spontaneous, intense periods of anxiety usually lasting less than an hour. Panic disorder is characterised by sudden episodes of terror, usually accompanied by palpations, tachycardia, sweating, weakness, dizziness or feeling faint (Rogers *et al.* 2004). More frightening, the person may experience nausea and/or chest pain, or even feel unable to breathe properly. These attacks frequently produce a sense of unreality along with an intense fear of impending doom (Barlow 2002).

A significant feature of panic disorder is its unpredictability. Individuals with this disorder experience episodes of intense anxiety which occur very unexpectedly, even during sleep. This makes it difficult to predict their occurrence and may lead to the avoidance behaviour often associated with this condition (Barlow 2002). Despite generally lasting a very short time (five or six minutes) people who experience such attacks describe them as terrifying (Gauthier 1999). Fear of further attacks often leads those who experience them to avoid situations or places where escape is difficult if a panic attack ensues. In such cases the individual may be diagnosed with panic disorder with agoraphobia. Salkovskis (1991), as cited in Rogers *et al.* (2004), identified the presence of safety behaviours in people with panic disorder. The behaviours identified were avoidance, escape, and subtle avoidance. Ironically, these same behaviours result in maintaining the disorder by preventing the individual from confronting their fear and realising that the feared catastrophe or disaster does not happen.

POST-TRAUMATIC STRESS DISORDER (PTSD)

The defining characteristic of this disorder is the onset of anxiety symptoms after a traumatic event. PTSD usually follows an unusually traumatic event such as rape, war, physical or sexual abuse, car or air accident or other stressful events. The traumatic event that triggers the disorder, according to the DSM-IV-TR (APA 2000) must be significant, that is, there must have been a chance that the person could have died or sustained considerable bodily injury. Some people may simply witness a tragic event and develop post-traumatic stress disorder (Frisch and Frisch 2006).

Although it has existed through the centuries, PTSD has only been diagnosed as a specific disorder in the last three decades (Gauthier 1999). The symptoms of PTSD include reliving the traumatic event that gave rise to this disorder. There may be avoidance of reminders of the trauma, numbing of emotions and heightened arousal (Gauthier 1999). Individuals with PTSD may have flashbacks or nightmares and often feel detached from others (Shives 2005); and they may be irritable, have sleep disturbance and poor concentration (APA 2000).

OBSESSIVE COMPULSIVE DISORDER

Obsessive compulsive disorder (OCD) is one of the most complex anxiety disorders (Saunders and Wills 2003) and is frequently misunderstood. OCD is a relatively common mental illness with a reported prevalence of around one to two per cent of the population (de Silva and Rachman 1998; Wilkinson *et al.* 2000; Thompson 2000). OCD is characterised by recurring intrusive thoughts and images (obsessions) which lead to repeated behaviours (compulsions). Typically a person with OCD experiences a recurrent and distressing need or urge (obsession) to carry out a needless activity (compulsion) repeatedly. The person may try to resist this compulsion, which results in a build-up of tension that is relieved only when they perform the desired task. Unfortunately the drop in anxiety levels following the performance of the task is short-lived and the desire (obsession) to perform the ritual (compulsion) soon returns. Soon a perpetual cycle is established that dominates many or all aspects of the person's life.

When obsessions become a major preoccupation and rituals (compulsive activities) are being repeatedly performed, to the detriment of normal daily functioning, they may be considered pathological (Rogers *et al.* 2004; Saunders and Wills 2003; Wilkinson *et al.* 2000). Why people carry out such extreme rituals is generally incomprehensible to others. Obsessions generally are unpleasant thoughts, impulses or images, all of which are anxiety-provoking, and compulsions neutralise the anxiety caused by the obsession. For example, a common obsession involves fear of contamination; consequently constant hand washing relieves the anxiety associated with fearing contamination. Examples of other common obsessions and compulsions are shown in Figure 14.2.

Figure 14.2 Common obsessions and compulsions

Obsession	Compulsion
Thoughts that things must be in a specific order or sequence	Repetitive behaviours such as ordering
Persistent doubts	Checking behaviours
Contamination	Hand washing behaviours
Violent or sexual imagery	Praying or counting behaviours

It is believed that up to eighty per cent of patients with OCD may also have a concurrent depression (Barlow 2002).

PHOBIC DISORDERS

According to the DSM-IV-TR (APA 2000) people with this anxiety disorder experience excessive fear coupled with intense anxiety associated with exposure to certain objects or situations. Even thinking about the phobic object or situation can cause anxiety and consequently the feared object or situation is avoided. Phobic disorders include agoraphobia, social phobia or social anxiety disorder, and specific phobias. Agoraphobia and social phobias are often the most debilitating phobic disorders as it is difficult to avoid all social interaction and it is also difficult to avoid places where escape is not always easy.

Agoraphobia

The DSM-IV-TR (APA 2000) defines agoraphobia as anxiety about, or avoidance of, places or situations from which escape might be difficult (or embarrassing) or in which help may not be available in the event of having a panic attack or panic-like symptoms. As with many other anxiety disorders this fear leads to avoidance of many situations. While the stereotypical agoraphobic is unable to leave their home (Saunders and Wills 2003), many people with agoraphobia get out and about but avoid specific situations where they feel escape is not easy. For example, if going to the cinema with a friend the agoraphobic person may prefer to drive themselves as they can then have the option of leaving if they feel anxious. In this case, the person is not avoiding the cinema but avoiding being unable to leave, if a panic attack ensues. The agoraphobic individual thus fears making a fool of themselves in public. Approximately sixty per cent of phobias fall into the realm of agoraphobia and two-thirds of those with agoraphobia are women (Wilkinson *et al.* 2000).

Social Phobia/Social Anxiety Disorder

Social phobia is an extreme fear of socialising or social situations. It is a fear or intense dread of being embarrassed or humiliated during social interaction, which causes the sufferer to be intensely anxious. It can cause physical symptoms such as sweating, hot/cold flushes, blushing, headaches, shaking or an upset stomach (Mayo Health Clinic 2005). For some people the physical symptoms reach the level of a full-blown panic attack (Heckleman and Schneier 2000).

Unfortunately, social phobias interfere with day-to-day life much more than many other phobic disorders. We may be able to avoid snakes or even heights reasonably easily but social interactions are very difficult to avoid completely. Social phobias are also quite resistant to treatment. This phobia can become very constant and debilitating. Socially phobic individuals go to great lengths to avoid social interactions or at least the aspect of social activity they most fear, for example public speaking or performing on stage (Varcolis 2002). If feared situations cannot be avoided they are endured with considerable discomfort.

Social phobias can result in significant impairment of academic, occupational, professional and social functioning (Leahy and Holland 2000). Social phobia patients may have very significant avoidance habits, restricting their functioning and resembling agoraphobia. However in social phobia the avoided situations always involve social interactions and the fear of negative appraisal. Thus people with a social phobia are more comfortable when alone, while patients with agoraphobia are often more at ease in the company of others.

Specific Phobias

A specific phobia is an irrational fear of a specific place or object. Exposure to the feared situation results in high levels of anxiety or fear. Examples of specific phobias are snakes, dogs, heights, social situations, etc. (APA 2000). Specific phobias are very common and often cause few problems as people avoid the feared object or situation. However if the feared object or situation must be confronted regularly (e.g. a nurse who fears blood) then the person may find coping with this difficult. A few common specific phobias are given in figure 14.3.

Figure 14.3 Some examples of common specific phobias

Feared Objects/Situations	Clinical Title
Enclosed spaces	Claustrophobia
Flying	Aerophobia
Heights	Acrophobia
Open spaces	Agoraphobia
Spiders	Arachnophobia

ASSESSMENT

As stated previously, it is unusual to see anxiety as a stand-alone disorder in inpatient psychiatric facilities. However, mental health nurses may come across people with a wide range of anxiety disorders in the community, either through the primary care system or in specialised mental health clinics. Assessment is of vital importance to establish the extent of the anxiety and its impact on the person's physical, occupational and social functioning. A detailed assessment of the person's activities of living taking a biopsychosocial perspective will provide the mental health nurse with a detailed picture of the person and provide a framework for intervention. If the person is in hospital, it generally means that the anxiety disorder has seriously impacted on the person's life, for example they may be engaging in suicidal behaviour or neglecting self-care needs such as nutrition. In these cases these problems and others that impact on the patient's physical health status must be dealt with first.

Several assessment tools such as the hospital anxiety scale (Zigmond and Snaith 1983) and the fear questionnaire (Marks and Mathews 1979) can assist the nurse to quantify the person's anxiety. More simple assessments such as a visual analogue scale (see Rogers *et al.* 2004) or rating anxiety on a simple one to ten rating scale are very useful in disorders such as OCD and phobias. In the treatment of phobias and OCD, the development of a hierarchy of fear (see across) is generally the first step in the treatment programme. Mental health nurses play a key role in assisting the individual to develop this hierarchy and to explain the treatment interventions that will be used. Diary writing can also help the individual with anxiety to link their feelings to what is happening around them or to establish triggers to their anxiety and should be encouraged.

TREATMENT OF ANXIETY DISORDERS

Generally the first step in the treatment programme (following assessment) is educating the individual about anxiety and helping them to understand how the physical and psychological manifestations of anxiety produce their symptoms. Education is of particular importance when utilising specific intervention methods, such as exposure, and the development of a therapeutic nurse–patient relationship is imperative to the success of any intervention. Figure 14.4 gives a brief overview of the interventions that are commonly used in the treatment of the various anxiety disorders discussed in this chapter. Most of the principles used in the treatment of the anxiety disorders generally come from a cognitive behavioural perspective.

Cognitive behaviour therapy (CBT) is generally the treatment of choice for people with an anxiety disorder. According to Frisch and Frisch (2006) the goal of CBT in this instance is to help the individual to identify the sources of their anxiety. Through various techniques, the clinician assists the person in developing alternative mechanisms to deal with their anxiety and equip them with realistic problem-solving techniques to deal with anxiety-provoking situations as they arise. The clinician also engages in cognitive restructuring which challenges the individual's coping mechanisms and beliefs about their ability to cope. Westbrook *et al.*'s (2007) text can be referred to for a more comprehensive introduction to CBT. The main component of CBT in treating anxiety disorders is exposure to feared stimuli. Apart from exposure, CBT involves other behavioural components such as muscle relaxation, breathing exercises, modelling, thought stopping and homework.

Figure 14.4 Overview of interventions used in the treatment of anxiety disorders

Anxiety Disorder	General Interventions
Generalised Anxiety Disorder	• Relaxation techniques such as deep breathing • Avoiding stimulants such as caffeine • Confronting avoidance through dialogue regarding fear and anxiety • Techniques to help the individual accept uncertainty • Exercise • Setting realistic goals • Improving self-esteem • Helping individual to manage their anxiety and developing alternative skills to manage stress and anxiety
Panic Disorder	• Relaxation techniques such as deep breathing • Helping the individual to ascertain the triggers to their panic attacks, e.g. through diary keeping • Helping the individual prevent the onset of panic through relaxation techniques • Helping the individual to manage their anxiety generally and to develop alternative ways to manage their stress and anxiety
Post-Traumatic Stress Disorder	• Management of concurrent problems such as depression or alcohol or drug dependence • Eye movement desensitisation and reprocessing • Exposure to the traumatic event through imagery • Examining feelings of guilt, shame or anger that may be present either in group or individual therapy
Obsessive Compulsive Disorder	• Exposure and response prevention • Challenging beliefs that promote behaviour
Phobias	• Systematic desensitisation • Cognitive restructuring and modelling (social phobia) • Relaxation techniques • Improving esteem • Helping the individual to manage their anxiety generally and to develop alternative ways to manage their stress and anxiety

Source: Westbrook *et al.* 2007; Shives 2005; Rogers *et al.* 2004

Muscle Relaxation
Many forms of relaxation have been used in treating anxiety problems over the years and continue to have an important place in treating these disorders. The theory behind muscle relaxation is that muscles cannot relax and tense at the same time, so relaxing the muscles results in reducing tension. Relaxation is presented as a method of counteracting the patient's physiological responses to anxiety (e.g. palpitations, sweating, etc.). Like all skills, much practice is required to master this relaxation technique (Leahy and Holland 2000; Varcolis 2002).

Breathing Exercises
Breathing exercises are a useful part of relaxation therapy. The respirations of the anxious patient tend to be rapid and shallow and there is often a chronic pattern of 'over breathing' (Varcolis 2002).

Modelling
This approach involves the therapist becoming a role model for the client. In this way the client learns by imitation. The therapist themselves frequently does the modelling, but they could also have another person model the behaviour or show a video in which the desired behaviour is modelled (Varcolis 2002).

Thought Stopping
There are a number of thought-stopping techniques that clients find useful. One method involves the client shouting, 'stop' when they have an undesired thought (e.g. when a person with OCD has an obsessional thought). After some time the client learns to stop such thoughts without shouting aloud. Another technique involves placing a rubber band on the client's wrist and instructing them to snap it when they have an undesirable thought. Both these techniques teach the client to dismiss any undesirable thought processes.

Exposure
According to Westbrook *et al.* (2007:131) 'exposure to anxiety-provoking stimuli leads to the anxiety response gradually dying away as the person gets used to the situation'. There are several different types which are used primarily in the treatment of phobias and obsessive compulsive disorder.

Systematic Desensitisation
This is a form of exposure in which the individual with a phobia is gradually exposed to their feared object or situation over a period of time. The exposure can either be done in vivo (i.e. in real life) or the person can be asked to imagine that they are in contact with the phobic scenario (in vitro exposure). Prior to conducting the therapy the individual is asked to construct a hierarchy of fear. This is usually a ten-point scale with the lowest anxiety-provoking situation at the bottom rising to the most anxiety-provoking (i.e. panic) situation at the top.

Using relaxation techniques the individual is asked to expose themselves to the feared object until their anxiety levels are reduced by fifty per cent. Before and after exposure, anxiety levels are taken generally using a visual analogue scale. Gradually the individual becomes desensitised to the feared situation, moving on to the next point in the hierarchy of fear as they progress through the therapy.

Exposure and Response Prevention
This form of exposure is primarily used in the treatment of OCD. While being very similar to systematic desensitisation, this therapy asks the individual with OCD to resist the temptation to complete the compulsion when they are troubled with obsessional thoughts. The main difference between this and systematic desensitisation is that during the therapy the individual is asked not to practise relaxation techniques or to take anti-anxiety medication. By doing this the individual not only becomes desensitised to the feelings of anxiety, they also learn, over time, to realise that their belief that something terrible will happen if they do not carry out their compulsion is ill-founded. The patient is asked to construct a hierarchy of fear and to work through the hierarchy generally over two-hour sessions. They are also encouraged to learn to relax and to use exercise etc to manage their anxiety outside the therapy.

Other Forms of Exposure
These include introceptive exposure, and flooding. Introceptive exposure involves the client confronting the physical symptoms of anxiety (Craske and Barlow 2000). If the patient fears cardiovascular symptoms, for example, interceptive exercises may require them to run around for a few minutes; this will induce the cardiovascular symptoms and the client learns that although these symptoms may be uncomfortable they are not dangerous and don't, contrary to their belief, result in disastrous consequences.

Flooding is full-on or direct exposure to the feared object or situation. Exposing an individual client with a fear of spiders directly to spiders is a form of flooding (Gauthier 1999).

Eye movement desensitisation and reprocessing is generally indicated in the treatment of post-traumatic stress disorder and was first introduced by Shapiro (2001). This treatment involves the therapist helping the individual to become desensitised to the distressing memory while helping them to reprocess that particular memory through eye movement and other forms of external stimulus. A more detailed explanation of the therapy is available at the website www.emdr.com/index.htm.

Homework
The homework ethic has long been promoted in cognitive therapy. Homework involves repeating exposures that were conducted in therapy or conducting variations of them outside therapy (Hubbert *et al.* 2006). Homework compliance has been associated with positive outcomes for up to two years after treatment (Park *et al.* 2001).

Pharmacotherapy

A variety of drugs are available for the medical management of anxiety disorders, and an overview of the most common is given in Figure 14.5. For a more comprehensive explanation of their indications, doses, interactions and side effects, see the *British National Formulary* or Healy (2005).

Figure 14.5 Examples of drugs used to treat anxiety

Type	Class	Example/Notes
Selective serotonin reuptake inhibitors (SSRIs)	Antidepressants	Citalopram (Cipramil) and Escitalopram (lexapro) are used to treat panic disorder and GAD respectively. Sertraline (Lustral) is licensed to treat OCD. Paroxetine (Seroxat) is licensed to treat a wide variety of anxiety disorders.
Trycyclic antidepressants	Antidepressants	Clomipramine (Anafranil) is specifically indicated in the treatment of OCD.
Reversible monoamine oxidase inhibitors	Antidepressants	Moclobemide (Manerix) is used in the treatment of social phobia.
Benzodiazepines	Anxiolytics	Diazepam (Valium); alprazolam (Xanax). Indicated in the short-term treatment of severe anxiety; may help the person to feel relaxed; may induce sleep when given at night. Associated with tolerance, and dependence.
Beta adrenoceptor blocking drugs	Beta blockers	Propranolol (Inderal) is more often used in the treatment of cardiovascular disease; in anxiety these are generally indicated for the treatment of the somatic symptoms of anxiety such as palpitations, tremor or rapid pulse.

CONCLUSION

The anxiety disorders are among the most common mental health disorders. Individuals with anxiety disorders experience high levels of anxiety which impact on their personal, occupational and social functioning. People with anxiety disorders are rarely seen in the acute setting; however, anxiety as a symptom is present in a number of illnesses. People with anxiety disorders employ a wide range of maladaptive coping mechanisms to deal with the unpleasant anxiety feelings and often avoid confronting the situations or objects that provoke anxiety. This chapter has examined a number of the more common anxiety disorders and given an overview of the treatment measures. Mental health nurses can utilise the principles of CBT to assist people with anxiety to manage their symptoms.

Reflective Questions

1. Think of the strategies you as an individual use to manage your anxiety. How could you use these strategies to help people with anxiety disorders?
2. A client in your care states that they 'can't learn how to relax'. What strategies could you use to help this individual to learn and practise relaxation techniques?
3. You have been asked to give a presentation about systematic desensitisation to a group of individuals living in the community. What factors might you take into consideration before delivering the presentation?
4. How can you as a mental health nurse utilise the principles of CBT in the management of anxiety disorders?

References

American Psychiatric Association (APA) (2000) *Diagnostic and Statistical Manual of Mental Disorders* (DSM-IV-TR) (4th edn: text revision). Washington DC: APA.

Barlow, D. (2002) *Anxiety and its Disorders: The Nature and Treatment of Anxiety and Panic.* London: Guilford Press.

Beck, A. T., Emery, G. and Greenberger, R. L. (1985) *Anxiety Disorders and Phobias: A Cognitive Perspective.* New York: Basic Books.

British National Formulary (BNF) (2007). London: British Medical Formulary and Royal Pharmaceutical Society of Great Britain.

Brown, T. A. and Barlow, D. H. (1992). 'Diagnostic co-morbidity among anxiety disorders. Implications for treatment and DSM-IV'. *Journal of Consulting and Clinical Psychology*, 60, 835–44.

Clarke, L. A., Watson, D. and Mineka, S. (1994) 'Temperament, personality and the mood and anxiety disorders'. *Journal of Abnormal Psychology*, 103, 103–116.

Craske, M. G. and Barlow, D. H. (2000) *Mastery of Your Anxiety and Panic* (3rd edn). San Antonio: Psychological Corporation/Graywind Publications.

de Silva, P. and Rachman, S. (1998) *Obsessive Compulsive Disorder: The Facts.* Oxford: Oxford Medical Publications.

Eysenck, H. J. (1967) *The Biological Basis of Personality.* Springfield: Charles C. Thomas.

Frisch, N. C. and Frisch, L. E. (2006) *Psychiatric Mental Health Nursing.* Canada: Thompson.

Gauthier, J. G. (1999) 'Bridging the gap between biological and psychological perspectives in the treatment of anxiety disorders'. *Canadian Journal of Psychology*, 40 (1), 1–11.

Gray, J. A. and McNaughton, N. (1996) 'The neuropsychology of anxiety: reprise', in D. A. Hope (ed.), *Nebraska Symposium on Motivation, Vol. 43:*

Perspectives on Anxiety, Panic, and Fear. Lincoln: University of Nebraska Press.

Healy, D. (2005) *Psychiatric Drugs Explained.* Edinburgh: Churchill Livingstone.

Heckleman, L. R. and Schneier, F. R. (2000) 'Diagnostic issues' in R. L. Leahy and S. J. Holland (eds), *Treatment Plans and Interventions for Depression and Anxiety Disorders.* London: Guilford Press.

Hubbert, J., Ledley, D. and Foa, E. (2006) 'The use of homework in behaviour therapy for anxiety disorders: integration of between sessions (homework). Activities into psychotherapy'. *Journal of Psychotherapy Integration,* 16(2), 128–39.

Kendler, K. S., Neale, M. C., Kessler, R. C., Heath, A. C. and Eaves, L. J. (1992) 'The genetic epidemiology of phobias in women: the interrelationship of agoraphobia, social phobia, situational phobia and simple phobia'. *Archives of General Psychiatry,* 49: 273–81.

Kendler, K. S., Walters, E. E., Neale, M. C., Kessler, R. C., Heath, A. C. and Eaves, L. J. (1995) 'The structure of genetic and environmental risk factors for six major psychiatric disorders in women; phobia, generalized anxiety disorder, panic disorder, bulimia, major depression, and alcoholism'. *Archives of General Psychiatry,* 52, 374–82.

Kessler, R. (1999) 'Comorbidity of unipolar and bipolar depression with other psychiatric disorders in a general population survey', in M. Tohen (ed.), *Comorbidity in Affective Disorders,* New York: Marcel Dekkes Inc., pp. 1–25.

Lang, A. J. and Stein, M. B. (2001) 'Anxiety disorders: how to recognize and treat the medical symptoms of emotional illness'. *Geriatrics,* 56(5), 24–34.

Leahy, R. L. and Holland, S. J. (2000) *Treatment Plans and Interventions for Depression and Anxiety Disorders.* London: Guilford Press.

Marks, I. M. and Mathews, A. M. (1979) 'Brief standard self-rating for phobic patients'. *Behaviour Research and Therapy,* 17: 59–68.

Mayo Health Clinic (2005) *Phobias.* Mayo Health Clinic Publications.

Park, J. M., Mataix-Cols, D., Marks, I. M., Ngamthipwatthana, T., Marks, M., and Araya, R. *et al.* (2001) 'Two-year follow up after a randomized controlled trial of self and clinician-accompanied exposure for phobia/panic disorders'. *British Journal of Psychiatry,* 178, 543–8.

Rogers, P., Curran, J. and Gournay, K. (2004) 'The person with an anxiety disorder', in I. Norman and I. Ryrie (eds), *The Art and Science of Mental Health Nursing: A Textbook of Principles and Practice.* London: Open University Press.

Salkovskis, P. M. (1991) 'The importance of behaviour in the maintenance of anxiety and panic: a cognitive account', in Rogers *et al.* (2004).

Sartorius, N., Ustua, T. B., Lecrubier, Y., and Wittchen, H. U. (1996) 'Depression comorbid with anxiety; results from the WHO study on psychological disorders in primary health care'. *British Journal of Psychiatry,* 30, 38–43.

Saunders, D. and Wills, F. (2003) *Counselling for Anxiety Problems.* London: Sage Publications.

Shapiro, F. (2001) *Eye Movement Desensitization and Reprocessing: Basic Principles, Protocols and Procedures* (2nd edn). New York: Guilford Press.

Shives L. R. (2005) *Basic Concepts of Psychiatric—Mental Health Nursing* (6th edn). Philadelphia: Lippincott Williams and Wilkins.

Thompson, P. H. (2000) 'Obsessive compulsive disorders: pharmacology treatment'. *European Child and Adolescent Psychiatry*, 9, 1/76–1/84.

Turner, T. (2003) *Anxiety*. London: Churchill Livingstone.

Varcolis, E. (2002) *Foundations of Psychiatric Mental Health Nursing: A Clinical Approach*. London: W. B. Saunders Company.

Westbrook, D., Kennerley, H. and Kirk, J. (2007) *An Introduction to Cognitive Behaviour Therapy: Skills and Applications*. London: Sage.

Wilkinson, G., Moore, B. and Moore P. (2000) *Treating People with Anxiety and Stress: A Practical Guide for Primary Care*. Abingdon: Radcliffe Medical Press.

Yates, W.R. (2005) *Anxiety Disorders*, www.emedicine.com/med/topic152htm. Last updated 2005. Accessed October 2006.

Zigmond, A. S. and Snaith R. P. (1983) 'The hospital anxiety and depression scale'. *Acta Psychiatrica Scandinavica*, 67, 361–70.

15
Care of the Person with Suicidal Behaviour

Louise Doyle

The extent of suicide and suicidal behaviour in Ireland has become a serious public health issue and a major cause for concern. Many people are directly affected by suicide and suicidal behaviour whether in a personal or a professional capacity. The family and friends of those who have died by suicide are left with substantial grief, often complicated with guilt and self-recrimination while mental health professionals charged with their care often feel a sense of failure at not having prevented this conclusive action.

This chapter will discuss the prevalence of suicide and suicidal behaviour in Ireland and will outline both the protective and the risk factors for suicide, including a consideration of suicide across the lifespan. The salient points of suicide risk assessment will be discussed along with the nursing care of a client engaging in suicidal behaviour.

NOMENCLATURE AND LANGUAGE OF SUICIDE

Before considering the extent of suicidal behaviour in Ireland it is important to briefly consider the nomenclature and language of suicide and suicidal behaviour. The term 'suicide' is universally understood and is commonly taken to mean the act of killing oneself intentionally.

However, when attempting to define and describe 'suicidal behaviour' the waters are muddied as there is much debate among researchers and clinicians about terminology, and there is no clear consensus regarding the use of a common term. Commonly used terminology includes deliberate self-harm (DSH), parasuicide, attempted suicide, non-fatal suicidal behaviour, self-injurious behaviour and self-mutilation. Some of these terms are used interchangeably, but for the purpose of this chapter the definitions used will be consistent with those employed in the *National Strategy for Action on Suicide Prevention* (HSE *et al.* 2005). In this document, suicidal behaviour is an umbrella term and is defined as the spectrum of activities related to suicide, including suicidal thinking, self-harming behaviours not aimed at causing death and suicide attempts (Commonwealth Department of Health and Aged Care (Australia) 1999). Some concepts specifically associated with suicidal behaviour are:

- **Suicidal ideation**: vague, fleeting thoughts about wanting to die.

- **Suicidal intent:** thoughts about a concrete plan to die by suicide.
- **Suicidal threat:** the expression of a person's desire to end his/her life.
- **Suicidal gesture:** intentional self-destructive behaviour that is clearly not life-threatening but does resemble an attempted suicide.
- **Self-mutilation:** considered to be any incident where an individual has attempted to deliberately alter or destroy body tissue without suicidal intent (i.e. cutting, burning, scratching, hitting, biting, pinching) (Favazza 1989).
- **Deliberate self-harm (DSH):** the various methods by which people deliberately harm themselves, including self-cutting and taking overdoses. Varying degrees of suicidal intent can be present and sometimes there may not be any suicidal intent, although an increased risk of further suicidal behaviour is associated with all DSH (HSE *et al.* 2005).

It is also important to briefly consider the language used to describe suicide. Suicide in Ireland was decriminalised in 1993. It is therefore inappropriate and unhelpful to continue using terms such as 'commit' when describing suicide, as this term has an obvious association with crime. Rather, terms such as 'died by suicide' can help to describe a death by suicide in a manner that is not value-laden. The Irish Association of Suicidology and the Samaritans, in their *Media Guidelines for the Portrayal of Suicide* (2006), suggest appropriate language to use when describing deaths by suicide.

SUICIDE AND SUICIDAL BEHAVIOUR IN IRELAND

Suicide rates in Ireland have increased from 6.9 per 100,000 in 1982 to 11 per 100,000 in 2005 (HSE 2006). Kelleher (1996) argues that this rise in suicide rates is genuine and is not a result of more accurate reporting or reclassification of unnatural deaths. On closer examination it is apparent that the increase in Irish suicide rates in the latter part of the last century was largely as a result of a striking rise in suicide in young men, among whom the increase has been four-fold since 1990. Suicide is now the most common cause of death for men aged 15–24 years (Aware 1998). While the overall female suicide rate has increased slowly since 1980, the rate of suicide among young women aged 15–24 years more than doubled in the 1990s, albeit from a low base rate. However, there is still a large gender variation in suicide rates in Ireland, with a male/female ratio of 4.5:1. This increase in suicide rates in young people has resulted in Ireland now having the fifth highest suicide rate in Europe in the 15–24 year age group.

The rates of deliberate self-harm (DSH) have also increased. It is widely accepted that there is a strong link between deliberate self-harm and suicide. The recently published *National Strategy for Action on Suicide Prevention* (HSE *et al.* 2005) emphasises that a history of one or more acts of deliberate self-harm is the strongest predictor of repeated suicidal behaviour, both fatal and non-fatal. The Report of the National Database on Deliberate Self-Harm (NSRF 2006) highlights that in 2005 there were approximately 11,000 presentations with deliberate self-harm to emergency departments. Of these presentations, almost half (46 per cent) were by people under thirty years of age. The trend in deliberate self-harm in Ireland is different from the suicide trend as the male/female ratio is reversed to some degree, standing at a ratio of 1:3 men to women.

SUICIDE ACROSS THE LIFE SPAN

Patterns of suicidal behaviour differ across the lifespan, peaking in adolescence/early adulthood and again in the older person. The factors affecting a person's decision to end their life can change as they move from childhood, through adolescence, adulthood and on to older age. A brief consideration of some of the patterns and factors affecting these patterns is outlined in this section.

Childhood

Suicide and suicidal behaviour in childhood is uncommon in Ireland and the suicide rate for children is lower than in any other age group. Suicidal behaviour in children is more impulsive than in adults. They are less likely to engage in suicidal behaviour that involves planning, such as hoarding and ingesting drugs. As with all age groups, depression is linked to suicidal behaviour in children. In particular, feelings of inferiority and low self-esteem are often present (Stillion and McDowell 1996). A risk factor specific to childhood is the *expendable child syndrome* (Sabbath 1969). Parents of expendable children communicate low personal regard, withdrawal of love, hostility and even hatred. Expendable child syndrome can activate a wish to die and it is not unusual for the child to consider suicide as a way to stop being a burden to the parent. These children may feel responsible for their parents' negative emotions and feel they should be punished for the role they play in making their parents unhappy.

An immature view of death is also a risk factor for childhood suicidal behaviour. It is generally believed that children under seven years of age have an immature view of death. They think of death as being a transient and reversible state. Children between the ages of seven and twelve develop an increasing understanding of the facts of death. By the age of twelve, almost all children understand that death is universal, inevitable and final. Research has shown that suicidal children have less well-defined concepts of death and are less likely to understand the finality of death (Carlson *et al.* 1994). Suicidal children have experienced more frequent and earlier loss than others. Many of these children have lost parents through death or divorce before the age of eleven. Conduct disorders, bullying and school-related problems are also related to childhood suicidal behaviour. The family environments of suicidal children are less healthy and more likely to be dysfunctional. Incidence of parental conflict including physical violence is greater than usual in the homes of these children. A relationship also exists between childhood suicide and child abuse, especially sexual abuse (Stillion and McDowell 1996).

Adolescence

Adolescence is a transitional period during which individuals experience many physical, emotional and social changes. As children move into their teens, the incidence of a range of mental health problems increases. In particular, suicidal behaviour often emerges during adolescence and in its broadest sense is relatively common in this group. For completed suicide, the rate in Ireland for 15–19-year-olds during the years 1999 to 2003 inclusive was 12.5 per 100,000 (HSE 2006). This rate was significantly higher for males (20.4 per cent) than for females (4.5 per cent). The National Suicide Research Foundation (2006), however, reports that the trends in deliberate self-harm are reversed, with females having a much higher rate (606 per 100,000) than males (303 per 100,000) in 2005. This means that 1 in 165 Irish adolescent girls was treated in hospital as a result of deliberate self-harm in 2005. Community studies of Irish adolescent suicidal behaviour would suggest that the actual extent of self-harm is much greater, with hidden, unreported self-harm a real issue (Sullivan *et al.* 2004).

Many factors associated with adolescent suicidal behaviour are consistent with those throughout the lifespan and they include mental illness. In particular, eating disorders, depression, substance abuse, anxiety disorders and personality disorders are all associated with adolescent suicidal behaviour. Problems that often emerge during adolescence can also contribute to suicidal behaviour. These might include examination pressure, transition from school to college/employment and issues regarding sexual identity. Impulsivity has been noted to be particularly associated with adolescent suicidal behaviour (Hawton *et al.* 1982), as has poor problem solving skills: adolescents have had fewer life experiences to draw upon than adults and therefore do not have the same repertoire of options available to them (Stillion and McDowell 1996).

Adulthood

The highest suicide rate in Ireland occurs in young adult males. For the period between 1999 and 2003 the rate of suicide was highest in males aged 20–24 years (20.9 per 100,000) and 24–29 years (20.3 per 100,000). The highest rate of suicidal behaviour for males also occurs in adult males, with a rate of 392 per 100,000 for the 20–24 age group in 2005 (NSRF 2006). As with all age groups, depression is significantly associated with suicidal behaviour in adults. Depression may be precipitated by trigger factors that occur particularly in adulthood, such as changing roles (from student to wage earner), early career stresses, lack of intimate interpersonal relationships, 'age 30' evaluation and 'mid-life' evaluation (where life choices are evaluated) and, for women, post-natal depression and post-natal psychosis. Furthermore, factors such as long-term unemployment, single status (marriage acts as a protective factor), increase in substance abuse and being a convicted prisoner are all associated with higher rates of suicidal behaviour and are also more associated with males.

Older People

The demographics of suicide in the older person in Ireland differ from suicide demographics internationally. In Ireland, suicide rates are highest for young men while internationally the suicide rate is highest in the older population. However, suicide among older people in Ireland is still high (16.1 per 100,000 for the 60–64 year age group 1999–2003) and is on the increase (HSE 2006). Suicidal ideation and self-harming behaviour is less common in later life than among younger groups. Conwell and Duberstein (2005) identify that self-destructive acts in the older person often have a greater lethality, which results from a number of factors such as greater physical illness and frailty, fewer warnings given of suicidal plans, the use of more lethal means and the fact that many older people live alone or are isolated. This means that they are less likely to be discovered in time if they do attempt suicide. In Ireland, 45.3 per cent of older people over 65 years live in rural areas and approximately 27 per cent of older people in this age range live alone (HSE and DoHC 2006). The resulting social isolation with concomitant loneliness and lack of social integration is associated with suicidal behaviour in older adults. Other factors associated with suicidal behaviour in this age group include mental health problems (particularly depression), feelings associated with retirement, diagnosis of a terminal illness, bereavement (particularly widowhood) and being more accepting of death (Stillion and McDowell 1996).

RISK AND PROTECTIVE FACTORS FOR SUICIDE

Throughout the literature many studies have tried to identify the predictors of suicide from various theoretical perspectives, but no universally accepted model explains suicide conclusively. Suicide is generally considered to be a complex phenomenon, the causes of which are likely to involve a combination of psychological, biological, social and environmental factors. However, one of the most famous theories is the sociological theory of 'anomie' developed in the seminal work *Le Suicide* by the renowned French sociologist Durkheim (1897), which was translated into English in 1952. This explanation of suicide is concerned partly with societal norms and the affects of these norms upon individuals. Societal norms have changed considerably in Ireland over the past twenty years as witnessed by increases in single-parent families, separation/divorce, crime and alcohol dependency. These social changes appear to contribute to the rise in suicide.

There are both risk factors and protective factors that may increase or decrease a person's level of suicide risk. However, there are problems when relying on risk factors which attempt to identify those at greatest risk of suicide as these factors are known characteristics of vulnerable groups of people who have taken their own lives rather than of each individual (Cooper and Kapur 2004). Commonly identified risk and protective factors are outlined below.

Risk Factors
- Age and gender: suicide in Ireland is most common in adolescents and young adults but is high and is increasing in the older person. Males are more likely to die by suicide in Ireland but females are more likely to engage in suicidal behaviour.
- History of mental health problems: the most noteworthy causal factor related to suicide is mental illness. In particular, affective disorders, psychotic disorders and substance abuse are all associated with an increased suicide risk.
- History of previous self-harm: a history of previous self-harm or attempted suicide indicates an increased risk of further suicidal behaviour.
- High suicidal intent: indicated by the persistence of suicidal ideation, the presence of a suicide plan including the choice of a highly lethal suicide method, access to means of suicide and plans for death (will changes, family farewell etc) (Cooper and Kapur 2004; Kutcher and Chehil 2007).
- Hopelessness: the inability to see any hope for the future is associated with higher suicide risk.
- Medical history: a history of a physical illness increases suicide risk and is highly correlated with the presence of depression. Some physical illnesses associated with a higher suicide risk include multiple sclerosis, Huntington's disease, dementia and HIV/AIDS (Kutcher and Chehil 2007).
- Family history of mental illness or suicide.
- Loneliness and social isolation.
- Unemployment.
- Life events including bereavement and loss, abuse (past or present), legal/financial problems, relationship problems, loss of parents through separation or death during childhood (Cooper and Kapur 2004).

Protective Factors
- Absence of mental illness.
- Employment.
- Having children in the home/sense of responsibility to family.
- Pregnancy.
- Strong religious beliefs.
- High life satisfaction.
- Positive coping skills.
- Positive problem-solving skills.
- Positive social support.
- Positive therapeutic relationship.

(Kutcher and Chehil 2007.)

SAD PERSONS SCALE

There are many tools that can help mental health professionals assess the risk of suicide and suicidal behaviour. These include the 'tool for assessment of suicide risk' (TASR) (Kutcher and Chehil 2007) and the Beck scale for suicidal ideation (BSI) (Beck and Steer 1991). Patterson *et al.* (1983) have developed an easy-to-use scale to help health professionals assess suicide risk by identifying the presence of risk factors. This scale is known as the SAD PERSONS scale (SAD PERSONS is an acronym based on the first ten letters of the common suicide risk factors). A score of one is given for the presence of each risk factor and the closer the score is to ten, the more 'at risk' the person is considered to be.

- **Sex**: males are more likely than females to die by suicide.
- **Age**: certain age groups are more associated with suicide, e.g. adolescence/early adulthood and older age.
- **Depression**: mental illness and in particular depression is the biggest risk factor for suicide. Symptoms of depression such as feelings of worthlessness, helplessness and hopelessness are all associated with a higher suicide risk.
- **Previous attempt**: a history of attempted suicide or self-harm is significantly associated with further suicide attempts.
- **Ethanol (alcohol) use**: the rate of suicide is higher among those who are alcohol dependent than among the general population.
- **Rational thought loss**: those whose judgement and rational thought are impaired are more likely to die by suicide. This includes the presence of psychosis, e.g. hearing command hallucinations or experiencing paranoid delusions.
- **Social supports lacking**: those who lack social support, social integration and are isolated are at greater risk.
- **Organised plan**: the presence of an organised suicide plan is an indicator of higher suicide risk. The more organised the plan, the greater the risk.
- **No spouse**: those who are single, divorced, widowed or separated are at greater risk for suicide. This is particularly so for males.
- **Sickness**: the presence of chronic, debilitating, severe and painful illnesses increases suicide risk.

This scale can be helpful to mental health nurses by ensuring the collection of relevant psychosocial history which can contribute to an assessment of suicide risk. However, this scale, like other suicide assessment scales, should only be used in *combination* with other methods of identifying suicide risk. Shea (1999) highlights that use of this scale alone to assess suicidality may cause health professionals to underestimate actual suicide risk. This is illustrated in an example provided by Shea (1999) where a middle-aged woman scores only one point on the above scale as she is suffering from post-partum psychosis and is hearing voices. Her score of one would suggest a low suicide risk, but the voices she is hearing are command hallucinations which are telling her to kill herself in order to protect her newborn child. This example illustrates the need to assess not risk factors alone but how these factors affect the person concerned.

RISK ASSESSMENT

Suicide risk assessment is complex and requires consideration of a number of factors in a number of ways. This section will outline the salient points of suicide risk assessment for mental health nurses. A fuller discussion of suicide risk assessment is provided in Kutcher and Chehil (2007). As previously identified, risk factors are the characteristics of a large sample of people who have died by suicide. However, the presence of such factors does not necessarily alert the mental health professional to an immediate danger of suicide or to the fact that a client *is* at higher risk, but it does indicate that there is good reason to suggest that the client *may be* at higher risk (Shea 1999). Similarly, the presence of protective factors does not necessarily suggest that a client is not at risk of suicide. It is important therefore to undertake an individual suicide risk assessment which, while considering the presence of risk and protective factors, also takes into account a person's individual characteristics and the presence of warning signs of suicide.

Warning signs of suicide differ from risk factors: warning signs imply near-term risk whereas risk factors suggest risk over much longer periods. Many risk factors are static and enduring (e.g. psychiatric illness) whereas warning signs are episodic and variable (e.g. thoughts of suicide, behaviours preparing for suicide). Rudd *et al.* (2006) have defined a suicide warning sign as the earliest detectable sign that indicates heightened risk for suicide in the near term (i.e. within minutes, hours or days). Some of the main immediate and less immediate warning signs of suicide as developed by the American Association of Suicidology (Rudd *et al.* 2006) are as follows.

Warning signs of suicide

Immediate signs:
- Threatening to hurt or kill themselves.
- Looking for ways to kill themselves, e.g. seeking access to pills.
- Talking or writing about death, dying or suicide.
- Making 'final' arrangements. Saying goodbye. Tidying up affairs. Making a will.

Less immediate signs:
- Hopelessness.
- Rage, anger, seeking revenge.
- Acting recklessly or engaging in risk activities seemingly without thinking.
- Feeling trapped — as if there is no way out.
- Increasing alcohol or drug use.
- Withdrawing from friends, family or society.
- Anxiety, agitation, unable to sleep or sleeping all the time.
- Dramatic changes in mood.
- No reason for living; no sense of purpose in life.

Warning signs, however, are not always present and when they are they may not be obvious and may only be observed in retrospect. Kutcher and Chehil (2007) identify that many suicidal individuals may not voice suicidal thoughts or plans of self-harm to their healthcare provider. Furthermore, Cooper and Kapur (2004) stress that it is important to be aware of the misleading demeanour of the 'smiling depressive', a sudden calmness after the person has been depressed without evidence of resolution of their problems. In many of these cases, the individual has made up their mind to die by suicide and this decision has resulted in them *appearing* happier and calmer. It is therefore important to directly question the client regarding the presence of suicidal thoughts or plans for suicidal behaviour. Many health professionals appear reluctant to approach the issue of suicide with a client, fearing that it may increase the likelihood of them engaging in suicidal behaviour. On the contrary, Kutcher and Chehil (2007) suggest that clients may feel relieved that they have been given 'permission' to talk about the topic and to discuss honestly and openly how they have been feeling.

UNCOVERING SUICIDAL IDEATION AND BEHAVIOUR

When undertaking a nursing assessment of *any* client it is important to consider the risk of suicide. However, this is even more so for those who are at a heightened risk of suicide as determined by the presence of risk factors. The ability to assess suicide risk is an important skill for all nurses in all settings. Community mental health nurses, nurses working in in-patient settings and those working in hostels in the community are required continuously to assess the bio/psycho/social functioning of clients in their care, and this includes the assessment of suicide risk. Suicide risk assessment needs to be an ongoing process as a client's degree of suicidality is not a static quality but may fluctuate quickly and unpredictably (Shives 2005). One of the basic prerequisites prior to undertaking a nursing assessment is the establishment and development of a good nurse/client relationship. Disclosing personal thoughts such as thoughts of suicide or self-harm may be threatening to the client for many reasons, including that they may believe suicide to be a form of weakness or they may believe they will be 'locked up' if they do articulate their feelings (Shea 1999). It is essential, therefore, that a relationship is established between the nurse and the client that is non-judgemental and is based on warmth and empathy. Developing such a relationship allows the client to feel safer in disclosing their thoughts of suicide or self-harm. Kutcher and Chehil (2007) have identified some ways in which the suicide assessment can be broached in a general way before asking more specific questions about suicide. These are outlined across.

Uncovering suicidal ideation and behaviour

The empathic statement:
- I can see how difficult things have been for you lately ...
- It seems that things have been hard for you and that it has been difficult to cope ...
- You seem to be having a hard time ...

The gentle inquiry:
- I wonder if you would help me understand how this has been for you?
- Can you share your concerns with me?
- Can you tell me about what has been happening?
- How have things been for you lately?

Asking the question:
- Have you ever thought about harming yourself?
- Have you ever tried to do anything to yourself that could have seriously harmed you or killed you?
- Have you been thinking about harming yourself?

Source: Kutcher and Chehil (2007)

NURSING PRINCIPLES FOR A CLIENT WHO IS SUICIDAL

The nursing care of a client who is suicidal centres on two main principles: keeping the person safe and engaging with the person.

Client Safety
Schultz and Videbeck (2005) have identified some basic principles to ensure the physical safety of a client in an in-patient setting. These include:
- Knowing the whereabouts of the client at all times.
- Being aware of sharp objects (glass, knives, etc.) or other items that could potentially be used to harm oneself (lighters, bleach, etc.).
- The client's bed should be situated near the nurses' station to facilitate observation.
- Staying with the client when they undertake certain self-care activities, e.g. bathing, shaving.
- Being aware of a client who could be 'cheeking' their medication and hoarding it.
- Undertaking frequent checks on the client but in an irregular manner so the client cannot predict the pattern of observation.

If a client has been assessed as a high suicide risk, they may be placed under 'special' observation. Special or one-to-one observation is when the person is placed under the continuous observation of a nurse. During this period of observation the nurse remains within arm's length of the client at all times. The main rationale behind the use of such a practice is that it ensures the client's safety and minimises their ability to cause harm to themselves. This special observation also helps to ensure that the client actually *feels* safe. Special observation is prescribed by a doctor and the period of time that a person remains under this high level of observation varies but the decision to discontinue this practice should be taken after a thorough suicide risk assessment.

While the practice of special observation is widespread in psychiatric in-patient facilities, its effectiveness is questioned by many. Cutcliffe and Barker (2002) argue that the therapeutic value of such special observation has long been questioned and describe it as a crude, custodial form of intervention to meet the highly complex needs of this client group. Furthermore, they argue that it does little to address the crux of the client's problems that led them to feel suicidal in the first place. Cleary *et al.* (1999) identify how nursing dilemmas arise from this practice, particularly in relation to patient privacy (e.g. in the toilet) as the nurse must keep the patient within sight. While there is little doubt that the practice of special observation is custodial in nature, the therapeutic effect it has on a client depends to a large extent on the nurse undertaking the observations. Studies have identified how, despite their close proximity, some nurses make little or no attempt to engage with the client while undertaking observation and many patients report that nurses did not talk to them at all during the observation period (Fletcher 1999; Jones *et al.* 2001). Engaging with a client who is suicidal or is self-harming is a crucial nursing role and should be central to all nursing interventions.

Engaging with the Client

Cutcliffe and Barker (2002) stress the importance of both engagement and inspiring hope with a client who is suicidal. Engagement is concerned with establishing a human connection with the person. This connection, in the form of the therapeutic relationship, is essential for a client who is feeling suicidal. Conveying caring, acceptance and understanding is important in this process. A non-judgemental attitude is crucial as the person needs to know that the nurse is not judging their behaviour or blaming them for self-harming. Acceptance and tolerance are also particularly important to a person who is experiencing feelings of worthlessness and hopelessness. Furthermore, if a true therapeutic relationship exists based on empathy and caring, the person will feel more comfortable disclosing their thoughts of suicide/self-harm. Cutcliffe and Barker (2002) suggest that the act of truly engaging with and caring for a person can in itself inspire hope in someone who is experiencing suicidal thoughts. If a person senses that the nurse 'caring' for them is uninterested or judgemental this can reinforce feelings of worthlessness; however, a nurse who demonstrates genuine caring can have a positive effect on self-esteem and feelings of hopelessness. Caring for a person who is suicidal can be a difficult process and keeping the person safe is obviously of utmost importance. However, this need not be done to the exclusion of therapeutic involvement with the client. As Cutcliffe and Barker (2002:618) identify, 'only through engaging with the person will the nurse come to understand the nature of the person's needs, and what might need to be offered to address them'.

SPECIFIC INTERVENTIONS FOR THOSE WHO SELF-HARM

While the nursing care principles of keeping the client safe and therapeutic engagement are very relevant for those who engage in deliberate self-harm, there are more specific interventions that mental health nurses can utilise with this client group.

First, however, it is essential that nurses are aware of their own feelings and responses to these clients. Those who regularly engage in low-lethality self-harming behaviour often induce feelings of frustration, anger and resentment in those charged with their care. These feelings can then contribute to the formation of negative attitudes towards those who self-harm (see Chapter 16). Kutcher and Chehil (2007) identify the importance of not letting negative or ambivalent feelings towards clients interfere with clinical care. Some interventions identified in the literature specifically for those who self-harm include:

- A no-harm contract: the client agrees in an oral or written contract with the health professional not to engage in self-harming behaviours. The effectiveness of these contracts, however, has not been demonstrated in the literature.
- Harm minimisation: the client is given the opportunity to reduce the severity of the self-harm by being taught how to harm themselves safely. This can include behaviours such as holding ice in their hands, punching a pillow or snapping an elastic band against their wrist. However, Noonan (2004) has identified how this technique can perpetrate the client's need to feel an immediate physical response to a psychological stressor.
- Distraction techniques: the client is actively distracted from their urge to self-harm by engaging in more positive activities such as taking a walk, listening to music, etc.

Other interventions for this client group include problem-solving techniques and dialectical behaviour therapy. A further consideration of interventions can be found in Chapter 16.

POSTVENTION

Despite the best efforts of mental health professionals, some individuals do die by suicide both in in-patient settings and more commonly in the community. Kutcher and Chehil (2007) have identified four principles that are important when this happens: support; learn; counsel; and educate.

Support

Providing support to those colleagues who have been affected by a client's suicide is important and this support should come not only from colleagues but also from health service management in the form of debriefing if appropriate. Feelings of self-blame and failure to help the client may be particularly associated with the aftermath of a client suicide.

Learn

Learning from the experience of a client's suicide is an important part of the process and this should occur in a multidisciplinary format and should be non-judgemental and supportive.

Counsel

Many mental health nurses will have been working not only with the client who died but also with their family members. In this case it is important to provide support for those who have been bereaved by suicide. Nurses can act as a resource to put the family in touch with specific support groups, such as Console, that help family members of those who died by suicide.

Educate

The death of a person by suicide can provide an opportunity for mental health professionals to educate others with regard to suicide and recognising the warning signs. This may be particularly relevant if the person who died by suicide was involved in a group, e.g. school, college, hostel, etc.

CONCLUSION

Suicide and suicidal behaviour is not uncommon in Ireland and mental health nurses in a range of settings regularly come into contact with those who engage in suicidal behaviour. Understanding the factors that influence a decision to take one's own life and the ability to assess clients for suicidal thoughts and behaviours is crucial to the mental health nurse's role. Utilising practical interventions to keep the client safe, and therapeutic interventions to engage with the client, the mental health nurse can make a real difference in meeting the needs of this vulnerable client group.

Reflective Questions

1. What do you believe are the contributory factors to suicide among young people in Ireland?
2. How might you assess a severely depressed person for suicide risk?
3. What are your opinions about the practice of special observation for clients who are suicidal?
4. Examine your opinions about self-harm and your responses to clients who present with repeated self-harming behaviour.

References

Aware (1998) *Suicide in Ireland — A Global Perspective and A National Strategy.* Dublin: Aware Publications.

Beck, A. and Steer, R. (1991) *Manual for the Beck Scale for Suicidal Ideation.* San Antonio: Psychological Corporation.

Carlson, G. A., Asarnow, J. R. and Orbach, I. (1994) 'Developmental aspects of suicidal behaviour in children and developmentally delayed adolescents', in G. G. Noam and S. Borst (eds), *Children, Youth and Suicide: Developmental Perspectives.* San Francisco: Jossey-Bass.

Cleary, M., Jordan, R., Horsfall, J., Mazoudier, P. and Delaney, J. (1999) 'Suicidal patients and special observation'. *Journal of Psychiatric and Mental Health Nursing,* 6, 461–7.

Commonwealth Department of Health and Aged Care (Australia) (1999). *LIFE Strategy.* Australia: CDHAC.

Conwell, Y. and Duberstein, P. (2005) 'Suicide in older adults: determinants of risk and opportunities for prevention', in K. Hawton (ed.), *Prevention and Treatment of Suicidal Behaviour: From Science to Practice.* Oxford: Oxford University Press.

Cooper, J. and Kapur, N. (2004) 'Assessing suicide risk', in D. Duffy and T. Ryan (eds), *New Approaches to Preventing Suicide: A Manual for Practitioners.* London: Jessica Kingsley.

Cutcliffe, J. R. and Barker, P. (2002) 'Considering the care of the suicidal client and the case for "engagement and inspiring hope" or "observations"'. *Journal of Psychiatric and Mental Health Nursing,* 9, 611–21.

Durkheim, E. (1952) *Suicide: A Study in Sociology.* Oxfordshire: Routledge Classics.

Favazza, A. R. (1989) 'Why patients self-mutilate'. *Hospital and Community Psychiatry,* 40, 137–45.

Fletcher, R. F. (1999) 'The process of constant observation: perspectives of staff and suicidal patients'. *Journal of Psychiatric and Mental Health Nursing,* 6(1), 9–14.

Hawton, K., O'Grady, J., Osborn, M. and Cole, D. (1982) 'Adolescents who take overdoses: their characteristics, problems and contacts with helping agencies'. *British Journal of Psychiatry,* 140, 124–31.

Health Service Executive (HSE), National Suicide Review Group and Department of Health and Children (2005) *Reach Out — National Strategy for Action on Suicide Prevention 2005–2014.* Dublin: HSE.

Health Service Executive (HSE) (2006) National Office for Suicide Prevention *Annual Report 2005.* Dublin: HSE.

Irish Association of Suicidology and the Samaritans (2006) *Media Guidelines for the Portrayal of Suicide.* IAS.

Jones, J., Ward, M., Wellman, N., Hall, J and Lowe, T. (2001) 'Psychiatric inpatients' experiences of nursing observations. A United Kingdom perspective'. *Journal of Psychosocial Nursing,* 38(12), 10–19.

Kelleher, M. J. (1996) *Suicide and the Irish*. Cork: Mercier Press.

Kutcher, S. and Chehil, S. (2007) *Suicide Risk Management. A Manual for Health Professionals*. Massachusetts: Blackwell Publishing.

National Suicide Research Foundation (NSRF) (2006) *Report of the National Database on Deliberate Self-Harm*. Cork: NSRF.

Noonan, I. (2004) 'Therapeutic management of suicide and self-harm', in I. Norman and I. Ryrie (eds.), *The Art and Science of Mental Health Nursing: A Textbook of Principles and Practice*. Berkshire: Open University Press.

Patterson, W. M., Dohn, H. H., Bird, J. and Patterson, G. A. (1983) 'Evaluation of suicidal patients: The SAD PERSON Scale'. *Psychosomatics*, 24(4), 343–9.

Rudd, M. D., Berman, A. L., Joiner, T. E., Nock, M. K., Silverman, M. M., Mandrusiak, M., Van Orden, K. and Witte, T. (2006) 'Warning signs for suicide: theory, research and clinical applications'. *Suicide and Life-threatening Behavior*, 36 (3) 255–62.

Sabbath, J. C. (1969) 'The suicidal adolescent: the expendable child'. *Journal of the American Academy of Child Psychiatry*, 8, 272–89.

Schultz, J. M. and Videbeck, S. L. (2005) *Lipponcott's Manual of Psychiatric Nursing Care Plans*. Philadelphia: Lipponcott, Williams and Wilkins.

Shea, S. C. (1999) *The Practical Art of Suicide Assessment: A Guide for Mental Health Professionals and Substance Abuse Counselors*. New Jersey: John Wiley and Sons.

Shives, L. R. (2005) *Basic Concepts of Psychiatric–Mental Health* Nursing (6th edn). Philadelphia: Lipponcott, Williams and Wilkins.

Stillion, J. M. and McDowell, E. E. (1996) *Suicide Across the Life Span*. Washington DC: Taylor and Francis.

Sullivan, C., Arensman, E., Keeley, H. S., Corcoran, P. and Perry, I. J. (2004) *Young People's Mental Health: A Report of the Results of the Lifestyle and Coping Survey*. Cork: National Suicide Research Foundation.

16
Explaining and Treating Personality Disorders

Jim Maguire

Initially, personality disorder was a relatively neglected area of psychopathology but since the 1970s it has become the focus of attention of an ever-growing body of empirical research. Yet personality disorder often seems to defy classification. Obviously, the term implies abnormal personality, but personality itself is a concept that is not easily defined. It is commonly accepted that personality refers to regular and consistent (rather than occasionally occurring) behaviours, perceptions, thought patterns and feelings.

The aim of this chapter is to define, classify and discuss the aetiology of personality disorders, and discuss treatment approaches and nursing care for people with this type of disorder.

Kneisl *et al.* (2004:480) defined personality as the 'individual qualities, including habitual behaviour patterns, that make a person unique'. Personality consists of personality traits, specific features or behavioural patterns that make up an individual's overall personality. They are evident early in childhood, develop over time and become very stable in adulthood to uniquely define a person's personality. If these traits evolve in a manner that is maladaptive, causing the person for example to be manipulative, insensitive, anxious, excessively dependent or withdrawn, so that relationships with others are problematic, then a personality disorder has developed.

Personality disorder is therefore an umbrella term to describe rigid, stereotyped behaviour patterns that persist throughout a person's life. People with personality disorder characteristically lack insight into the impact of their behaviour on the environment and fail to accept responsibility or consequences for their behaviour. The *Diagnostic and Statistical Manual of Mental Disorders* or DSM-IV-TR (APA 2000) distinguishes personality disorders from other mental disorders, classifying them as Axis II disorders.

238 Clinical Application to Practice

DSM-IV-TR criteria for a diagnosis of personality disorder:
1. An enduring pattern of inner experience and behaviour that deviates markedly from the expectations of the individual's culture. This pattern is manifested in two or more of the following areas:
   - Cognition (i.e. ways of perceiving and interpreting self, other people and events).
   - Affectivity (i.e. the range, intensity, lability and appropriateness of emotional response).
   - Interpersonal functioning.
   - Impulse control.
2. Inflexible and pervasive across a broad range of personal and social situations.
3. The enduring pattern leads to clinically significant distress or impairment in social, occupational, or other important areas of functioning.
4. The pattern is stable and of long duration and its onset can be traced back at least to adolescence or early adulthood.
5. The enduring pattern is not better accounted for as a manifestation or consequence of another mental disorder.
6. The enduring pattern is not due to the direct physiological effects of a substance (e.g. a drug of abuse, a medication) or a general medical condition (e.g. head trauma).

The Mental Health Act 2001 also distinguishes between mental illness and personality disorder, stating that the involuntary admission of a person with personality disorder is not authorised. Kendall (2002) claims it is impossible to conclude with confidence that personality disorders are, or are not, mental illnesses: there are ambiguities in the definitions and basic information about personality disorders is lacking.

CLASSIFICATION OF PERSONALITY DISORDERS

Many types of personality disorder are described in the literature. Figure 16.1 shows the three clusters or categories of personality disorders defined by the APA.

Figure 16.1 Personality disorder clusters (APA 2000) and lifetime population prevalence

Cluster A (Odd or Eccentric types or Schizophrenia-spectrum disorders)	Lifetime prevalence in population
Paranoid personality disorder	0.5—2.5%
Schizoid personality disorder	0.2—0.8%
Schizotypal personality disorder	2.5—3%

Cluster B (Dramatic, Emotional or Erratic types)	Lifetime prevalence in population
Borderline personality disorder	1—2%
Histrionic personality disorder	0.7—3%
Narcissistic personality disorder	< 1%
Anti-social personality disorder	2%
Cluster C (Fearful or Anxious types)	**Lifetime prevalence in population**
Avoidant personality disorder	2%
Dependent personality disorder	0.3—2%
Obsessive-compulsive personality disorder	1—1.9%

INCIDENCE AND PREVALENCE

There are no reliable data on the global prevalence of personality disorders. This is because many people with such disorders have no insight and never seek help from mental health services. Also, personality disorders exist on a continuum of severity where many are sub-clinical and never diagnosed. The median prevalence for any one personality disorder across six major studies was 12.9 per cent (Mattia and Zimmerman 2001). There are no Irish statistics available for the prevalence of personality disorders but these clients accounted for 2.5 per cent of all in-patient admissions (n=85) in mental health services in 2005 (MHC 2005). It is known that men are more likely to be diagnosed with obsessive-compulsive, narcissistic, anti-social, schizoid, schizotypal or paranoid personality disorders. Women are more likely to be diagnosed as having borderline, dependent or histrionic types (APA 2000).

Many of those who come into contact with mental health services are seeking treatment for relationship problems, depression or other co-morbid Axis I disorders, and the diagnosis of personality disorder is incidental. Some personality disorders have high co-morbidity with substance abuse, complicating treatment interventions (Serman *et al.* 2002). Clients may also have more than one personality disorder. Although children can sometimes have a personality disorder, the diagnosis is not usually made until they reach adulthood. Dependent personality disorder and borderline personality disorder are the most commonly seen personality disorders in clinical settings.

AETIOLOGICAL THEORIES

As with many disorders, aetiological theories offer suggestions as to causative factors and attempt to support those suggestions with research-based evidence. It must always be remembered that a multiplicity of factors influence personality and no two people experience the same influences on their personalities, be they biological, genetic/familial or psychosocial.

Biological and Genetic Theories

Biological or genetic factors may play a role in personality disorder. Reduced left-sided temporal lobe grey matter volumes have been found in clients with schizoid personality disorder (Kirrane and Siever 2000). Serotonin dysregulation has been found to be a factor in borderline and other personality disorders (Hansenne *et al*. 2002). It is also known that physical trauma to the brain, particularly to the frontal lobe area, can lead to dramatic personality changes (Damasio 1994). To date, no specific gene has been linked with personality disorder. Numerous studies demonstrate higher incidences of several traits of personality disorders in first-degree relatives (Torgersen *et al*. 2000; White *et al*. 2003). However, it is extremely difficult to determine whether such correlations are due to heredity or social/environmental factors or both.

Psychosocial Theories

Psychodynamic theories suggest that personality disorders are related to early life interactions with parents (Figure 16.2).

Figure 16.2 Psychodynamic beliefs about the relationships between personality disorders

Personality disorder type	Associated parental style in child's early life
Paranoid personality disorder	Rigid and over-controlling
Schizoid, schizotypal, antisocial, histrionic, narcissistic, dependent personality disorder	Emotionless and rejecting
Borderline personality disorder	Non-accepting or/and abusive
Avoidant and obsessive-compulsive personality disorders	Critical, especially about early bowel or bladder accidents

Erikson (1968) claimed that failure of an adolescent to establish his or her identity results in *identity diffusion*, in which the person has a poor sense of coherence, difficulty committing to roles and problems in intimate relationships. Some individuals deal with this by choosing a 'negative identity' with behavioural patterns that meet the criteria for personality disorder (Wilkinson-Ryan and Westen 2000).

Sexual and other types of childhood abuse are believed to be related to personality disorders, especially borderline personality disorder (BPD) (Zanarini *et al*. 2002). Early-onset childhood sexual abuse is so associated with BPD that BPD may be a complex type of post-traumatic stress disorder, according to McLean and Gallop (2003).

Social Learning Theory

This theory argues that the development of personality disorder may arise in those who fail or imperfectly learn social norms. Anti-social behaviour may be learned from and modelled by parents (Bowers *et al*. 2000).

THE NATURE OF CLIENTS WITH PERSONALITY DISORDERS

Personality disorders have been grouped into clusters for practical reasons. For treatment purposes, personality disordered clients with similar characteristics can be looked at together, although the essential differences of the disorders within a cluster will all be considered. Each type has personality traits that are particular to it, but there are some traits that are common to all people with a personality disorder. These include:

- lack of insight about the disorder and its impact on others
- a belief that all problems are caused by others
- failure to accept the consequences of their own behaviour.

These traits lead to maladjustment, inability to learn, repeated dysfunctional interactions and behaviours and a lack of remorse for actions. Like personality, personality disorders are very stable phenomena which are chronic and pervasive, affecting all aspects of the person's life.

CLUSTER A (PARANOID, SCHIZOID AND SCHIZOTYPAL PERSONALITY DISORDERS)

These clients rarely seek treatment but they are seen clinically as their behaviours and beliefs often cause them to come into contact with mental health services. The common features of these so-called *odd* or *eccentric* disorders are distrust and social detachment. These clients are considered the most disordered or different from what society considers normal people. They are poor at emotional engagement and are often considered to be detached or cold. They have few or no friends. Schizoid and schizotypal personality disorder differ from schizophrenia in terms of severity, the latter being more severe.

Characteristics of Cluster A Personality Disorders
Paranoid personality disorder:
- Suspiciousness — makes communication and rapport difficult.
- Inflexibility — no insight and is unwilling to try new things or change.
- Hostility — safety issues must be considered and there may be a history of trouble with the law and others.
- Withdrawal — isolates him/herself, though some hold down jobs, getting by through use of rigid pre-planned responses.

Schizoid personality disorder:
- Emotional withdrawal — does not desire close personal relationships; tends towards solitary occupations. Tends to be unaffected by criticism or praise. Takes pleasure in few, if any, activities.
- Thought disorder — not a major feature; has elaborate fantasies.

Schizotypal personality disorder:
- Mood shifts and anxiety — may be treated clinically for these conditions.
- Thought disorder — usually more severe than schizoid type; evidenced by loose associations; may experience derealisation, depersonalisation, grandiose ideation, suspiciousness, paranoia.
- Unkemptness — personal and environmental untidiness.
- Behaviour — odd, eccentric, solitary.

CLUSTER B (BORDERLINE, HISTRIONIC, NARCISSISTIC AND ANTI-SOCIAL PERSONALITY DISORDERS)

These are the dramatic-emotional personality disorders. Key features are irresponsibility, manipulative behaviours, intense emotions and rages, impulsiveness, lability, self-centredness, a need for instant gratification and attention and a poor ability to make or sustain friendships. People with cluster B personality disorders live very much in the here and now, acting often with little consideration of the consequences of their actions.

Borderline Personality Disorder (BPD)
BPD is the most well-described personality disorder. Hennessey and McReynolds (2001) described it as one of the most intrusive illnesses known. People with BPD are highly emotional and often run into conflict with others. Their impulsivity and unpredictability lead them into situations that are dangerous for themselves and others. The term borderline relates to the opinion that, although cluster B clients tend to remain in touch with reality, those with BPD live psychologically somewhere on the border between reality and psychosis. Key characteristics include:
- Impulsiveness — sudden, irrational decisions that cause them to lose a job, a partner or everything they own.
- May get into trouble with the law due to impulsive criminality such as shoplifting.
- Deliberate self-harm (DSH) — another feature of impulsiveness. Injuries may be superficial or life-threatening.
- Boredom.
- Fear — fear of abandonment and, paradoxically, of engulfment, so they may reject someone just as that person begins to offer them what they seemed to desire.
- Unrealistic expectations — especially of relationships. The inevitable disappointments can lead to violent rows or excessive clinging and demanding behaviour.
- All or nothing thinking — seeing people as either all good or all bad at a particular time.

BPD is thought to originate from dysfunctional childhood events. The child fails adequately to resolve conflicting feelings in association with development of autonomy, instead fearing both abandonment and over-involvement. People with BPD often meet the criteria for the presence of one or more other personality or mental disorder.

Histrionic Personality Disorder

People with histrionic personality disorder are attention-seeking and manipulative. They dramatise ordinary events and 'act out' when demands are not being met quickly enough. Acting out may involve tantrums, promiscuity, complaints, or unreasonable demands; behaviours which appear to others to be selfish and immature. The person may regress to earlier life behaviours in order to attain the attention of others. Again, there are relationship difficulties, mood variations and unreasonable expectations from others, especially authority figures.

Narcissistic Personality Disorder (NPD)

These are highly dependent on the praise and admiration of others. Key characteristics include:

- Grandiosity and arrogance — exaggerates and boasts about real or desired abilities and achievements. This self-promoting behaviour is thought to be a consequence of low self-esteem.
- Attention-seeking — another consequence of low self-esteem. Craves partners and friends who will admire and praise them and who can elevate their status in the eyes of others.
- Insincerity — cares little for the feelings of others. Ignores those perceived to be unaccomplished or of no use to them.

Anti-social Personality Disorder (ASPD)

Anti-social personality disorder is also known as *sociopathy* or *psychopathy*. Characteristics include:

- Manipulative behaviours — bullying, exploitive sexual relationships and promiscuity. Can be charming and disarming, feigning total interest in others to win them over.
- Intelligence — this, with their charm, can enable them to attain positions of power and influence.
- Insensitivity to others — blame others when confronted; disrupt and flout rules or laws. Rash, impulsive risk-takers; engage in petty or serious crimes.
- Remorselessness — can readily discard people when deemed to be no longer of use to them.
- Instability — usually unable to work consistently at a particular job and move on frequently, often leaving a trail of debts behind them.

It is not surprising that the first time people with ASPD come to the notice of authorities is often when the police become involved. Sometimes mental health services are the first contact, but this is usually due to a concurrent mental disorder or suicide attempt. Due to their lack of insight these clients rarely self-refer. The manipulative, splitting behaviours they engage in while in clinical settings pose substantial challenges for health professionals. Childhood conduct disorders such as attention deficit hyperactivity disorder (ADHD) present like early versions of ASPD and have been linked to it (Hill 2003).

CLUSTER C (AVOIDANT, DEPENDENT AND OBSESSIVE-COMPULSIVE PERSONALITY DISORDERS)

These, the *anxious–fearful* personality disorders, are characterised by non-assertiveness, worries, fears, indecisiveness, self-deprecating behaviours and withdrawal.

Avoidant Personality Disorder
The main characteristics of avoidant personality disorder are:
- Anxiety and ineptitude in social situations.
- Fear of rejection or shame, often causing them to interpret benign gestures or comments by others as ridicule.
- A craving for attention and affection.
- Over-seriousness and hypersensitivity.
- Loneliness, with few or no friends.

Dependent Personality Disorder
Characteristics include:
- A craving for attention and affection.
- Clinging behaviour and fear of being alone — inability to find a supportive relationship causes intense anxiety. May offer to do almost anything, even unpleasant tasks, for the person whose approval they seek.
- Lack of confidence.
- Poor decision-making skills.
- Tend to agree with things out of fear of disapproval.

Obsessive-Compulsive Personality Disorder (OCPD)
In OCPD the preoccupation with order, lists, detail and organisation impinges less severely on everyday life than it does for the client with obsessive-compulsive disorder (OCD). The main characteristics of OCPD are:
- Seriousness — excessive pedantry; stubbornness; over-conscientious; conformist.
- Preoccupations — with tidiness, rules, cleanliness and impulsive urges.
- Rigidity — meticulousness, sometimes accompanied by incongruent slovenliness in some other aspects of their lives. Their lives are full of rules and rituals and they tend to be hoarders of useless objects. They are suited to some types of work that involve routines, perfection and repetition. However, rituals and fear of errors may incapacitate them in work.

PERSONALITY DISORDER NOT OTHERWISE SPECIFIED

The DSM-IV-TR (APA 2000) reserves this category for personality disorders that do not fall easily into any of the other types. These personality disorders have features of more than one type. Examples are passive-aggressive personality disorder and self-defeating personality disorder.

NURSING CARE AND TREATMENT APPROACHES TO PERSONALITY DISORDERS

Many clients with personality disorder are never treated clinically. The person has no insight into his/her disorder and therefore may never seek help. One is more likely to know them in everyday life as the odd or eccentric neighbour, the person who has repeated skirmishes with the police, 'the black sheep' of a family or the ruthless (and often successful) politician, movie star or business person. Efforts to point out problematic aspects of their lives will usually be dismissed or cause offence.

Those with personality disorder who are involved with mental health services are likely to have BPD, paranoid or schizotypal personality disorder, or to have presented with another (usually Axis I) disorder. Responsiveness to treatment for people with personality disorders is described as moderate or modest at best. Those who are least responsive are the anti-social and narcissistic types (Comer 2004).

Treatment approaches for personality disorders include biological or medical treatments and psychosocial interventions. The choice of treatment modality depends on the client's motivation for insight and change. Figure 16.3 summarises the main approaches.

Figure 16.3 The main interventions used for personality disorder

Behaviour therapy	A therapy that involves substituting desirable behaviour responses for undesirable ones.
Object relations therapy	Therapy based on psychodynamic assumption that the desire for human relationships is the main motivation for behaviours.
Cognitive behaviour therapy (CBT)	Therapies that help people recognise, understand and change their faulty thinking patterns.
Dialectical behaviour therapy (DBT)	A type of CBT where the therapist combines modelling of more appropriate ways of interpreting and reacting to situations with social skills training.
Psychodynamic-psychoanalytic therapy	Therapies that seek to uncover traumatic events in the client's past life in order to understand the inner torment
Eye movement desensitisation	A relatively new form of exposure therapy where clients

and reprocessing (EMDR) (Brown and Shapiro 2006)	move their eyes rhythmically from side to side whilst flooding their minds with images of objects and situations they usually try to avoid.
Social interventions	*Group, couples or family therapy* Focus on a range of topics such as self-harm, avoidance, manipulation, substance abuse, emotions and interpersonal skills. *Therapeutic communities* Residential, self-run communities where clients experience mutual helping, tolerance and confrontation.
Pharmacological treatments (see end of this chapter)	Mainly SSRIs, anxiolytic, neuroleptic and anticonvulsant medications.

One of the main purposes of an intervention programme for personality disorders is client education. An education programme should address:
- The nature of the personality disorder and its effects on the client and others.
- Warning signs for when the client needs help, and who to seek it from.
- Coping strategies for the many challenges that arise because of their disorder.

NURSES' ATTITUDES TO PERSONALITY DISORDER

Bowers *et al.* (2000) summarise research on this issue and conclude that nurses tend to express negative judgements about patients who are seen as hostile, unco-operative, complaining and manipulative, who suffer from chronic or stigmatised illnesses, who self-harm, or who make staff feel ineffective. Personality disordered patients fit several of these characteristics.

NURSING ASSESSMENT

A comprehensive nursing assessment approach for a client with personality disorder includes the physical, emotional, cognitive, social and spiritual domains.

Figure 16.4 Five domains of nursing assessment

Domain	Assessment
Physical	Activities of daily living, appearance, behaviours and body language, physical illness, substance abuse, safety, self-harm.
Emotional	Hostility, impulsiveness, suspiciousness, anxiety, self-esteem, guilt, intolerance, passivity, anger, hopelessness.
Cognitive	Insight, problem solving, judgement, delusions, altered thinking.
Social	Social skills, manipulation, relationships, secretiveness, grudges, illegal activities, attention seeking, confidence.
Spiritual	Meaning and purpose in life, beliefs.

NURSING CHALLENGES

These are common to several types of personality disorder.

Manipulation

Clients with personality disorder are often manipulative. They engage in behaviours, such as criticising, praising, blaming, devaluing and bribing, that have the tendency to 'split' staff. The nursing and other staff must be aware of manipulative behaviours and act to counter them. This involves challenging the client's splitting statements where one staff member is praised and others are not. An effective strategy is to point out that what the client is saying contradicts earlier statements by the client or actions by the staff.

Some strategies to deal with manipulation are outlined below:
- Having a cohesive group of professionals who communicate well with each other.
- Looking at how interpersonal problems arise as a result of manipulative behaviours.
- Teaching delayed gratification through group work, role-play and behavioural techniques such as counting before acting/saying.
- Using agreed behavioural contracts.
- Being non-judgemental and fair.
- Responding in a manner that causes the client to focus on his/her own intentions and behaviours.
- Setting appropriate and agreed limits for the client's behaviour.
- Teaching alternative behaviours when the client feels anxious.
- Asking the client what he is really looking for when he behaves inappropriately.

Boredom

Clients often use this complaint to opt out of activities that may be threatening or limiting to them. Clients may leave arranged activities before they are over, which needs to be explored and challenged. A full programme of therapeutic activities should be in place to minimise opportunities for boredom. When the client makes efforts to participate more fully, he should be praised for doing so.

Relationship Problems

Clients with a personality disorder often experience great difficulties in their personal/social relationships. Emotional responses may be intense and smothering, or blunted and restricted. The nurse should assess the nature of the client's relationships, discussing them with the client either individually or in group sessions. Unhelpful emotional responses should be identified and alternative strategies to delay impulsive, inappropriate responses should be discussed and rehearsed. Role-play, behaviour therapy, CBT, drama groups and didactic sessions are all techniques that may be useful. Clients may need to be reassured that it is acceptable to display appropriate emotions in certain situations and they may need to discover which emotions are appropriate. It may also be useful to engage family members or other significant people at an intermediate or later stage of the treatment programme for counselling, couples therapy, or family therapy.

Impulsiveness

Impulsiveness is taking action based on whims or sudden desires rather than careful thought. It leads to many different problems in the lives of people with personality disorders and their friends and families. Clients speak, act, abuse alcohol or drugs, resign from their job, make financial decisions or walk out of home or relationships without considering the consequences. They may also come to the attention of the legal system.

The nurse must help the client to become aware of these rash actions and their consequences. Safety is the primary concern as clients are likely to harm themselves or others financially, emotionally, psychologically or physically through impulsive actions. Usually, the client is angry or anxious before making such decisions, so the nurse can assist them in identifying situations and precipitants that increase these emotions with the aim of the client learning to make alternative responses that are more productive and appropriate. Taking time out or using delaying or relaxation techniques may be useful. Most clients have one or two major impulsive patterns such as alcohol abuse or dangerous driving, so these can be prioritised for intervention. Resources within the multi-disciplinary team (MDT) (counsellors, social workers) and the community (nurses, self-help groups, parole officers, and friends) may be important players in the treatment plan. A behavioural contract is often found to be useful.

Challenges in Cluster A Personality Disorders

Mistrust or Suspiciousness

The clients with Cluster A personality disorders that mental health nurses are most likely to encounter are the paranoid type and, to a lesser extent, the schizotypal type. These clients have had lifelong experiences of mistrusting other people, who exclude them as a consequence, which reinforces their mistrust. They are also usually very rigid in their perception of the world but they are capable of learning to be well-adjusted in their behaviour and social relationships. Therefore, the nurse needs to be patient, yet confident that she/he can make a difference in these clients' lives. The nurse should approach the client with an open, non-threatening style and should be very aware of the signals he/she may convey through pauses, tone of voice, the nature and pace of questions and all aspects of body language. There should be no sudden movements or surprises. A key worker or primary nurse system of care will help as the client is likely to deal mainly with one member of the nursing staff, thus getting the time needed to learn to trust and relax in the nurse's presence. The nurse should acknowledge the client's reality while not agreeing with what the client says or does if his/her speech or actions are inappropriate. Mistaken beliefs should be gently explored while presenting/prompting more accurate interpretations of events or statements. This often involves reassuring the client that the intentions of others are not malicious or that other people are not discussing the client.

Anger and Aggression

It is reasonably foreseeable that the suspicious, mistrustful or paranoid client may be angry or aggressive. The nurse's primary concern is to try to prevent anger and aggression and many of the techniques he/she may use have already been described. In the event of anger or aggression, the nurse should remain calm and not reflect the client's anger. The client should have their feelings acknowledged but limits must be made clear in relation to how anger is expressed. It is inappropriate for the client to frighten other clients or staff with displays of verbal or physical aggression and the client must be tactfully informed of this. The nurse should try to remove the client to a less public area while ensuring through backup and positioning that their own safety is not compromised. The nurse should be non-judgemental, non-patronising and truthful. A walk in the hospital grounds or a cup of tea in a quiet room may be sufficient in some situations. In other cases, where the safety of the client or others is a risk, it may be necessary to suggest time-out, or even intervene against the person's wishes to medicate, hold or seclude the client. (For further discussion of the management of violence and aggression see Chapter 20.)

When the crisis is past, staff should always ensure that there is some form of debriefing that includes the client. This session can be used for a constructive exchange of views on what happened and it is an opportunity for planning how repeat incidents can be avoided. The client is encouraged to identify precipitant events and alternative responses that could be used in the future. Sometimes a person with personality disorder displays their anger by non-co-operation, avoidance, impatience, ignoring, resentment or sarcasm. This is known as passive-aggressive behaviour. The behaviour must be explored with the client to help the nurse and the client to determine what is truly going on. The client is assisted to focus on the source of his impatience or anger and how his passive aggression is unhelpful to himself and others.

Vagueness, Thought Disorder and Distractibility

These characteristics are most prominent in schizotypal personality disorder. The nurse or therapist tries to focus the client on realistic and useful thoughts and dismiss the others. Asking the client to repeat or summarise what he is saying is a useful technique for distractibility or vagueness. Time-keeping exercises and routines may also introduce some order in these clients' lives.

Challenges in Cluster B Personality Disorders

People with borderline personality disorder are often encountered in the clinical setting. They sometimes pose perplexing and seemingly intractable challenges for friends, family and mental health professionals. These challenges include self-mutilation, suicide attempts, impulsiveness, manipulation, attention seeking, unstable relationships, anger, unpredictability/impulsiveness, poor judgement, irresponsibility and disruptiveness, coupled with poor self-esteem and feelings of emptiness and loneliness.

Sometimes the apparent lack of success of many standard nursing interventions causes nurses to despair, particularly in the presence of BPD. Nurses must be careful not to stereotype people with BPD as beyond help or requiring expert, specialist interventions. Fundamental nursing skills such as being respectful and patient, listening attentively, being non-judgemental, setting fair limits and being there for the client will eventually establish a therapeutic rapport which is a key element for progress (Bowers *et al.* 2000).

There are, however, some specialist interventions that have been found to be particularly helpful with many clients with BPD (and other personality disorders). These psychotherapies are outlined in Figure 16.3. It is well described that BPD can diminish over time, as if the client 'grows out of it' (Paris 2002; Brown and Shapiro 2006) but it is also known that psychotherapy can accelerate this remission (Perry *et al.* 1999; Paris 2002).

Deliberate Self-harm

This is a common feature of BPD. Self-destructive behaviour usually poses low-risk lethality but some clients seriously disfigure or even kill themselves. This type of auto-aggression may take the form of cutting, burning, biting or hitting oneself or pulling out one's hair. Clients with BPD do not view these behaviours as very problematic. Rather, they see them as helpful in that the self-induced pain makes them feel real and in touch with themselves again. Many clients describe feelings of immense relief during and after self-injury. Others, because of feelings of shame or guilt, believe that this self-injurious behaviour is deserved and absolving. A thorough nursing assessment should include assessment of the risk for self-harm or suicide. Risk assessment scales have been devised that can assist with this aspect of assessment and are discussed further in Chapter 15.

Nurses should endeavour to establish a trusting relationship with the client. This involves being honest, fair, firm at times, being a good listener and being non-judgemental. The client should be reassured that they are now in a safe environment with people who care for their well-being. The client's property must be checked for potentially harmful objects, which should be removed.

Where the client persists in these self-injurious behaviours, it may be necessary to place the client under close or constant observation. A psychiatric intensive care unit (PICU) or high observation/intensive care area (ICA) is usually the most suitable setting. Where the client succeeds in self-harming, the nurse should attend to the physical injury and to the heightened emotional state of the client. It is important to be kind, attentive and non-critical while not reinforcing the behaviour in any way. Self-injurious behaviour may be almost relentless and is very stressful on clients and staff. Nurses must be very self-aware to detect when they are reaching a point where their coping is less effective and take appropriate measures. The tired, stressed nurse is at risk of being harsh, judgemental or traumatised, resulting in damage to the all-important nurse–client relationship.

The nursing skills necessary for clients with histrionic (or hysterical) personality disorder (HPD) are often similar to those for BPD. Clients are grandiose and overly emotional. They seek out treatments and attention so they often present to mental health services voluntarily. HPD is very challenging because of dramatic, switching emotions, tantrums, impulsiveness, dishonesty and grandiosity. Clients will often pretend that an intervention has worked when it has not. Group therapy and other psychotherapeutic interventions can be helpful.

Narcissistic Personality Disorder
This is quite resistant to treatment. Specialist cognitive behavioural and psychodynamic therapies offer some possibilities for enabling the client to learn to become aware of the views and feelings of others and to be less self-preoccupied and manipulative.

Mood changes and feelings of emptiness are common features of cluster B personality disorders and nurses have an important role to play in assessing and intervening where clients are experiencing abnormal moods. These interventions are discussed in Chapter 12.

Challenges in Cluster C Personality Disorders
Social withdrawal, low self-esteem and fear of being alone are features of cluster C disorders. It is important to confront clients about their negative beliefs and help them learn to replace such thoughts with more self-affirming ones. The nurse should emphasise the positive in the client's life: personal achievements, friendships and interests. The client must be encouraged to interact with others. Group sessions with other clients are challenging but potentially rewarding for those with low self-esteem and self-confidence. These clients are always watchful for behaviours or comments that affirm their low opinions about themselves, so the nurse must strive to demonstrate kindness and understanding. Manipulation is also a feature of these personality disorders, so the nurse must balance kindness and encouragement with firmness and consistency.

Those with obsessional-compulsive traits have additional needs for intensive behaviour and cognitive therapy to address the obsessional thoughts and the actions they take as a consequence. This is addressed more thoroughly in Chapter 14.

PHARMACOLOGICAL INTERVENTIONS

Pharmacological treatment, if used, should serve only as an adjunct to psychosocial treatments. Modest successes are reported in studies using selective serotonin reuptake inhibitors (SSRIs) such as paroxetine in the reduction of suicidal ideation, impulsivity and depression (Soloff 2000). Soloff recommends low-dose neuroleptics for acute global symptom management. Clinicians are inclined to use SSRIs, neuroleptic agents, and anticonvulsants when the client has symptoms that have traditionally been responsive to such agents.

CONCLUSION

Personality disorders are perhaps the most challenging disorders nurses will encounter in their working lives. The collective despair and negative feelings (Nehls 2000) that sometimes prevail among mental health professionals in the face of these challenges is understandable in light of the intransigence of most personality disorders and the, at best, moderate outcomes of treatment. Personality disordered clients tend to be stigmatised by the very people charged with helping them. The need for nurses and others to be self-aware is therefore paramount. It is important for nurses to remember that the inappropriate behaviours of many clients can diminish with proper interventions and with time, and that clients who improve are often well able to accurately describe which interventions were most helpful and to name the carers who didn't give up on them.

Reflective Questions
1. Examine the attitudes and beliefs you and your nursing colleagues hold with regard to clients with personality disorder. How might they enhance or obstruct the formation of a therapeutic nurse–client relationship?
2. Which aspects of the in-patient milieu that you have experienced are suitable or unsuitable for therapeutic care of clients with personality disorder?
3. How useful is the organisation of personality disorders into diagnostic clusters?
4. Discuss the evidence for and against classifying personality disorders as something other than mental illness.

References
American Psychiatric Association (APA) (2000) *Diagnostic and Statistical Manual of Mental Disorders* (DSM-IV-TR) (4th edn: text revision). Washington DC: APA.

Bowers, L., McFarlane, L., Kiyimba, F., Clark, N. and Alexander J. (2000) *Factors Underlying and Maintaining Nurses' Attitudes to Patients with Severe Personality Disorder — Final Report to National Forensic Mental Health R&D*. London: City University.

Brown, S. and Shapiro, F. (2006) 'EMDR in the treatment of borderline personality disorder'. *Clinical Case Studies*, 5(5): 403–20.

Comer, R. (2004) *Abnormal Psychology* (5th edn). New York: Worth Publishers.

Damasio, A. (1994) *Descartes' Error: Emotion, Reason and the Human Brain*. New York: Avon Books.

Erikson, E. (1968) *Identity: Youth and Crisis*. New York: WW Norton.

Government of Ireland (2001) *Mental Treatment Act 2001*. Dublin: Stationery Office.

Hansenne, M., Pitchot, W. and Ansseau, M. (2002) 'Serotonin, personality and borderline personality disorder'. *Acta Neuropsychiatrica*, 14(2), 66–70.

Hennessey, M. and McReynolds, C. (2001) 'Borderline personality disorder: psychosocial considerations and rehabilitation implications'. *Work: Journal of Prevention, Assessment and Rehabilitation*, 17, 97–104.

Hill, J. (2003) 'Childhood trauma and depression'. *Current Opinion in Psychiatry*, 16(1), 3–6.

Kendall, R. (2002) 'The distinction between personality disorder and mental illness'. *The British Journal of Psychiatry*, 180, 110–15.

Kirrane, R. and Siever, L. (2000) 'New perspectives on schizotypal personality disorder'. *Current Psychiatry Report*, 2, 62–6.

Kneisl, C. R., Wilson, H. S. and Trigoboff, E. (2004) *Contemporary Psychiatric-Mental Health Nursing*. New Jersey: Prentice Hall.

Mattia, J. and Zimmerman, M. (2001) 'Etiology and development', in J. Livesley (2001) *Handbook of Personality Disorders: Theory, Research and Treatment*. New York: Guildford Press.

McLean, L. and Gallop, R. (2003) 'Implications of childhood sexual abuse for adult borderline personality disorder and complex posttraumatic stress disorder'. *American Journal of Psychiatry*, 160, 369–71.

Mental Health Commission (MHC) (2005) *Annual Report*. Dublin: MHC.

Nehls, N. (2000) 'Recovering: a process of empowerment'. *Advances in Nursing Science*, 22, 62–70.

Paris, J. (2002) 'Implications of long-term outcome research of the management of patients with borderline personality disorder'. *Harvard Review of Psychiatry*, 10, 315–23.

Perry, J., Bannon, E. and Ianni, F. (1999) Effectiveness of psychotherapy for personality disorders. *American Journal of Psychiatry*, 156, 1312–21.

Serman, N., Johnson, J., Geller, P., Kanost, R. and Zacharapoulou, H. (2002) 'Personality disorders associated with substance use among American and Greek adolescents'. *Adolescence*, 37 (148), 841–54.

Soloff, P. H. (2000) 'Psychopharmacology of borderline personality disorder'. *Psychiatric Clinics of North America*, 23(1), 169–92.

Torgersen, S., Lygren, S., Oien, P. A., Skre, I., Onstad, S. and Edvardsen, J. (2000) 'A twin study of personality disorders'. *Comprehensive Psychiatry*, 41, 416–25.

White, C. N., Gunderson, J. G., Zanarini, M. C. and Hudson, J. I. (2003) 'Family studies of borderline personality disorder: a review'. *Harvard Review of Psychiatry*, 11, 8–19.

Wilkinson-Ryan, T. and Westen, D. (2000) 'Identity disturbance in borderline personality disorder: an empirical investigation'. *American Journal of Psychiatry*, 157, 528–41.

Zanarini, M. C., Yong, L., Frankenburg, F. R., Hennen, J., Reich, D. B. and Marino M. F. and Vujanovic, A. A. (2002) 'Severity of reported childhood sexual abuse and its relationship to severity of borderline psychopathology and psychosocial impairment among borderline inpatients'. *Journal of Nervous and Mental Disease*, 190(6), 381–7.

17

Childhood and Adolescent Mental Health Problems

Gordon Lynch

A quarter of our population are under 18 years old (DoHC 2006) and all adults have lived through childhood and adolescence. Yet, of the 8,000 nurses working in mental health the number of nurses working in child and adolescent mental health services (CAMHS) can be counted in tens. This chapter presents an overview of the most common and specific mental health problems that are encountered in CAMHS and the role of nurse therein.

DEVELOPMENT OF CHILD AND ADOLESCENT MENTAL HEALTH SERVICES

The first CAMHS clinic in Ireland was opened by the Lucena services (then called St John of God's) in 1955. Further services were developed in the 1970s by the Mater in Dublin and in the west by the health boards. It was during this period that the first nursing appointments were made. Over the years, restructuring has brought changes, but as of 2005, the Health Service Executive (HSE) is responsible for all CAMHS in the south of Ireland (the Lucena and Mater services are still providers on the HSE's behalf in parts of Dublin and surrounding areas).

The 2006 strategic policy document *A Vision for Change* (DoHC 2006) for all mental health services in the Irish Republic initiated the resourcing of CAMHS to provide services for those under the age of 18, as mandated by the 2001 Mental Health Act. It suggests that there should be a comprehensive network of CAMHS clinics throughout the country (one per 50,000 of the population) each with a multi-disciplinary team including two nursing posts.

NURSING IN CAMHS

Nurses in CAMHS undertake specialised training and work in various settings: clinics, the community, clients' homes, residential settings, in liaison posts in general hospitals, and in specialised areas such as addiction services. Crucially, they are part of multi-disciplinary teams in which they independently assess, plan, implement and review therapeutic programmes and work as equals with other disciplines. It is not unusual for nurses to be working simultaneously with an individual child, his/her parent/s, teacher/s, the school authorities and other professionals working with the child, such as speech and language therapists, among others.

YOUNG PEOPLE AND MENTAL HEALTH

One in five young people may have mental health difficulties (Mental Health Foundation 1999), ten per cent may have a diagnosable mental health disorder (Meltzer *et al.* 2000) and two per cent will, at some stage, have difficulties that may necessitate residential treatment. Difficulties may manifest in ways that are never recognised and many young people with mental health problems never have contact with any service. Many end up in other services such as the judicial, social welfare or special education services.

Mental health needs of young people are largely entrusted to parents or carers and the mainstream education system. Any child can have mental health issues, but those who have suffered through neglect or abuse (emotional, physical or sexual) are more likely to have difficulties. Nurses in CAMHS become involved when difficulties arise, though most services should also have preventative and educational functions led by nurses. Community care services (social work departments) are responsible for the safety and welfare of children. All professionals working with children are mandated by *Children First* (DoHC 1999) to take responsibility for reporting information concerning abuse or neglect of young people. *Children First* also provides for co-operation between social work departments and other professionals and agencies working with children at risk.

Many symptoms or manifestations of problems are also characteristics of an emotionally well child. It is the intensity, duration and combinations of particular characteristics that turn them into symptoms which can interfere with the young person's progress into mature adulthood. The prevalence of problems varies significantly. Disorders of perception (e.g. schizophrenia, schizo-affective disorder) are not frequently encountered among children and younger adolescents but feature more among 16- and 17-year-olds. Difficulties relating to anxiety, socialisation, communication, behaviour and concentration are more frequent in CAMHS.

Childhood problems can manifest themselves in adult life either in the same or in another guise. A childhood anxiety may become a lifelong burden. Concentration and attention difficulties can spawn angry, anti-socialised behaviour in the face of repeated failure and negative responses. Delinquency, depression, low self-esteem and other mental health difficulties may manifest in adulthood. Common sense and research tell us that early intervention is more likely to have a lasting benefit and may reap benefits in terms of prevention (Sanders and Markie-Dadds 1996).

OVERVIEW OF THE PRESENTATIONS TO CAMHS

Mental health difficulties do not always neatly comply with the diagnostic criteria of DSM-IV-TR (APA 2000) or ICD-10 (WHO 1992). Problems are complex manifestations of a number of causal factors and diagnostic categories are attempts to put order and accessibility into a diverse and unordered reality. See Figure 17.1 for an overview of presentations to CAMHS.

Figure 17.1 Overview of presentations to CAMHS

Type of Problem	Examples	Interventions
Mood	• Depression • Suicide • Self-harm/para-suicide	• Safety • CBT • IPT (Interpersonal therapy) • SSRIs • Combined therapies
Emotion	• Anxiety (generalised, separation ...) • Panic attacks • Phobias, fears ... • School refusal • Post-traumatic stress disorder • Acute stress reactions	• Behaviour therapy • CBT • Educational support • SSRIs, Clomipramine (not as first choice or sole treatment)
Behaviour	• Oppositional defiant disorders • Mixed disorders of emotion and behaviour	• Parent training • Behavioural therapy • Family therapy
Attention	• Attention Deficit Hyperactivity Disorder • Attention Deficit Disorder	• Stimulant medication • Parent training • Behavioural therapy • Combined therapies
Eating Disorders	• Anorexia Nervosa • Bulimia	• Family therapy • Behavioural therapies • CBT
Substance Misuse	• By young person • By parent/carer	• Family therapy • Multi systemic family therapy • Education/skills programmes (preventative) • Family therapy
Autistic Spectrum	• Autism • Asperger's Syndrome	• Intensive behavioural programmes • Strengths-based therapies

Type of Problem	Examples	Interventions
Psychotic Disorders	• Schizophrenia • Manic/bipolar disorders	• Neuroleptics • Clozapine (cautiously with resistant symptoms) • Lithium • Supportive and strengths-based therapies

DEPRESSION, SUICIDE AND SELF–HARMING BEHAVIOUR

It is now universally acknowledged that children as young as six suffer the same symptoms and distress (altered only in the context of their age and developmental profile) as adults (Puig-Antich 1986).

Depression

Features of depression are documented in Chapter 12. In addition, we should be alert to specific issues that may present in children and adolescents:

- Irritability — a common manifestation of depression in children and adolescents.
- Academic decline.
- Withdrawal from sport and hobbies.
- Alcohol and substance abuse and anti-social behaviour (Basu 2004).

Twin studies have demonstrated a substantial genetic risk loading (Akiskal and Weller 1989; Kolvin and Sodowski 2001). Depressed children are more likely to have parents with depression, and family dysfunction contributes to the risk.

Suicide

While suicide is not common before puberty (Barker 2004) it cannot be ruled out as a risk. In adolescence it is an increasing phenomenon, males being at greatest risk (Hawton and van Heering 2000).

Self-harming Behaviour

Sometimes described as *cries for help*, para-suicide and self-harm include minor overdoses, self-mutilation and threats of suicide. These are more frequent among adolescent girls than boys. These behaviours are indeed a signal of distress and although often lacking real suicidal intent they do carry a risk of death. Self-harming behaviour is often done secretly, yet is clearly a signal of some distress and carries substantial safety risks. Self-harming behaviours frequently develop an addictive quality and it is not uncommon to hear someone describing the relief they bring.

Causes are multiple and include:

- attachment difficulties

- genetic factors
- social and family and life events
- separation
- loss and bereavement.

Management/Treatment

Treatment of young people with depression must include immediate:

- provision for their safety
- CBT
- interpersonal therapy
- SSRI (or other medication) if no response to psychological therapies within six weeks
- combined therapies (psychological and pharmacological).

In severe cases a residential admission may be indicated. In many cases, education, advice and support of immediate carers is frequently an efficient way of addressing safety issues and may bring longer-term therapeutic value to the individual and their family by strengthening bonds and demonstrating care and empathy. A valuable nursing role includes providing this kind of support to families during times of crises. The existence and/or the extent of suicidal ideation must be monitored continuously throughout any intervention and risk factors must be minimised. Liaising with adult mental health services may help to address parents' own issues.

EMOTIONAL DISORDERS

Emotional disorder in childhood encompasses anxiety and mood disorder and refers to conditions where disordered emotion is a central feature (Kovacs and Devlin 1998). Emotional disorders in adulthood probably had their onset in childhood. Untreated emotional disorder re-occurs and carries increased risk of lifelong disability and suicide (Flisher 1999; Costello *et al.* 2002). Anxiety and depression are frequently linked (Kolvin and Sadowski 2001). Attention and behaviour difficulties associated with depression and other emotional problems are well documented (Fonesca and Perrin 2001; Brooks–Gunn *et al.* 2001; Verhulst 2001).

Anxiety

Anxiety is a normal part of a child's or adolescent's life. If anxiety levels are frequently and significantly out of keeping with the situation and inappropriate to the developmental age there may be a problem. When children suffer such severe and pervasive levels, the term 'anxiety disorder' can apply. It is the most common disorder of childhood (Coghill 2003). For illustrative purposes we should look at a few areas particularly relevant to children and adolescents.

Separation Anxiety

Closely associated with attachment, ICD-10 describes this anxiety disorder as an excessive anxiety concerning separation from those whom the child is attached to (WHO 1992). Examples include fear of going to sleep, especially alone, fear when a parent goes out, and fear of leaving a carer to attend school. It is often associated with sleep disturbance, appetite disturbance, nightmares and very marked somatic symptoms ranging from sweaty palms and palpitations to abdominal pain, vomiting and headache.

Phobias

Phobias cause extreme stress and fear, are not logically based and are out of proportion when faced with some situations or events (see Chapter 14). Children, especially younger children, may not always have much insight into the irrationality of their fears. Many children have fears of all kinds of things, such as dogs or thunder. With support and reassurance from their parent/carers, these fears usually pass. When they do not readily pass and their degree is clinically abnormal, they may meet the criteria for a diagnosis of phobic anxiety.

School Refusal

School refusal or phobia is characterised by an extreme reluctance to go to school. There is an element of separation anxiety and the resistance may be extreme and seem insurmountable to the family or carers. However, once in school the child usually settles. Underlying causes and dynamics tend to be complex and often feature:
- attachment issues
- family dynamics
- generalised anxiety.

The focus of treatment is twofold: early intervention to get the child into school; exploring and addressing the underlying issues.

It must be clear to the child that 'they will go to school' without negotiation. This may involve handing over a seemingly distressed child at the school gate. The child, parents and teachers may need support and guidance. As school attendance is re-established the child and the family's broader issues can be explored. However it must be noted that a child may have good reason for refusing to go to school — bullying by peers or teacher might well be a reason for reluctance to attend.

Panic Attacks

Panic attacks are more common among older children and adolescents and often associated with phobic states. They are usually unexpected and recurring and accompanied by physical symptoms. They are frightening and disabling, particularly when they first occur. A diagnosis of panic disorder can be helpful to the sufferer as it describes a condition that also happens to other people and can be addressed.

Post-traumatic Stress Disorder (PTSD)

PTSD does occur in children and adolescents. In children, the perception of events as dangerous can in itself be traumatising. Road traffic accidents, earthquakes, explosions and all kind of natural and man-made disasters are frequent precipitants of PTSD. So also are assaults, burglaries in the family home (even if the child was not present) and other deliberate human actions. A very profound PTSD can emerge in responses to chronic or repeated trauma including abuse and bullying. For children, sexually traumatic events may include developmentally inappropriate sexual experience without threatened or actual violence or injury (APA 2000).

Features of PTSD include:
- re-experiencing the traumatic event
- avoidance of associated stimuli (APA 2000)
- disturbed sleep pattern, nightmares, bed-wetting and soiling occur more frequently in children and adolescents.
- hypervigilance and an exaggerated startle response
- irritability, anger, lability
- concentration difficulty
- PTSD in children is often associated with depression, panic attacks, phobias, generalised anxiety.
- alcohol and substance abuse is common in adolescence.

Management/Treatment of PTSD

PTSD cannot be treated while the trauma continues to be perpetrated. Therefore the source of the trauma must be addressed and this usually involves liaison with other agencies/colleagues. Short-term emotional support to the child/adolescent and the parent(s)/carer(s) is a necessary part of the treatment; this can include practical support. In the longer term the use of therapies that allow the individual to work through the precipitating trauma and contextualise it are effective. Trauma-focused cognitive behavioural therapy (CBT) is widely and effectively used.
- Eye movement de-sensitisation and reprocessing (EMDR) is a specialised therapy with evidential support.
- Debriefing following trauma is not an effective treatment.
- Drug treatments should not be routinely prescribed.

CONDUCT DISORDER

The APA (2000) describes conduct disorder as a persistent and repetitive pattern of behaviour involving aggressive and non-aggressive behaviour, deceitfulness and serious rule violation. ICD-10 stresses repetitive, persistent patterns of anti-social, aggressive or defiant behaviour (WHO 1992). People with conduct disorders tend to under-achieve academically, often failing to complete school or achieve literacy. Difficulties with authority result and non-compliance leads to exclusion from school and training programmes and, in later life, periods of unemployment. Contact with forensic services is frequent.

Causes include:

- social factors
- family issues
- educational difficulties
- emotional neglect, emotional and physical abuse
- attachment issues
- trauma and loss.

Parenting has profound effects and adults who have not negotiated their own journey into mature adulthood are less likely to instil in their own children the qualities required to develop as responsible adults. Part of maturity is recognising appropriate behaviour and responding appropriately. Parents who see their child as a threat to themselves tend to respond in a negative and punitive manner. This adversely affects behavioural development but so also does an absence of structure, authority or control. Families under stress, without money and without social supports are at greatest risk. Co-morbidity with other difficulties such as ADHD and educational difficulties is common. Thirty-three per cent of people diagnosed with conduct disorder have been shown to have dyslexia or a specific reading disorder (Rutter *et al.* 1976).

Management/Treatment

Parent training is effective and two-thirds of children under ten will benefit (Wolpert *et al.* 2002). Less complex presentations have better outcomes. However, the following adverse factors can influence the effectiveness of parent training:

- age
- co-morbidity
- severity of conduct problems
- parental conflict
- exposure to violence
- socio-economic disadvantage.

Rules or limits should be clear, reasonable and easy to understand. Limits are the foundations to freedom. Imagine a garden where a child plays and which has no wall, fence or visible boundary. The child cannot know how far to go in safety. A clear boundary allows the child freedom and safety within the defined limits. Rules and limits on general behaviour are the same.

Parent training alone is less effective with older children. Socialised conduct disorder in adolescence is more likely to respond to multi-modal therapies. These may include behavioural management and effective diversionary or skills-based responses. The most effective interventions are intensive and require close co-ordination between many agencies. Multi-systemic therapy is delivered in an integrated and co-ordinated manner involving contact with all aspects of the individual's life. It is the most effective treatment for delinquent adolescents in reducing recidivism and improving individual and family functioning (Wolpert *et al.* 2002).

Psychological interventions are better than physical ones. Incarceration is a counter-effective treatment for anti-social behaviour. However, containment of the behaviours is an essential element in treating conduct disorder. The message that behaviour can be contained is in itself therapeutic and reassuring. In extreme cases it is necessary to provide the physical containment in which a therapeutic programme can unfold. Physical containment needs to be carried out in a nurturing and well-structured manner where the milieu itself (the day-to-day living and routine) is therapeutic. Individual programmes are integrated into the milieu. Parents may bring their child's challenging behaviour to health professionals to be 'fixed'. The holistic approach of professional nursing ensures that the response to a referral is broad and inclusive of all the aspects of the child's life — especially the family.

ADD/ADHD

Attention deficit disorder/attention deficit hyperactivity disorder is perhaps the most popularly known (and a somewhat controversial) disorder of childhood and adolescence. It is characterised by:
- a marked difficulty maintaining attention
- impulsivity
- high activity levels.

ADD/ADHD referrals feature predominantly in the work of a CAMHS clinic. Whether it is viewed as a disorder that someone has or as a spectrum of characteristics, criteria for diagnosis are laid down in WHO (1992) and APA (2000). The DSM-IV-TR invokes a broader range of diagnostic criteria, which lend themselves to more frequent diagnosis. Most clinicians follow the lead of Eric Taylor (Taylor *et al.* 1994) and take both sets of criteria into account:
- The symptoms are pervasive and are definitely identified in at least two different settings. (Home and school are most frequently used but clinic-based observation groups and other settings are also fine.)
- The symptoms were present before the child's seventh birthday.
- The symptoms must be present for at least six months and are not accountable by the child's developmental stage e.g. a three-year-old will normally have less ability to maintain attention than an eleven-year-old.
- The symptoms significantly affect the child's functioning, e.g. education, socialisation.

There are many possible contributory factors.
- genetics
- environment
- cognitive development.

Twin studies have shown a genetic susceptibility (Schacher and Tannock 2002) and Eric Taylor suggests a dramatically increased risk with first-degree relations of a child with a diagnosis of ADHD. Learned behaviour patterns also have a role. There is also a cultural construct around ADHD. In Nigeria, for example, the concept of ADHD is hardly recognised as society, families and the education system accommodate themselves to a broader range of children's behaviours (Akpen 2005).

Management/Treatment
- Parent training and behaviour management programmes.
- School-based psycho-educational and behavioural programmes.
- Pharmacological interventions (usually stimulant medication).

Education is a typical part of a nursing role within CAMHS. Guidance towards an understanding of the difficulties being experienced facilitates progress. Parenting programmes are usually delivered by nurses and another team member. Different models share basic guiding principles, including:
- structure and predictability
- focus on positives
- re-enforcement
- avoiding draconian punishments
- ignoring minor behaviours.

CAMHS nurses and educational psychological services work together to devise programmes within schools to assist and support teachers who are containing hyperactive behaviours. There is evidence to suggest that diet modification and fish oils have some benefits, but research is inconclusive and the long-term effects of high doses of fish oils have not been addressed.

EATING DISORDERS

Anorexia Nervosa
Anorexia means loss of appetite. Anorexia nervosa is a serious illness with the highest mortality rate (ten per cent) of any psychiatric condition (Lewer 2006). A psychological disorder with physical symptoms, it is characterised by a relentless pursuit of weight loss involving:
- food avoidance
- induced vomiting/purging
- excessive exercising
- distorted body image.

Without intervention, starvation may occur, along with all the physical complications that this journey involves. There may be co-morbid psychological symptoms including depression and obsessive compulsive symptoms. It affects people of all backgrounds and ages, including pre-pubertal children. While more common among girls in early adolescence, it is also seen in boys. Attitudes to eating are influenced by family, culture, religion, friends, advertising, fashion, and more. Causation is complex and unique to each individual but frequently includes:

- family dynamics
- social influences.

Management/Treatment

Monitoring and maintaining physical health, including maintenance of a basic weight, are paramount. High levels of individual support and the cultivation of trust and an alliance are required. This is normally the remit of nursing staff and it demands high levels of skill and professionalism. In-patient or outpatient therapies involving the entire family have been most effective. The importance of developing a therapeutic alliance with a principal figure cannot be overstated. Long-term therapeutic programmes are the norm.

Bulimia Nervosa

Characterised by chaotic patterns of food avoidance, over-indulgence, induced vomiting and purging, bulimia is rarely pre-pubertal and is most common in older girls and young women (Lask and Bryant-Waugh 2000). There are overlaps with anorexia nervosa, but while weight gain may be avoided, there is rarely the same degree of weight loss, and symptoms are frequently concealed. In-patient treatment is not common. CBT and family therapy are indicated.

SUBSTANCE MISUSE

Substance misuse is addressed in Chapter 19 but needs to be looked at briefly in the context of CAMHS nursing. Substance misuse does impact on the development of many children and adolescents. Frequently the damaging effects are caused by the substance misuse of the adults who care for them, including excessive use of alcohol and prescribed and illicit drugs. Adolescents are frequent users of the same drugs and alcohol the adults in their lives use.

- Five times as many children are affected by parental alcohol problems as by parental drug abuse.
- Alcohol misuse has been identified as a factor in over 50 per cent of all child protection cases (Turning Point 2006).
- Alcohol and substance misuse impacts on every aspect of the lives of children and adolescents.
- Women who drink over 56 units of alcohol weekly have up to a thirty per cent chance of giving birth to a child with foetal alcohol syndrome (AHRSE 2003).
- Children of parents who abuse alcohol are more likely to experience violence, physical, sexual and emotional abuse, material deprivation and parental separation.

Young people's own substance misuse can also have harmful consequences. Generally young people referred to mental health services with alcohol or drug misuse problems are referred to specialised services such as the Community Addiction Services. Many such services are co-ordinated by nurses taking on front-line treatment and educational roles. CAMHS nurses need to be ever-vigilant for the possibility of substance misuse contributing to an overall presentation. Changes in personality, stealing, telling lies, academic decline, changed social patterns (often a move to friends who parents consider less desirable) can all be signs of substance misuse.

ASD (AUTISTIC SPECTRUM DISORDERS)

Autism itself falls within the remit of the disability services; however, assessment and diagnosis of autistic spectrum disorders (also known as pervasive developmental disorders) fall within the remit of CAMHS, along with the ongoing support and therapy for children and families who meet the criteria for an autistic spectrum disorder without having a diagnosis of autism. An autistic spectrum disorder is a complex developmental disability that affects the way the person communicates and relates to people around them (National Autistic Society 2007). It is generally characterised by:
- socialisation impairment
- communication difficulties
- specialised and overriding interests, to such a degree that they interfere with the individual's overall functioning
- ritualistic and compulsive behaviours.

The impairment in socialisation is often present from early infancy. Some parents observe, and others may identify in hindsight, the aloofness of the infant who avoids eye contact, does not raise their arms to be lifted and rejects physical and verbal overtures. Although many make great progress in their social development (with support, guidance and training for the individual and their parents/carers) there is generally a lifelong difference between people with ASD and the rest of the population in terms of social reciprocity and emotional empathy. Communication difficulties range from profound (a complete absence of speech) to mild (only a slight language deficit). There may always be a deficit in identifying nuances and subtleties of everyday conversation (literal interpretation).

Specialised interests may be overwhelming to parents/carers or they may be seen as eccentric. Frequently specific interests are extreme versions of normal behaviours. Boys frequently have extended phases of particular interest in dinosaurs, for example, but a boy with an ASD may pursue this interest at all times, to the detriment of his ability to function normally. Individuals may develop a remarkable knowledge of a subject, giving the false impression of great ability. People on the autistic spectrum have the same IQ range as the general population.

Asperger's syndrome can be described as a milder version of autism, in which speech delay or regression is not a feature. It is characterised by specific groups of symptoms which vary significantly from person to person and can be disabling.

Some people with Asperger's may become hugely successful in a specialised field even though they never develop the social skills to negotiate everyday tasks like exchanging niceties about the weather.

Causes are unknown, but genetic factors may play a part. Some evidence suggests that a minority of cases may be associated with conditions affecting neurological development such as maternal rubella, tuberculosis and encephalitis (National Autistic Society 2007). There is no established link with any vaccines.

Assessment

Assessment should be comprehensive and may involve nursing, psychological, psychiatric and speech and language input, including observation in school, the family home and clinic settings. Children with a severe autistic disability are usually spotted at early developmental check-ups by health professionals (public health nurses) if parents or carers have not already become aware themselves. Normal development is often reported until sometime during the second year of life. Milder variations may slip through until school. Children with Asperger's syndrome sometimes get to secondary school before problems are correctly identified. At the extreme end of the spectrum is classic autism, which is usually associated with very significant disability — limiting prospects of independent living.

Management/Treatment

Appropriate intervention early in life can, in many cases, maximise skills and abilities and allow people to achieve their full potential in life. Specialised education, structured support, parent/carer support and training and educational work with siblings and other extended family members all have a role with a focus on working to the strengths of the individual. Social skills training, while not shown to be effective with classic autism, has been shown to be of benefit to people with Asperger's syndrome.

NURSING ROLES AND INTERVENTIONS

Nurses are ideally placed in CAMHS teams to work at all levels, from primary care givers with roles in education, prevention, early intervention and liaison, to providing specialised therapies and clinical management. CAMHS nurses differ from colleagues in other fields by virtue of the extent of their involvement in:

- multi-disciplinary work
- family work
- liaison with education services
- co-working with other agencies
- play therapy
- advocacy
- strengths-based therapies.

Play is as important a part of nursing with younger children as is therapeutic conversation with people who have acquired verbal skills. Even at its most informal, a child's play is a window to their life experience, understanding and unconscious mechanisms. The vast majority of parents/carers, regardless of how cases first present, are deeply committed people who want the best outcome for their families. They frequently have skills, strengths and resources within themselves and around them that they have lost sight of or not yet been able to utilise. One of the most effective roles in CAMHS nursing is enabling children, adolescents and their families to identify and build on their solution-building strengths rather than seeing themselves as having problems that they depend on outside agencies to fix.

CONCLUSION

This chapter has presented an overview of the most common and specific mental health problems encountered in CAMHS. Children are not treated in isolation and their biological and/or caring family is nearly always part of a therapeutic input. This may range from support, education, psychotherapeutic interventions and collaboration with nurses and other members of the multidisciplinary team.

Reflective Questions
1. Why would nurses in CAMHS need to have a close working relationship with social workers in child protection?
2. Think of areas where the overlap between emotional and physical difficulties might be greater than those encountered by nursing colleagues in adult mental health services.
3. In what way might CAMHS and adult mental health nursing services jointly improve the service experienced by children and families?
4. Do you think that a search for a clear diagnosis is always the most helpful intervention with children and adolescents who present at CAMHS?

References
Akiskal, H. S. and Weller, E. B. (1989) 'Mood disorders and suicide in children and adolescents', in H. I. Kaplan and B. J. Sadock (eds), *Comprehensive Textbook of Psychiatry* (5th edn). Baltimore: Williams and Wilkins.

Akpen, U. (2005) 'Thoughts on Cultural Differences in Psychiatric Care — A Nigerian Perspective', paper delivered to Diversity in Child and Mental Health conference, Association for Child and Adolescent Mental Health (ACAMH IRL), St Patrick's Hospital, Dublin, 25 November 2005.

Alcohol Harm Reduction Strategy for England (AHRSE) (Prime Minister's Strategy Unit) (2003) *Interim Analytical Report*. UK: Cabinet Office.

American Psychiatric Association (APA) (2000) *Diagnostic and Statistical Manual of Mental Disorders* (DSM-IV-TR) (4th edn: text revision). Washington DC: APA.

Barker, P. (2004) *Basic Child Psychiatry* (7th edn). Oxford: Blackwell.

Basu, R. (2004) 'Mental health problems in childhood and adolescence', in I. Norman and I. Ryrie (eds), *The Art and Science of Mental Nursing*. Open University Press: Maidenhead.

Brooks-Gunn, J., Auth, J., Peterson, A. and Compass, B. (2001) 'Psychological processes and development of childhood and adolescent depression', in: I. Goodyear (ed.), *The Depressed Child and Adolescent* (2nd edn). London: Cambridge University Press.

Coghill, D. (2003) 'Current issues in child and adolescent psychopharmacology', *Advances in Psychiatric Treatment*, (9), 289–99.

Costello, E., Pine, D., Hammon, C., Morah, J. and Platsby, P. (2002) 'Development and natural history of mood disorders'. *Society of Biological Psychiatry*, (52) 529–42.

Department of Health and Children (DoHC) (1999) *Children First — National Guidelines for the Protection and Welfare of Children*. Dublin: Stationery Office.

Department of Health and Children (DoHC) (2006) *A Vision for Change: Report of the Expert Group on Mental Health Policy*. Dublin: Government Publication Office.

Flisher, A. (1999) 'Annotation: mood disorder in suicidal children and adolescents; recent developments'. *Journal of Child Psychology and Psychiatry*, 40 (3) 315–24.

Fonesca, A. C. and Perrin, S. (2001) 'Clinical phenomenology, classification and assessment of anxiety disorders in children and adolescents', in W. K. Silverman and P. D. A. Treffers (eds) *Anxiety Disorders in Children and Adolescents: Research, Assessment and Intervention*. London: Cambridge University Press.

Government of Ireland (2001) *Mental Health Act 2001*. Dublin: Stationery Office.

Hawton, K. and van Heering, K. (2000) *Suicide and Attempted Suicide*. Chichester, UK: Wiley.

Kolvin, I. and Sodowski, H. (2001) 'Childhood depression: clinical phenomenology and classification', in I. Goodyear (ed.), *The Depressed Child and Adolescent* (2nd edn). London: Cambridge University Press.

Kovacs, M. and Devlin, B. (1998) 'Internalising disorders in childhood'. *Journal of Child Psychology and Psychiatry*, 39(1), 47–63.

Lask, B. and Bryant-Waugh, R. (2000) *Anorexia Nervosa and Related Eating Disorders in Childhood and Adolescence* (2nd edn). Brighton: Psychology Press.

Lewer, E. (2006) 'Nursing children and young people with eating disorders', in T. McDouggall (ed.) *Child and Adolescent Mental Health Nursing*. Oxford: Blackwell.

Meltzer, H., Gatward, R., Goodman, R. and Ford, T. (2000) *The Mental Health of Children and Adolescents in Great Britain*. London: Stationery Office.

Mental Health Foundation (UK) (1999) *Bright Futures*. London: Mental Health Foundation.

National Autistic Society (2007) *What is Autism?*, www.nas.org.uk/.

Puig-Antich, J. (1986) 'Psychological markers: effects of age and puberty', in M. Rutter, C. A. and P. B. Izard (eds) *Depression in Young People: Developmental and Clinical Perspectives*. New York: Guilford.

Rutter, M., Graham, P., Chadwick, O. F. (1976) 'Adolescent turmoil: fact or fiction?' *Journal of Child Psychology and Psychiatry*, 17: 35–76.

Sanders, M. and Markie-Dadds, C. L. (1996) 'Triple P: a multi level family intervention programme for children with disruptive behaviour disorders', in P. Cotton and H. Jackson (eds) *Early Intervention and Prevention in Mental Health*. Melbourne: Australian Psychological Society.

Schacher, R. and Tannock, R. (2002) 'Syndromes of hyperactivity and attention deficit', in M. Rutter and E. Taylor (eds) *Child and Adolescent Psychiatry* (4th edn). Oxford: Blackwell.

Turning Point (2006) *Bottling it up: The Effects of Alcohol Misuse on Children, Parents and Families*. London: Turning Point.

Taylor, E., Doepner, M., Seargent, J., Asherson, P., Banaschewski, T., Buitelaar, J. and Coghill, D. (1994) 'European guidelines for hyperkinetic disorder – first upgrade'. *Journal of European Child and Adolescent Psychiatry*, (13) 1–130.

Verhulst, F. C. (2001) 'Community and epidemiological aspects of anxiety disorders in children' in: W. K. Silverman and P. D. A. Treffers (eds) *Anxiety Disorders in Children and Adolescents, Research, Assessment and Intervention*. London: Cambridge University Press.

Wolpert, M., Fuggle, P., Cottrell, D., Fonagy, P., Phillips, J., Pilling, S., Stein, S. and Target, M. (2002) *Drawing on the Evidence — Advice for Mental Health Professionals working with Children and Adolescents*. Division of Clinical Psychology (Faculty for Children and Young People), Leicester: British Psychological Society.

World Health Organisation (WHO) (1992) *The ICD-10 Classification of Mental and Behavioural Disorders. Clinical Descriptions and Diagnostic Guidelines*. Geneva: WHO.

18
Care of the Older Person with Dementia

Brian Keogh

Caring for the older person with dementia is a complex process and requires a diverse portfolio of interpersonal and clinical skills. In Ireland there are currently 38,000 people living with dementia, which is expected to increase to 70,115 people in 2026 (Alzheimer Society of Ireland 2006). According to O'Shea (2007) this will make dementia a national health priority. The increasing number of older people living in Ireland means that more and more psychiatric nurses will be employed to care for this population, arguably — given the multifaceted skills required to care for this group — making it an area where they can excel. Although mainly associated with older people, dementia can affect people at any age. This chapter discusses dementia and the older person and its implications for psychiatric nursing practice. The different types of dementia are outlined as well as the pharmacological treatments available. Nursing interventions are discussed, placing an emphasis on communication skills and other non-pharmacological approaches.

DEMENTIA AND THE OLDER PERSON

Dementia is an umbrella term that describes a range of conditions that involve memory impairment and other deficits in cognitive functioning. The ICD-10 (WHO 1992) defines dementia as a syndrome, which is caused by a progressive disease of the brain, characterised by disturbance of higher-order functions such as memory, thinking, orientation, understanding, speech, language and judgement. These cognitive functions are frequently accompanied by other behaviours such as decline in emotional control, socially accepted behaviours or volition (WHO 1992). According to the DSM-IV-TR (APA 2000) there are twelve different types of dementia which are classified by their underlying cause(s):

- dementia of the Alzheimer's type
- dementia with Lewy bodies
- vascular dementia
- frontotemporal dementia
- dementia due to Parkinson's disease
- dementia due to Huntington's disease
- dementia due to Creutzfeldt–Jakob Disease

- substance-induced persisting dementia
- dementia due to other general medical conditions
- dementia due to human immunodeficiency virus
- dementia due to multiple aetiologies
- dementia not otherwise specified.

According to Bolla et al. (2000) four main types of dementia account for ninety per cent of presented cases of dementia:
- Alzheimer's disease
- dementia with Lewy bodies (DLB)
- vascular dementia
- frontotemporal dementia.

These types of dementia will be discussed in greater detail in this chapter.

CAUSES OF DEMENTIA

According to the Dementia Services Information and Development Centre (DSIDC 2003), research into establishing an exact cause of dementia is slow. However, they do identify that age is a major risk factor. While the incidence of dementia increases as we age, making older people more vulnerable to the condition, this does not mean that all older people will develop dementia. Other causes are linked to the type of dementia that the person presents with, making Alzheimer's disease, the presence of Lewy bodies, damage to the vascular system and changes in the frontotemporal brain structure all overall causes of dementia.

Other disorders that damage the central nervous system (e.g. Parkinson's disease and Huntington's disease) may also make people with these conditions more vulnerable to dementia. Prolonged substance abuse and some general medical conditions such as HIV infection or head injury may also increase the risk. Finally, genetics may also have a role to play in the development of dementia with chromosome defects associated with the development of Alzheimer's disease (Alzheimer's Disease Society 2003).

ALZHEIMER'S DISEASE

Alzheimer's Disease (AD) is by far the most common form of dementia, accounting for approximately sixty per cent of all dementias (NICE 2004). The DSM-IV-TR criteria for AD are listed below:
- Multiple cognitive deficits.
- Includes memory impairment and one or more of the following deficits in cognitive functioning:
  1. Aphasia (inability to talk or to understand speech).
  2. Apraxia (disorder of voluntary movement).
  3. Agnosia (inability to recognise objects despite intact sensory function).
  4. Disturbance in executive functioning (e.g. inability to make plans, impairment in judgement).

- Gradual onset and continual decline.
- Cognitive impairments cannot be better explained by delirium, other conditions or other mental disorders.
- The deficit in cognitive functioning causes impairment in social and occupational functioning and is a marked decline in the person's previous level of functioning.

Causes of AD

Munoz and Feldman (2000) suggest that the exact causes of AD are unknown: however, several theories have been put forward:

- Structural abnormalities: Alzheimer's disease is characterised by the increased number and density of neurofibrillary tangles and senile plaques. These microscopic alterations in brain tissue are found as part of normal ageing but to a greater extent in patients with AD.
- Chronic inflammatory disease: there is some evidence to suggest that the brains of people with AD have a mild active inflammation.
- Head trauma: damage to the brain may be linked to the development of AD.
- Genetic factors: there appears to be a familial pattern with AD, which would suggest that genetics may play a role in the development of the disease. Researchers are also investigating the link between AD and a gene found on chromosome 21.
- Ageing: ageing is an important risk factor for the development of AD, with the incidence increasing with age.

(Adapted from Munoz and Feldman 2000)

Clinical Features and Clinical Progression of AD

Clinical presentation and progression of AD varies from individual to individual, with independent variables such as the age and general physical health of the person influencing the progression of the disease. Initially memory loss, especially for recent events, is the first clinical feature noticed. This can be distressing for the person as they are often aware of their lapses in memory.

At this stage attempts are made to disguise memory loss through confabulation. This occurs when false or 'made up' memories replace forgotten events. Confusion and disorientation also occur and this may initially worsen during stressful times or when the person is away from familiar surroundings.

Personality changes may also be evident at this time, with the person becoming irritable and aggressive, a trait that often precedes admission to hospital. The person's speech is generally affected (aphasia) and the person forgets the names of familiar objects (agnosia) and people. The person with AD will often refer to objects as 'it' or to people as 'them' and may find it difficult to express themselves articulately, even during simple conversations. Socially accepted behaviours may also be forgotten and the person with AD may become dis-inhibited or sexually inappropriate.

As the disease progresses confusion and disorientation worsen, impacting on the person's ability to carry out a wide range of activities of daily living. Judgement and logic are lost and the person with AD becomes dependent on carers for most self-care needs and requires constant supervision. The person's memory also deteriorates, impacting on their ability to recall recent and distant events. Names of adult children or their husband/wife etc. may be forgotten, resulting in upset for family members. Behaviours such as wandering, aggression and problematic vocalisations such as shouting may also be present. These can be a result of confusion, stresses in the person's environment or unmet physical, psychological or social needs such as hunger, anxiety or boredom.

Occasionally delusions, hallucinations, illusions and depression are also present. The progressive nature of the disease is evident as the person with AD demonstrates reduced cognitive ability, eventually becoming unresponsive and totally dependent on others for their physical, psychological, social and spiritual needs.

VASCULAR DEMENTIA

Vascular dementia differs from AD in that the progressive deterioration of the disease occurs in a step-like fashion unlike the downward linear progression of AD. The cause of this type of dementia is major cerebrovascular disease. This results in the person experiencing 'mini-strokes' which impact on their cognitive abilities in a variable and distressing manner. The person with vascular dementia experiences periods of confusion interspersed with periods of lucidity, making the progression of the disorder highly unpredictable and causing great stress to the individual and their family. As the disease progresses, periods of lucidity become less frequent and the confused periods may become more pronounced. Vascular dementia occurs more often in men (Nazarko 2006) and life expectancy can be shorter than with other forms of dementia. The causes are linked to arteriosclerosis, cerebral emboli, cerebral haemorrhage (Desira and Martin 2004) and hypertension (Nazarko 2006).

DEMENTIA WITH LEWY BODIES (DLB)

Lewy bodies are tiny deposits of protein that develop in the brain and which are thought to interfere with important neurotransmitters required for healthy brain function. They are also found in patients with Parkinson's disease. According to Nazarko (2006) this form of dementia is very difficult to diagnose as its clinical features can be confused with AD or Parkinson's disease. This form of dementia is characterised by fluctuating cognitive impairment peppered with periods of increased confusion (McKeith and Fairbairn 2001), Parkinsonian features, falls and psychotic symptoms such as hallucinations and delusions (Martin 2006). Extreme care needs to be taken when treating these symptoms as patients with DLB exhibit a heightened sensitivity to neuroleptic drugs (Walling 2004).

FRONTOTEMPORAL DEMENTIA

Previously known as Pick's disease, this type of dementia, according to Martin (2006) is less commonly diagnosed than AD, vascular dementia or LBD. It occurs when there is damage to the frontal and temporal areas of the brain and is more common in middle age (Goward 2000). Personality changes, behavioural problems, social disinhibition and aphasia are initial features with memory loss and other characteristic features of dementia occurring as the disease progresses (Townsend 1999).

DIAGNOSING DEMENTIA

There is no one definitive test for dementia and a diagnosis of dementia is made following extensive clinical examination, which aims to rule out other physical or mental disorders that may account for the patient's symptoms. Psychiatric disorders such as depression or neurological disorders such as epilepsy may account for the patient's memory loss and confusion, while a chest infection, undiagnosed diabetes or vitamin deficiencies may also mimic the symptoms of dementia (Ouldred 2004).

In older people the symptoms of depression can often be confused with dementia, making accurate assessment and intervention a key priority. Nurses caring for older people must be aware that people with dementia are more prone to depression and targeting the depressive symptoms may improve the quality of life for the older adult with dementia. Diagnostic technology such as computed axial tomography (CAT), magnetic resonance imaging (MRI) and positron emission tomography (PET) may also assist the clinician in making a diagnosis.

PHARMACOLOGICAL INTERVENTIONS

Currently, there are no drugs available that can reverse or stop the basic physiological processes that contribute to the development of dementia. Many of the medications are used for managing the behavioural symptoms of dementia such as agitation and aggression. Currently the most successful treatment of dementia has been achieved through the use of drugs that inhibit acetylchoinesterase (Nordberg and Svensson 1998), a neurotransmitter associated with memory and cognition. Drugs such as Donepezil, Rivastigmine and Galantamine are licensed to treat mild to moderate AD. These drugs are thought to enhance cognitive functioning in patients who are in the earlier stages of the disease, consequently slowing down its progression; however, the overall course of the disease remains unaffected. Memantine is indicated in moderate to severe AD and affects the transmission of glutamate, another neurotransmitter involved in memory and learning. A summary of the drugs used in the treatment of dementia appears in Figure 18.1. For further information on side effects, cautions, interactions and doses please consult the *British National Formulary*.

Figure 18.1 Summary of pharmacological treatments of dementia

Drug	Cautions	Side effects
Donepezil hydrochloride (Aricept)	Patients at risk of developing peptic ulcers Asthma Chronic obstructive pulmonary disease	Sick sinus syndrome Nausea Vomiting Diarrhoea Fatigue Insomnia Muscle cramps Headache Dizziness Bradycardia
Rivastigmine (Exelon)	Renal impairment Mild to moderate hepatic impairment Gastric or duodenal ulcers Monitor body weight	Asthenia Anorexia Weight loss Nausea Vomiting Drowsiness Abdominal pain Confusion
Memantine hydrochloride (Ebixa)	History of convulsions Renal impairment	Constipation Headache Dizziness Vomiting Confusion Fatigue
Galantamine (Reminyl)	Cardiac disease Electrolyte disturbance Patients at risk of developing peptic ulcers Chronic obstructive pulmonary disease	Nausea Vomiting Diarrhoea Abdominal pain Dyspepsia Syncope Dizziness Confusion

Response to these drugs is measured by improved cognition and global scores (Nordberg and Svensson 1998), and these tests are administered two to four months after establishing the therapeutic dose (BNF 2007). Approximately half of people taking these drugs will show an improvement (BNF 2007). The drugs should be discontinued in those thought not to be responding. Specialists may repeat the cognitive assessment four to six weeks after the drug has been stopped and if significant deterioration occurs during this short period, consideration should be given to restarting therapy. Patients with dementia generally exhibit a broad range of behaviours that can be treated symptomatically. However, careful consideration has to be given to any decision to give psychotropic drugs to older people and they should be avoided if at all possible. Drugs such as Resperidone and Olanzapine should be avoided in older people with dementia, as they are associated with an increased risk of stroke in this population (BNF 2007).

Doses of medications for the elderly are generally one-half to two-thirds lower than usually prescribed. Older people have a decreased ability to absorb and metabolise drugs, which make them vulnerable to side effects and toxicity, often worsening the symptoms that the drug was prescribed for in the first place. Consequently, in the management and care of people with dementia it should be noted that 'the best treatment option might be non drug therapies' (Beattie 2003:119).

PRINCIPLES OF CARE FOR THE OLDER PERSON WITH DEMENTIA

Policy documents such as *An Action Plan for Dementia* (National Council for Ageing and Older People 1999) have strived to implement a comprehensive care package aimed at ensuring that people with dementia are cared for in the community with supports from the person's general practitioner, the public health nursing services, social services and other supports such as from the voluntary sector. The majority of people with dementia are cared for at home by relatives; however, some require hospital admission and may need to be cared for in long-term facilities.

As dementia is a progressive disorder, nursing care is aimed at maintaining the person's independence while focusing on their strengths and supporting them during difficulties (Kitwood 1997). Nursing care is underpinned by effective communication skills, while ensuring individualised and person-centred care. Following a comprehensive nursing assessment, interventions need to be designed that are cognisant not only of the person's basic physical needs, but of their need for social interaction, appropriate intellectual and physical stimulation and psychological support.

This section divides nursing interventions into three subsections: strategies for improving communication with older people with dementia; interventions targeted at confusion, disorientation and behaviours that challenge; and interventions aimed at specific activities of daily living.

Assessment
Assessment of the individual with dementia is essential to developing a plan of care that reflects the needs and wants of the person in terms of their biological, psychological, social and spiritual perspectives. Several factors will have to be considered prior to conducting the assessment and it should be noted that the assessment is not a unique event, but something that will occur in response to the progression of the illness and other factors such as the physical health of the

person. The location of the assessment should be given due consideration and assessing the person at home will allow the nurse to examine the person in their own environment as well being more convenient for the person. Assessment on admission to hospital may be traumatic for the person with dementia with a concomitant reduction in the person's functioning and an increase in levels of confusion and agitation. Admission to hospital is often a consequence of a family crisis where the primary carer(s), for a multitude of reasons, feel that they can no longer care for the individual. Family members must be included in the assessment and the process must be carried out with tact and sensitivity utilising the nurse's interpersonal and observational skills. Attempts must be made by the nursing staff undertaking the assessment to put the person at ease while eliciting the required information.

Assessment of the older person with dementia is complex and requires the comprehensive collection of information about all aspects of the person's life. The Royal College of Nursing describe an assessment based on essential care components. Within each category the nurse assesses the older person based on their ability or disability and their need for nursing care (RCN 2004). The essential care components are presented in figure 18.2.

Figure 18.2 Essential care components (RCN 2004)

Component 1	Component 2	Component 3
Maximising Life Potential	Prevention and Relief of Stress	Promotion and Maintenance of Health
Personal fulfilment	Communication	Personal hygiene
Spiritual fulfilment	Pain control	Dressing
Social relations	The senses	Motivation
Sexuality	Memory	Sleeping
Cognition	Orientation	Mobility
	Loss, change and adaptation	Elimination
	Behaviour	Risk
	Relatives and carers	Eating and drinking
		Breathing
		Emotion

Rating scales are also used in the assessment of older people with mental health problems. These scales are used to complement the formal physical and mental assessment and are not meant to be diagnostic. Examples of some of the main scales used are shown in Figure 18.3.

Figure 18.3 Examples of rating scales used in clinical practice

Rating Scale	Purpose
Alzheimer's disease assessment scale/cognitive subscale (ADAS-cog) (Rosen et al. 1984)	A 70-item rating scale that measures for cognitive and non-cognitive symptoms of AD. A lower score indicates better function.
Mini mental state examination (MMSE) (Folstein et al. 1975).	A comprehensive assessment divided into 5 sections that measure orientation, memory (2 sections), attention, calculation and language, writing and drawing. A score of less than 26 may indicate cognitive impairment.
The geriatric depression scale (GDS) (Yesavage et al. 1983).	15-item tool for measuring depression in the older person, which can be administered quickly and has been used extensively in mental health care.
Clifton Assessment Procedures for the elderly (CAPE) (Pattie and Gilleard 1979)	Comprehensive assessment that aims to assess the person's functional capabilities in terms of the ADLs as well as their cognitive functioning.
Watson clock drawing test (Watson et al. 1993)	This test can screen for and assess the level of cognitive impairment. Participants are asked to draw and number a clock; there is variation in the scoring procedures used.

As well as physical needs and the level of assistance required to carry out activities of daily living, the nurse needs to assess for social and psychological factors that impact on the quality of life for the person in their care. The assessing nurse must try to establish a comprehensive picture of the person in terms of their likes and dislikes, hobbies and their personality before they became ill. Other important information that needs to be established from the assessment is the person's past and current medical problems and any prescribed pharmacological treatments. Factors that impact on the patient's safety must also be established, for example the nurse needs to know if the person is prone to agitation or aggressive outbursts, if there is a history of falls or if the patient wanders.

Communicating with Older People with Dementia

Effective communication skills are essential when caring for the person with dementia and they underpin every intervention with the person. They also form the basis of many of the interventions that can be used in a structured or informal way, such as reality orientation or reminiscence therapy. The advantages of both planned and unstructured interactions cannot be underestimated in terms of their impact on the cognitive function of the person and their response to health care interventions (Kiely *et al.* 2000).

Initially, communication skills are relatively intact in people with dementia; however, as the illness progresses, people with dementia are often unable to articulate their needs and may communicate by other means. Nurses need to be aware of these non-verbal communications and respond accordingly. For example, an increase in agitation may occur when a physical need like hunger or thirst is not met. According to Perry *et al.* (2005) there are several barriers to communication for people with dementia, especially in long-term care. These include the person's level of aphasia, the physical environment of the care facility and negative stereotyping of older people with dementia. They found that the people with dementia in their research communicated with nurses at a higher level of functioning than was expected and that a broad range of conversational strategies can be used when communicating with people with dementia (Perry *et al.* 2005). Some strategies for improving communication are:

- always referring to the person by name
- maintaining eye contact
- ensuring that hearing aids and glasses (as necessary) are worn by the person
- speaking in a clear and distinct voice, giving one piece of information at a time and providing additional time for the person to assimilate the information
- breaking down sentences or requests into more easily understandable steps
- always explaining your intentions prior to completing them, repeating them as necessary
- modifying the physical and the social environment to make it more conducive for conversation, e.g. minimising noise from radios or the television, sitting people close to each other to encourage conversation.

Other general communication strategies are contained in Chapter 8.

Reality Orientation

Reality orientation (RO) is an intervention aimed at reducing confusion in older people with dementia by orientating them to time, place and person. There are generally two types of RO: formal individual or group sessions; and informal RO aimed at constantly reminding the older person of the time and their whereabouts. Physical modifications of the environment in the form of large-faced clocks, calendars and signs indicating the location of toilets and bedrooms, etc. are made (Ross 2003) and when communicating with people with dementia, nursing staff are encouraged to give information about the time and the location. Structured RO involves individual or group sessions, which centre on time-related topics such as current affairs. It is important to ensure that structured RO sessions are aimed at the particular level of the individual taking part, and RO may not be suitable for all people with dementia.

Reminiscence Therapy

Reminiscence therapy involves the formal and informal recalling of events or memories from the past (Hong *et al.* 2005). This is a flexible form of therapy and can be used with people who have mild or severe dementia. Structured reminiscence, according to Hong *et al.* (2005), involves stimulating all five senses to prompt recollections and conversation about events or music from a particular time. Informal reminiscence can occur at any time; for example watching an old film or listening to an old record may evoke pleasant memories for an individual with dementia.

Validation Therapy

This form of therapy, developed by Feil (1993), aims to look for meaning in the actions of the older person with dementia. Feil believes that people with dementia sometimes retreat into a past world in an attempt to resolve difficult feelings. The goal of validation therapy is to 'validate' the person's experience and to accept the person's feelings in a non-judgemental and dignified manner. Validation therapy involves aspects of reminiscence therapy and communication skills are used to explore the person's experience and the emotions it evokes. For example if the person with dementia states that they have to leave the unit to go to work, an appropriate response might be to explore the occupation of the individual and their feelings surrounding it.

Needs-Driven Dementia Compromised Behaviour Model

Although more of an approach to care than a therapy, this model, developed by Algase *et al.* (1996), aims to alter our perceptions of behaviours associated with dementia. It proposes that behaviours previously conceptualised as 'challenging' (wandering, aggression and shouting) are in fact responses to environmental and individual factors (Kolanowski 1999). The aim of the model is to discover the meaning of the behaviour to the individual and to establish why it occurs. For example, physical aggression may be caused by the individual's inability to manage the stresses caused by being confused — reality orientation, validation and effective communication skills may help reduce the aggressive behaviour by targeting confusion.

Specific Interventions

Some nursing interventions to assist the person with dementia with some of the main activities of daily living affected are briefly outlined in the table below. Gitlin *et al.* (2003) suggest that making modifications to the physical, task and social environment may help the person with dementia to manage better their activities of daily living (ADLs). These modifications are reflected in some of the nursing interventions set out in Figure 18.4.

Figure 18.4 Summary of nursing interventions based on the ADLs

Activity of Daily Living	Problem	Nursing Interventions
Maintaining a safe environment/ mobilising	Wandering Falls Absconding Aggression	Assessment Observation Modification of the physical environment, e.g. adequate lighting, handrails, appropriate footwear, walking aids, etc. Effective communication skills
Eating and drinking	Will not eat or drink Difficulty eating and drinking	Find out person's food likes and dislikes and try to provide Meals on the run, e.g. sandwiches or high-calorie drinks Observe during mealtimes Modify physical environment, e.g. adapted cutlery, adequate lighting in the dining room, non-slip place mats Modify task, e.g. cut up food for the person Communication skills, e.g. encourage person to eat and remind them to eat Dietician advice if necessary Assistance with eating and drinking when necessary Fluid balance chart and weight chart to monitor progress
Cleansing and dressing	Will not wash Difficulty washing and dressing	Establish routine; attend to patient's needs when they are the least confused. Communication skills, explain all interventions. Respect the patient's need for privacy and dignity Prompt where necessary Assist when necessary Modify physical environment, e.g. slip-on shoes instead of lace-ups, zippers instead of buttons etc. Modify task environment, e.g. model what you want the person to do, lay out their clothes in order etc.

Activity of Daily Living	Problem	Nursing Interventions
Expression of sexuality	Uninhibited sexual behaviour	Individualised approach Recognise and accept patient's needs for intimacy and the need to be close to other people Orientation Providing privacy Treating the patient with dignity Limit setting if appropriate Responding appropriately (Higgins *et al.* 2006)
Elimination	Incontinence due to confusion or apraxia Constipation	Orientation Reminders Modify physical environment, e.g. adequate lighting, modified clothes, etc. Modify task environment, e.g. large signs for the toilets, etc. Look for non-verbal cues High-fibre diet Exercise Adequate fluids
Sleeping	Not sleeping Reversed sleeping pattern	Avoid cat napping during the day Structured activities during the day Exercise regime Modify physical environment, e.g. providing an environment that is conducive to rest Modify task environment, e.g. orientation etc. Establish routine
Working and playing	Boredom	Structured day for patient Activities based on the needs of the patient Cognitive stimulation, e.g. word games, reading, etc. Structured reality orientation groups Reminiscence therapy Exercise Outings Encourage visits from families

Clinical Scenario

John Smith, a retired senior civil servant, is a 72-year-old man with Alzheimer's disease who has been admitted to the local care of the older person unit for a period of assessment and treatment. Recently his elderly frail wife became unable to care for him at home due to his increasingly unpredictable behaviour. John had become hostile towards his wife, accusing her of stealing his belongings and trying to harm him. His diet was also neglected and he appeared to have lost weight. He was also refusing to wash and change his clothes. On admission to hospital John was irritable and aggressive, shouting at other patients and visitors to call the police, as he was being held captive.

The admitting nurse selected a quiet environment to complete the assessment and made sure that John and his wife were comfortable before proceeding with the nursing admission formalities. She maintained eye contact throughout the interview while speaking clearly and distinctly to John, repeating the questions when necessary. An MMSE examination score of 16 suggested cognitive impairment. A plan of care was drawn up with the main goal of returning John to his home environment with support from the community services. A multi-disciplinary team approach ensured that all of John's and his wife's needs were met. Interventions were aimed at maintaining John's independence while ensuring that he had a structured day, which helped to decrease his agitation and improve his appetite. The focus of his care was on individuality, cognitive stimulation and including John and his wife in the caring process. Appropriate practical information was given to John's wife to help her understand John's illness and referral to the local branch of the Alzheimer Society of Ireland meant that she was able to meet people who were looking after their loved ones with dementia in a friendly and supportive environment.

CONCLUSION

Population projections estimate that by the year 2011 there will be approximately 728,000 older people living in Ireland (NCAOP 2004). The vast majority of these will defy negative stereotypes of ageing and remain physically and mentally healthy throughout later life. Dementia affects about five per cent of all 65-year-olds (DSIDC 2003) and the majority of these people will be cared for at home. Psychiatric nursing care is often required because relatives are no longer able to care for the person with dementia for a variety of reasons. This vulnerable group of individuals requires nursing care that is underpinned by interpersonal skills, sensitivity and a commitment to an individualised approach.

Reflective Questions

1. Discuss ways in which you may be able to help an individual with dementia remain physically and mentally stimulated during a period of hospitalisation.
2. Think about the last time you helped an older person with dementia to carry out an activity of daily living. In what way could you have made this a more positive experience for that person?

3. Imagine you are an older person with dementia living in a nursing home. What aspects of care would be most important to you?
4. The wife of a hospitalised patient with dementia approaches you and asks, 'Will my husband get better?' What do you say to her?

References

Algase, D., Beck, C., Kolanowski, A., Whall, A., Berent, S., Richards, K. and Beattie, E. (1996) 'Need driven dementia compromised behaviour: An alternative view of disruptive behaviour'. *American Journal of Alzheimer's Disease*, 11(6), 10–19.

Alzheimer's Disease Society (2003) *Genetics and Dementia*. London: Alzheimer's Disease Society.

Alzheimer Society of Ireland (2006) *Dementia Manifesto 2007–2009*. Dublin: Alzheimer Society of Ireland.

American Psychiatric Association (APA) (2000) *Diagnostic and Statistical Manual of Mental Disorders* (DSM-IV-TR) (4th edn: text revision). Washington DC: APA.

Beattie, J. (2003) 'Quality use of medicines' in R. Hudson (ed) *Dementia Nursing: A Guide to Practice*. Oxford: Radcliffe Medical Press.

Bolla, L., Filley, C., and Palmer, R. (2000) 'Dementia DDx. Office diagnosis of the four major types of dementia'. *Geriatrics*, 55(1), 34–7.

British National Formulary (BNF) (2007). London: British Medical Formulary and Royal Pharmaceutical Society of Great Britain.

Dementia Services Information and Development Centre (DSIDC) (2003) *About Dementia*, www.dementia.ie/about_dementia.htm (last accessed 5 April 2007).

Desira, L. and Martin, G. (2004) 'Person centred approach to care of older people with mental health problems' in S. Kirby, D. Hart, D. Cross and G. Mitchell, G. (eds), *Mental Health Nursing: Competencies for Practice*. Bristol: Palgrave MacMillan, 209–25.

Feil, N. (1993) *The Validation Breakthrough: Simple Techniques for Communicating with People with Alzheimer's Type Dementia*. Baltimore: Health Professions Press.

Folstein, M., Folstein, S. and McHugh, P. (1975) 'Mini mental state: a practical method of grading the cognitive state of patients for the clinician'. *Journal of Psychiatric Research*, 12, 89–99.

Gitlin, L., Liebman, J. and Winter, L. (2003) 'Are environmental interventions effective in the management of Alzheimer's disease and related disorders? A synthesis of the evidence'. *Alzheimer's Care Quarterly*, 4(2), 85–107.

Goward, P. (2000) 'Dementia: a clinical overview'. *Nursing and Residential Care*, 2 (12), 568–70.

Higgins, A., Barker, P. and Begley, C. (2004) 'Hypersexuality and dementia: dealing with inappropriate sexual expression'. *British Journal of Nursing*, 13(22), 1330–4.

Hong, C., Heathcote, J. and Quinn, P. (2005) 'Part one: the value of reminiscence'. *Nursing and Residential Care*, 7(1), 27–9.

Kiely, D., Simon, S., Jones, R. and Morris, J. (2000) 'The protective effect of social engagement on mortality in long term care'. *Journal of the American Geriatrics Society*, 48(11), 1367–72.

Kitwood, T. (1997) *Dementia Reconsidered: The Person Comes First*. Buckingham: Open University Press.

Kolanowski, A. (1999) 'An overview of the needs driven compromised behaviour model'. *Journal of Gerontological Nursing*, 25(9), 7–9.

Martin, A. M. (2006) 'Dementia: key factors in recognition and support'. *Practice Nursing*, 17(1), 12–16.

McKeith, I. and Fairbairn, A. (2001) 'Biomedical and clinical perspectives' in C. Cantley (ed.) *A Handbook of Dementia Care*. Buckingham: Open University Press.

Munoz, D. and Feldman, H. (2000) 'Causes of Alzheimer's disease'. *Canadian Medical Association*, 11, 65–72.

National Council for Ageing and Older People (NCAOP) (1999) *An Action Plan for Dementia*. Dublin: NCAOP.

National Council for Ageing and Older People (NCAOP) (2004) *Population Ageing in Ireland: Projections 2002–2021*. Dublin: NCAOP.

National Institute for Health and Clinical Excellence (NICE) (2004) *Dementia: The Management of Dementia, Including the use of Antipsychotic Medication in Older People*, Dementia Scope Version 2. London: NICE.

Nazarko, L. (2006) 'Recognising the signs and symptoms of dementia'. *Nursing and Residential Care*, 8(1), 32–4.

Nordberg, A. and Svensson, A. (1998) 'Cholinesterase inhibitors in the treatment of Alzheimer's disease: a comparison of tolerability and pharmacology'. *Drug Safety*, 19, 465–80.

O'Shea, E. (2007) 'Implementing policy for dementia care in Ireland: the time for action is now'. NUIG: Irish Centre for Social Gerontology.

Ouldred, E. (2004) 'Screening for dementia in older people'. *British Journal of Community Nursing*, 9, 10, 434–7.

Pattie, A. and Gilleard, C. (1979) *Manual of Clifton Assessment Procedures for the Elderly (CAPE)*. Sevenoaks: Hodder and Stoughton.

Perry, J., Galloway, S., Bottorff, J. and Nixon S. (2005) 'Nurse–patient communication in dementia: improving the odds'. *Journal of Gerontological Nursing*, 31(4), 43–52.

Rosen, W. G., Mohs, R. C. and Davis, K. L. (1984) 'A new rating scale for Alzheimer's disease'. *American Journal of Psychiatry*, 141, 1356–64.

Ross, C. (2003) 'Managing cognitive impairment in older people'. *Nursing and Residential Care*, 5(11), 529–32.

Royal College of Nursing (RCN) (2004) *Nursing Assessment and Older People: A Royal College of Nursing Toolkit*. London: RCN.

Townsend, M. (1999) *Essentials of Psychiatric/Mental Health Nursing*. Philadelphia: F. A. Davis Company.

Walling, A. (2004) 'Dementia with Lewy bodies vs. Alzheimer's disease'. *American*

Family Physician, 69(11), 2688–90.

Watson, Y., Arfken, C. and Birge, S. (1993) 'Clock completion: An objective screening test for dementia'. *Journal of the American Geriatrics Society*, 41(11).

World Health Organisation (WHO) (1992) *The ICD-10 Classification of Mental and Behavioural Disorders. Clinical Descriptions and Diagnostic Guidelines.* Geneva: WHO.

Yesavage, J., Brink, T., Rose, T., Lum, O., Huang, V., Adey, M. and Leirer, V. (1983) 'Development and validation of a geriatric depression screening scale: a preliminary report'. *Journal of Psychiatric Research*, 17, 37–49.

19
Working with Addiction Problems

Gerard Moore

There are many forms of addiction and depending on your perspective addiction can be understood as a relationship with a substance or a form of behaviour. This chapter is concerned with addiction in relation to alcohol and drugs.

In the last decade Ireland has had the highest increase in alcohol consumption among EU countries. Between 1989 and 1999 this increase was 41 per cent per capita, while other EU countries showed a decrease in the same period. In 2002 alcohol consumption per adult in Ireland hit 14.2 litres whereas the EU average was only 9.1 litres per capita.

The increase in substance abuse disorders is reflected in the number of people seeking treatment. In 1971, 2.4 per cent of people attending Irish psychiatric units and hospitals were diagnosed with alcoholic disorders, and by 2006 this figure had risen to 4.8 per cent. During the same period other drug disorders had risen from 0.1 per cent to 0.8 per cent (Daly and Walsh 2006). This finding is supported by the *Activities of Psychiatric Units and Hospitals* report (Daly *et al.* 2006), which shows that alcoholic disorders have the second highest rate of first admissions in all Health Service Executive (HSE) areas, with rates ranging from 37.0 per 100,000 in the Dublin/Mid-Leinster region to 26.1 per 100,000 in the Dublin North-East region. There is also a relatively high rate of drug use in Ireland, generally estimated at 5.6 per thousand of the population (Moore *et al.* 2004).

This chapter presents an overview of addiction and outlines the causes, symptoms and treatments of addiction problems.

HISTORY OF ADDICTION

During the mid to late eighteen hundreds addiction was dominated by a moral/temperance model characterising addiction as a sin or a crime. The moral model merged into a temperance model of addiction in which the locus of control around addictive behaviour shifted from the individual to the legislators. In Ireland the Temperance Movement, which began in the 1850s, advocated total abstinence — taking the pledge. Social thinkers recognised that a country with a developing industrial network could only succeed with a sober workforce. The temperance model resulted in the introduction of the first laws on the consumption of alcohol.

From the 1920s a more enlightened approach towards addiction began to emerge, driven initially by individuals who experienced the impact of addiction on their day-to-day lives and the failure of religion or the law to provide an adequate solution. In the USA, following the failure of prohibition, the first self-help approach to addiction emerged in the form of Alcoholics Anonymous (AA). The emphasis focused on the individual and his/her relationship with alcohol and advocated lifelong abstinence through a system of peer support.

Advances in neurobiology created a better understanding of the relationship between the individual and a substance at a biological level and facilitated the development of medical treatments such as pharmacological interventions. This disease-orientated approach to addiction was evident in the 1945 Mental Treatment Act, which allowed individuals to be detained for treatment. The latter part of the century saw a more psychosocial approach to the treatment of people with addiction problems, resulting in a shift from hospital-based care to community care.

The introduction of the Mental Health Act 2001 affirms the health services' intention to treat as many substance users as possible on an outpatient basis and removed the possibility of the involuntary admission of a person solely because of an addiction problem. Figure 19.1 presents an overview of the models of addiction and the treatment approaches associated with each model.

Figure 19.1 Models of addiction and treatment approaches for addiction

Model	Examples	Emphasised Causal Factors	Implied Interventions	Appropriate Intervention Agency
Moral	Abuse as sin Abuse as crime	Spirituality Personal responsibility	Spiritual direction Moral suasion Social sanctions	Clergy Law enforcement agency
Temperance	Prohibition	Alcohol Drugs	Abstinence Prohibition	Abstainers Legislators
American Disease	AA NA	Irreversible Constitutional Abnormality of individual	Identification confrontation Lifelong abstinence	Peer support
Educational	Lectures Affective education	Lack of knowledge Lack of motivation	Education	Educators
Character-logical	Psychoanalysis	Personality traits dispositions Defence mechanisms	Self-image modification	Psychotherapists
Conditioning	Classical Operant	Conditioned response Reinforcement	Counter-conditioning Altered contingencies Relearning disenabling	Behaviour therapists

Model	Examples	Emphasised Causal Factors	Implied Interventions	Appropriate Intervention Agency
Biomedical	Heredity Brain	Genetic Physiological	Risk identification	Diagnosticians Physicians
Social learning	Cognitive therapy Relapse Prevention	Modelling expectancies Skill deficits	Appropriate models/goals Cognitive restructuring Skill training Self-control training	Cognitive behaviour therapists
General systems	Transactional analysis	Family dysfunction	Family therapy Recognition, peer support	Family therapist Support groups
Socio-cultural	Control of consumption	Environmental cultural norms	Supply side intervention Social policy Server intervention	Lobbyists/legislators Social policy makers Retailers/servers
Public health	WHO National academy of science	Interactions of host, agent and environment	Comprehensive Multifaceted	Interdisciplinary

UNDERSTANDING ADDICTION

Addiction is continued involvement with a substance or activity despite ongoing negative consequences (Donatella 2006) and occurs on a continuum where the behaviours initially provide pleasure or stability that is beyond the person's ability to achieve otherwise. Over time it becomes necessary to engage with the substance or activity to feel normal.

According to the World Health Organisation (WHO 2007) addiction to drugs or alcohol can be understood as repeated use of a psychoactive substance, to the extent that the user is periodically or chronically intoxicated, shows a compulsion to take the preferred substance, has great difficulty in voluntarily ceasing or modifying substance use and exhibits determination to obtain psychoactive substances by almost any means. Typically, tolerance is prominent and a withdrawal syndrome frequently occurs when substance use is interrupted. The life of the addict may be dominated by substance use to the virtual exclusion of all other activities and responsibilities. The term 'addiction' also conveys the sense that such substance use has a detrimental effect on society, as well as on the individual.

Current conceptualisation of drug-taking behaviour, in relation to all psychoactive substances, suggests three categories under which use can be defined:

- **drug use** simply refers to the taking of drugs.
- **drug abuse** refers to any harmful use even if it does not constitute sufficient markers for a diagnosis with DSM–IV-TR (APA 2000) criteria
- **dependence** refers to substance dependence as defined in the DSM-IV-TR or addiction as defined in the ICD-10 (WHO 1992).

Addiction is characterised by a number of psychological and physical markers which are common to all presentations regardless of the substance being used. These include:

- **Habit:** the repeated engagement in a behaviour that in addiction leads to the development of tolerance.
- **Tolerance:** the experience that a progressively larger dosage of the substance or more intense involvement in the behaviour is required to obtain the desired effect.
- **Compulsion:** an obsessive preoccupation with a behaviour that results in an overwhelming desire to repeat the experience.
- **Obsession:** the experience of ongoing preoccupation with an addictive substance or behaviour.
- **Denial:** a psychological mechanism employed to refuse to perceive that the addiction is self-destructive.
- **Withdrawal:** a series of temporary bio-psychosocial symptoms that occur when the substance user abstains from their addictive substance or behaviour.
- **Relapse:** the tendency to return to the addictive substance or behaviour after a period of abstinence or reduced consumption.

SUBSTANCES OF ABUSE

The main substances of abuse are outlined in Figure 19.2. However, many more substances and behaviours than are addressed here have the potential for abuse.

Figure 19.2 Substances of abuse

Substance	Chemical Content	Administration	Absorption	Residual Effect
Tobacco	Nicotine	Smoking, chewing, snuff, patches, gum, tablets	Immediate	Depression and fatigue
Alcohol	Ethyl alcohol	Oral, inhalant	Immediate	Dehydration, hangover, tolerance addiction

Substance	Chemical Content	Administration	Absorption	Residual Effect
Cannabis	THC (Delta 9-Tetra-hydrocannabinol)	Smoked Eaten Drunk	Rapidly carried via bloodstream from lungs to brain	Addictive, increased risk of MI, respiratory illness, cancer, depression, anxiety, memory loss, problems with social functioning and psychosis
Cocaine	Naturally occurring substance from coca plant	Snorted, injected or smoked	Inhibits the reabsorbing of dopamine	Mood swings, restlessness, irritability, paranoia, psychosis, hallucinations, damage to mucous membranes
Heroin	Morphine naturally occurring in seed pod of Asian poppy	Smoking, snorting and injecting	Euphoria, sleepiness	Addiction, liver damage, lung damage, secondary effects from shared injecting paraphernalia
LSD	Lysergic Acid Diethylamide Manufactured from lysergic acid found in ergot (fungus)	Oral tablets, capsules, blotting paper	Unpredictable effect, mood swings, delusions, visual hallucinations, raised BP and heart rate	Anxiety, fear, paranoia, flashbacks
Mushrooms	Psilocybin psychedelic drug similar to LSD. Naturally occurring	Eaten raw or cooked	Similar effect to using cannabis, can last up to 12 hours	Risk of eating wrong mushrooms, stomach pains, hallucinations, anxiety, panic attacks
Ecstasy	MDMA 3-4 methylenedioxy-methamphetamine. Synthetic drug	Tablet or liquid	Stimulant and hallucinogenic	Raised temperature, dehydration, liver and kidney failure, damage to serotonin neuron receptors

Substance	Chemical Content	Administration	Absorption	Residual Effect
Solvents and glue	Paint thinners, dry cleaning fluids, petrol, glue, gases including butane, propane, aerosols and medical gases, nitrates including poppers, amyl nitrate, audiovisual cleaning fluids, liquid air fresheners. All are man-made products intended for different use	Inhaled directly or via a crude device such as a plastic bag	Absorbed quickly and has a short-term anaesthetic effect, slows body functions, occasional stimulant effect	Nausea, headache, loss of consciousness, brain damage, liver and kidney damage, hearing loss, bone marrow damage
PCP	Polyclylidine. Synthetic IV anaesthetic	Snorted, smoked or injected	Mood changes, numbing of feelings, feeling invulnerable, aggression, violence, suicide	Memory loss, depression, thought disorder
Steroids	Anabolic androgenic steroids Man made	Oral or injected (cycling and stacking)	Cancer, liver tumours, raised BP, mood swings, acne, shrinking of testicles, development of secondary sexual characteristics	Paranoid jealousy, manic symptoms, delusions, risk from unsafe injecting behaviours

AETIOLOGY OF ADDICTION

Addiction can be understood both as a health and a social problem and its causes can be found in social, biological and psychological origins. Some of the factors that contribute to the development of addiction are outlined below.

Social Factors
- Social deprivation and stress have been associated with the development of substance abuse and dependence. Economic and social/cultural marginalisation are often viewed as factors that contribute to drug use and drug abuse. Lower working classes may use illegitimate means (such as drug behaviour and

criminal activity) to achieve status and wealth in society (Moore 2007). The high level of 'problematic' drug use in many working-class communities is a consequence of inequality, poverty and a lack of resources in areas of education and employment.

- Some studies contend that peer alcohol and drug use has a strong effect on substance abusers.
- Ireland's culture revolves largely around alcohol, which is a socially accepted recreational drug.

Biological Factors

- Drug dependence can be viewed as a chronic brain disease because it is reported to produce changes in the dynamic functioning of the brain (Qureshi et al. 2000).
- Genetics studies suggest that the predisposition to alcohol dependence runs in the family. Twin and adoption studies reveal inheritability estimates of forty to sixty per cent. If the individual inherits a set of predisposing genes and encounters the necessary environmental influences (precipitating factors), there is a high probability that substance abuse disorder will result. Furthermore, genetic factors seem to determine cannabis use, abuse and dependence, at least in studies conducted with rodents (Qureshi *et al.* 2000).
- Endorphins are the body's naturally occurring opioids, which make a person feel good. Drugs and alcohol can stimulate the production of endorphins, thereby increasing the feel-good factor.

Psychological Factors

- **Personality theory** supports the contention that some people are born with 'addictive personalities'.
- **Behavioural theories:** some studies suggest that conduct problems of childhood, e.g. deviance, misbehaviour and aggression, might be important behavioural risk factors for later substance abuse, particularly for boys.
- **Operant conditioning** is based on the premise of reinforcing behaviour that makes us feel good (intoxication) and avoiding unpleasant feelings (withdrawal).
- **Mental health problems:** depression, schizophrenia, suicidal behaviour are all associated with an increase in alcohol/drug addiction.

EFFECTS OF ALCOHOL ABUSE

Alcohol abuse has both short- and long-term effects on physical, social, and psychological health. These are outlined in Figure 19.3.

Figure 19.3 Biopsychosocial effects of alcohol addiction

Physical	Social	Psychological
Affects all systems of the body	Affects ability to participate in normal social activity	Affects self-concept and interferes with ability to form and maintain relationships
Gastro–intestinal Reflux, oesophagitis, gastritis, peptic ulcer, pancreatitis, cancer of larynx, pharynx, and oesophagus, diarrhoea and malabsoption, gastro-intestinal bleeding due to gastritis or peptic ulcer, Mallory Weiss syndrome, varices, Boorhave's syndrome	*Work* Lack of motivation, days lost, loss of job, effect on disposable income	*Changes in Self-concept* Belief in being an addict
Nutritional Deficiencies Vitamins A, B1, B6, Folic acid, C and D	*Home* Homelessness	*Mood Disorders* Deceased ability to self-regulate mood, experiences of guilt and denial of problems, depression, anxiety
Alcohol Liver Disease Fatty changes, acute alcoholic hepatitis, alcoholic cirrhosis	*Relationship Problems* Marital break-up	*Safety* Increased risk of deliberate self-harm and suicide
Nervous System Withdrawal delirium tremens, Wernicke's encephalopathy, Korsakoff's psychosis, delusion of jealousy, alcoholic hallucinations	*Crime* Involvement in illegal activity, e.g. underage drinking, drug use, drug trafficking, theft to support habit may result in criminal charges and/or imprisonment. Accidents and death as a result of road use under the influence of alcohol and/or drugs	
Cardio–vascular System Cardiomyopathy, hypertension, increased coronary artery disease, strokes	*Cross-addiction* Increased risk of use of other mood-altering drugs	
Endocrine System Pseudo–Cushing's syndrome, pseudo-thyrotoxicosis		

Physical	Social	Psychological
Metabolic Disorders Hypoglycaemia, gout, metabolic acidosis, effects on diabetics		
Pregnancy and Infant *Development Complications* Even moderate amounts of alcohol can have damaging effects on the developing foetus, including low birth weight and an increased risk of miscarriage. High amounts can cause foetal alcohol syndrome, a condition that can cause mental and growth retardation.		

TREATMENT INTERVENTIONS

Before discussing treatment interventions, it is important to understand the processes that occur in behaviour change. Clients experiencing addiction must first be willing to work on actively combating the addiction. This involves an inner recognition of the addiction as a problem. Prochaska *et al.* (1992) have identified a five-stage trans-theoretical model of change, which can be used by mental health workers to understand where the client is in relation to their willingness to change. The five stages of this model are outlined below.

Five-stage Model of Change
1. **Pre-contemplation stage** — individuals do not believe they have a problem and therefore are resistant to change. The role of treatment should be to help the person become aware of the possible and real harms they are inflicting on themselves through their substance misuse.
2. **Contemplation** — an ambivalent stage in which the individual is aware of the cost of their substance abuse but this is still outweighed by perceived benefits of continued use. The treatment task involves helping the individual understand their misperceptions.
3. **Preparation** — during this stage there is recognition of the need for change and small steps may be made towards it. Treatment approaches should include enabling the person to develop a realistic plan for changing their behaviour and encouraging them to move away from being ambivalent in relation to addiction.
4. **Action** — an active stage of change in which new behaviours are acquired. Interventions need to be supportive in that they enable the individual to hold onto their rationale for change and actively provide the person with the tools they need to take action.

5. **Maintenance** — this stage is all about allowing the individual to develop a sustainable lifestyle. Much supportive work in relation to relapse prevention is required.

Recognising that an individual has reached a turning point is important. Turning points are expressed as:
- existential crisis
- rock bottom
- rational decisions
- epiphany
- should stop/want to stop
- desire for a new identity.

A turning point can be understood as a point beyond which an individual is now willing to go. It is usually accompanied by some experience or event that serves to stimulate or trigger the decision, for example a health, family or work crisis. The decision to stop may be influenced by experiences that damage a person's sense of self, such as when the substance user's identity conflicts with, and creates problems for, other identities that are unrelated to substance use. The key to the recovery process lies in the realisation by the substance user that their damaged sense of self has to be restored together with a reawakening of their old identities and/or the establishment of new ones. Cognitive shifts are required. This relates to a sense of self that is continually formed and reformed through interaction with others in which individuals internalise the attitudes that others hold towards them. For the substance abuser there is a need to move away from an identity in which the individual realises that he exhibits characteristics that are unacceptable both to themselves and others. For this to happen there are two basic requirements:
- a motivation to stop based upon a desire to restore a spoiled identity
- a sense of a future that is potentially different from the present.

TREATMENT APPROACHES

There are two main treatment approaches to addiction. The more traditional abstinence-based model is centred on the addict giving up the substance. The harm reduction model takes a more pragmatic perspective on addiction and aims to enable the addict to reduce or control their consumption, thereby decreasing the harms associated with substance abuse. There are three steps common to both that need to be negotiated:
- detoxification
- recovery
- relapse prevention.

Assessment for Alcohol Misuse

Prior to engaging in treatment it is necessary to conduct a careful assessment of the individual's substance abuse history. A careful assessment is the guide to the treatment plan. Alcoholism is frequently accompanied by other substance abuse disorders (particularly nicotine), anxiety and mood disorders, and anti-social personality disorder. Although associated with considerable morbidity and mortality, alcoholism often goes unrecognised in a clinical or primary healthcare setting. Indicators of possible problem drinking/alcoholism are outlined in Figure 19.4.

Figure 19.4 Indicators of problem drinking/alcoholism

Symptoms	Signs
Recurrent intoxication, nausea, sweating, tachycardia	Heavy, regular alcohol consumption, heavy cigarette smoking
Amnesic episodes (blackouts)	Other substance abuse (e.g. cannabis, cocaine, heroin, amphetamines, sedatives, hypnotics, and anxiolytics)
Mood swings, depression, anxiety, insomnia, chronic fatigue	
Grand mal seizures, hallucinations, delirium tremens	Unexpected medication response (drug interactions)
Dyspepsia, diarrhoea, bloating, haematemesis, jaundice	Poor nutrition and personal neglect
Tremor, unsteady gait, parasthesia, memory loss, erectile dysfunction	Frequent falls or minor trauma (particularly in the elderly)
	Accidents, burns, violence, suicide
	Recurrent absenteeism from work or school
	Spontaneous abortion, child with foetal alcohol syndrome
	Increased vulnerability
	Alcoholic parent, childhood conduct disorder, anti-social personality disorder
	Negative life event

Several brief screening instruments are available to quickly identify problem drinking (see Figure 19.5). Alcohol addiction is a lifelong disease with a relapsing, remitting course. Because of the potentially serious implications of the diagnosis, assessment for alcoholism should be detailed. Treatment involves a variety of psychosocial methods with or without newly developed pharmacotherapies that improve relapse rates. Screening for problem drinking and alcoholism needs to become an integral part of the routine health-screening questionnaire for all adolescents and adults, particularly women of childbearing age, because of the risk of foetal alcohol syndrome (APA 2002). Alcoholism often goes undiagnosed;

the rate of screening for alcohol consumption in health care settings remains lower than fifty per cent. Individuals may also withhold information because of shame or fear of stigmatisation. This can lead to missed information about conditions and potential complications, unexpected alcohol withdrawal symptoms, drug interactions, and lost opportunities for prevention, including intervention during pregnancy to prevent damaging effects of alcohol on the foetus.

Figure 19.5 Alcohol screening tools

Tool	Used to assess:	Potential
CAGE (King 1986)	Lifetime use of alcohol	Four simple questions. Useful for quick on-the-spot assessment of alcohol use. Depends on skills of assessor to collect and interpret data.
MAST — Michigan Alcoholism Screening Test (Selzer 1971)	Lifetime use of alcohol	Short quick easy test that gives a broad picture of alcohol use.
SADQ — Severity of Alcohol Questionnaire (Stockwell et al. 1983)	Severity of an alcohol use problem	A more precise test that is reasonably easy to apply with minimum training. Gives reasonable information on severity of use.
AUDIT — Alcohol Use Disorders Identification Test (Babor et al. 1989)	Alcohol use during past 12 months	Gives a clear account of past 12 months of drinking. A useful tool for use with individuals who have a short history of alcohol misuse.
LDQ – Leeds Dependency Questionnaire (Riastrick et al. 1994)	The severity of an addiction	Useful in the assessment of both severity and duration of dependency.
ASI — Addiction Severity Index (McLellan et al. (1992)	The severity of an addiction	Gives accurate information on severity and can be a useful tool as an aid to planning interventions.
MAP – Maudsley Addiction Profile (Marsden et al. 1998)	Changes over time, and outcomes from treatment	Helpful tool both for assessing outcomes of treatment and tracking changes in an individual's presentation over time.

Detoxification

Whether detoxification is in hospital or through an outpatient programme will depend on the severity of the person's condition. For alcohol detoxification, alcohol is withdrawn and precautions taken against the development of delirium tremens. A benzodiazepine may be used and is normally given on a sliding scale with reductions introduced every 48 hours over a period of five to fourteen days. During the withdrawal phase, a detailed physical examination should be made and attention given to any organic conditions that require treatment. It is usual to prescribe vitamin supplements, but an adequate well-balanced diet is equally effective. Night-time sedation may be prescribed; however, the risk of cross-dependency should not be ignored.

The nursing management of detoxification should centre on observation for symptoms as they occur and include observation for delirium tremens (DTs) which can occur at any time from 48 hours to seven days after the last drink and usually first appear in the evening or at night. DTs are characterised by intense fear, restlessness, illusions, delusions, visual hallucinations, tremulousness, ataxia, hypertension, tachycardia and pyrexia. The mortality rate can be as high as ten per cent and death can occur due to cardiovascular collapse or self-injury.

Nursing management of detoxification
- Observation and recording of vital signs.
- Orientation.
- Monitor fluid balance — ensure minimum of 2.5 litres in 24 hours.
- Encourage dietary intake or supplements if necessary.
- Nurse in quiet, non-stimulating environment.
- Offer support and reassurance.
- Assist with personal hygiene.
- Gradual return to activities of daily living.
- Vigilance for seizures at all times.

Abstinence
For abstinence to be successful the substance user must also learn to restore a balance to their lifestyle through non-compulsive engagements in other behaviours and/or substances. This is both a physical and cognitive process in which the substance user adjusts to being free from the direct influence of their addiction.

Pharmacological Treatments
Thirty to sixty per cent of those with alcohol dependency syndrome maintain at least one year of abstinence with psychosocial therapies alone (Finney *et al.* 1996). However, more than twenty per cent of people achieve long-term sobriety even without active treatment (APA 1994). More effective therapies are clearly needed, and pharmacotherapeutic agents have recently emerged that can be used as adjuncts to psychosocial treatments.

The most promising of these medications are the opioid antagonist, naltrexone (Revia), and the anti-craving drug acamprosate (Campral), a glutamate antagonist. Several studies have shown that naltrexone reduces alcohol consumption and is effective, when combined with psychosocial treatment, in reducing relapse rates (O'Malley 1996; Anton *et al.* 1999). Acamprosate, used extensively in Europe and now being tested in the United States, appears to be safe and well tolerated and may almost double the abstinence rate among those recovering from alcohol dependence (Sass *et al.* 1996). Disulfiram (Antabuse), is another pharmacological agent used in the treatment of alcohol dependency syndrome. It blocks the metabolism of acetaldehyde and causes an unpleasant flushing reaction if taken with alcohol. Outcomes of patients who take disulfiram are improved when the drug is taken under supervision (Chick *et al.* 1992).

Long-term Maintenance of Abstinence

Considerable evidence shows that long-lasting neurobiological changes in the brains of alcoholics contribute to the persistence of craving. At any stage during recovery, relapse can be triggered by internal factors (depression, anxiety, craving for alcohol) or external factors (environmental triggers, social pressures, negative life events). Psychosocial treatments concentrate on helping patients to understand, anticipate, and prevent relapse.

Alcoholics Anonymous (AA) Facilitation Therapy

AA is a voluntary, worldwide fellowship of men and women from all walks of life who meet together to attain and maintain sobriety. The only requirement for membership is a desire to stop drinking. Similar fellowships exist for gambling (GA), narcotics abuse (NA), spouses of alcoholics (Al-Anon) and the children of alcoholics (Alateen). AA and similar self-help groups follow twelve steps that alcoholics should work through during recovery. This free programme is particularly supportive for those who are isolated or lonely, or who come from a heavy drinking social background.

Cognitive Behaviour Therapy (CBT)

A large multi-site study, Project MATCH, found that there was no difference in the efficacy of CBT, motivational enhancement treatment (MET) and twelve-step facilitation (TSF) during the year following treatment: however, MET was found to be most effective in those patients with high levels of anger, and TSF and AA involvement was particularly effective in patients from a heavy drinking social environment (Project MATCH 1997).

Methadone Treatment Programmes

Withdrawal from opiate use is normally treated with methadone. Methadone can be prescribed under a strict protocol as a maintenance (potentially lifelong) programme for opiate users. Figure 19.6 outlines the methadone dosage threshold for users of this drug.

Figure 19.6 Methadone dosage threshold

Methadone Dosage Threshold	Potential Recipients	Rationale
Low	Regular low dosage for pre-contemplative to contemplative stage. Administered under supervision with harm reduction input aimed at engaging user in regular treatment	Some tolerance by the treatment providers of continued use during this stage of treatment. Objective is to encourage the drug user to engage in harm reduction and reduce the harmful consequences of drug use
Medium	Regular prescription administered under supervision with harm reduction interventions aimed at enabling user to stabilise and regularise daily life and improve general health status	There is recognition that stabilisation may take a period of time and has to keep pace with drug user's ability to change. Occasional slips are tolerated and the user is encouraged to examine each slip and make significant lifestyle changes
High	Regular dosage for committed abstainers from illicit substances, administered under supervision. Social and psychological supports available on individualised bases. May include self-administration	At this level the drug user is expected to remain drug-free: continued use of drugs may result in treatment regime being terminated

Motivational Interviewing

Motivational interviewing is an effective strategy for engaging and treating patients. It is defined as a client-centred directive method for enhancing intrinsic motivation to change by exploring and resolving ambivalence (Miller and Rollnick 2002). Interventions designed to increase motivation among substance abusers, such as motivational enhancement therapy, may be helpful in reducing early drop-out from treatment. This includes directly addressing discomfort with disclosure as well as encouraging gradual disclosure that begins with more comfortable, less threatening discussion topics. There are four basic principles:

1. Expressing empathy — this involves communicating acceptance and understanding.
2. Develop discrepancy — enabling the person to discern whether there is discrepancy between their goals and their behaviour.
3. Roll with resistance — the mental health worker has to accept resistance as natural and assist the individual in overcoming ambivalence.
4. Support self-efficacy — this involves expressing the belief to the substance abuser that they have the ability to change and supporting them in this belief.

The harm reduction model and motivational interviewing fit together, allowing the mental health worker to develop a consistent approach based on a careful assessment of the individual which helps to gain an understanding of where they are in relation to the trans-theoretical five-stage model of change (Prochaska *et al.* 1992).

ALTERNATIVE APPROACHES TO TREATMENT

The harm reduction model in relation to opiate use includes some controversial approaches to treatment which are not currently part of the services provided in Ireland for addiction.

Drug Consumption Rooms

This normally refers to supervised safe drug-taking facilities for the administration of drugs, which are provided by statutory or state-recognised agencies. Supervision is provided by trained staff operating as part of a multidisciplinary team. They aim to reduce harm for both the drug user and the wider community. The goals of harm reduction are achieved by supervising injections in a controlled setting, ensuring safety and quick responses to overdoses, providing sterile injecting equipment and condoms, collecting used needles and syringes and providing counselling and primary health care. Safe injecting facilities use a humanitarian approach and function on a background of medical ethics: reducing mortality, reducing morbidity, alleviating suffering and trying not to damage the patient by the measures taken (Haemmig 2003).

Naloxone Provision

Every year two per cent of people who inject heroin die, which is six to twenty times the rate expected in peer controls of those who do not use drugs (Sporer 2003). Some jurisdictions have introduced naloxone, a specific opiate antagonist, as a harm reduction measure. Naloxone has been sold over the counter in Italy for more than ten years and has been distributed through needle exchange programmes since 1995 (Simini 1998).

Heroin Provision

Pharmaceutical heroin (diamorphine) provision has been considered and trialled as a treatment approach to injecting drug users. It attracts people who might not otherwise be inclined into treatment, reducing illicit drug use, undercutting the black market and protecting the physical health and social functioning of the injecting drug users.

TREATMENT SETTINGS

Addictions can be treated in a variety of treatment settings (see Figure 19.7). Decisions about the most appropriate setting for an individual should be based on a thorough needs assessment; however, the setting available may be dictated by the geographic location of the individual.

Figure 19.7 Treatment settings for addiction

Setting	Service Available
GP	Detoxification, health screening, pharmacological interventions and supportive therapy
Primary care	Health screening, assessment, health education
Mental health OPD	Screening, mental health assessment, outpatient detoxification, supportive counselling
Home care team	Home detoxification programme, mental health screening, supportive counselling
In-patient acute unit	Detoxification, mental health screening, treatment of co-morbid conditions, supportive counselling
Addition treatment unit	Individual and group psychotherapy
Drug addiction services – outpatient	Screening, methadone maintance programmes, harm reduction programmes, supportive counselling
Drug addiction services – residential	Detoxification, group and individual therapy, life and work skills rehabilitation programmes
Therapeutic community	Residential care, supportive therapy, life skills training
Private services	Group and individual psychotherapy in residential and non-residential settings
Voluntary services	Harm reduction services, support for homelessness, screening for infectious diseases, supportive therapy in group and individual settings both residential and non-residential Various grades of hostel and residential support are available depending on whether the individual is currently clean and sober or using
Fellowships	12-step programmes

RECOVERY

Recovery is a process that enables the former substance user to rebuild their lives and regain independence. The recovery process can be both long and arduous, involving numerous attempts at treatment before a successful change is achieved. The following characteristics are common to most treatment programmes. However, all treatment programmes tend to have individual characteristics and one element of the whole package may be given stronger emphasis than another.

- Experienced, qualified professional staff.
- Flexible arrangements for in-patient and outpatient appointments.
- Assessment and treatment for medical impact of substance abuse — may be provided by an off-site agency.

- Engagement of concerned persons in the treatment process, e.g. partners, family members, friends or employers.
- A broad team of heath professionals, which may include outreach workers, nurses, doctors, social workers, educators, psychologists, pharmacists and psychotherapists.
- Flexible approaches to treatment including individual, couple and group options.
- Encouragement and access to engage in peer support and twelve-step fellowships.
- Quick and easy access to relapse prevention and aftercare support groups.
- Commitment to research, training and development.

CONCLUSION

Substance abuse is a relatively common health and social problem in Ireland and one with which the mental health nurse will be familiar from a variety of settings. Although new mental health legislation discourages the in-patient treatment of addiction on an involuntary basis, the co-existence of addiction with mental health problems in the form of dual diagnoses results in many clients with substance abuse being treated in mental health settings. As a result, it is imperative that the mental health nurses develop the skills and expertise to care for this client group and to work therapeutically with them.

Reflective Questions
1. Using the chart of addiction treatment approaches, discuss the approach mostly likely to be successful in changing attitudes towards substance abuse.
2. With reference to your experience, make a list of the positive and negative experiences that substance use has had on your life.
3. List and describe the services for substance abuse that have been available to mental health service users in your clinical practice areas.
4. If you were the Minister of Health and Children what services would you introduce for managing and treating substance use in Ireland?

Useful Websites
www.drugsalcohol.info
www.dancesafe.org
www.nida.nih.gov
www.hrb.ie
www.drugscope.org.uk
www.alcoholconcern.org.uk
www.nacd.ie
www.forward-thinking-on-drugs.org

References

American Psychiatric Association (1994) *Diagnostic and Statistical Manual of Mental Disorders* (4th edn). Washington DC: APA.

American Psychiatric Association (APA) (2000) *Diagnostic and Statistical Manual of Mental Disorders* (DSM-IV-TR) (4th edn: text revision). Washington DC: APA.

American Psychiatric Association (2002), www.aafp.org/afp/20020201/441.html, downloaded 6 June 2007.

Anton, R. F., Moak, D. H., Waid, L. R, Latham, P. K., Malcolm, R. J. and Dias, J. K. (1999) 'Naltrexone and cognitive behavioural therapy for the treatment of outpatient alcoholics: results of a placebo-controlled trial'. *American Journal of Psychiatry*, 156, 1758–64.

Babor, T., De la Fuente, J., Saunders, J. and Grant, M. (1989) *AUDIT, The Alcohol Use Disorder Identification Test: Guidelines for Use in Primary Care.* Geneva: World Health Organisation.

Chick, J., Gough, K., Falkowski, W., Kershaw, P. Hore, B. and Mehta, B. (1992) 'Disulfiram treatment of alcoholism'. *British Journal of Psychiatry*, 161, 84–9.

Daly, A. and Walsh, D. (2006) *Irish Psychiatric Units and Hospital Census 2006.* Dublin: Health Research Board.

Daly, A., Walsh, D., Ward, M., and Moran, R. (2006) *Activities of Irish Psychiatric Units and Hospital 2005.* Dublin: Health Research Board.

Department of Health and Children (DoHC) (2002) *Interim Report of the Strategic Task Force on Alcohol.* Dublin: Stationery Office.

Donatella, R. J. (2006) *Access to Health* (9th edn). San Francisco: Pearson Education.

Finney, J. W., Hahn, A. C. and Moos, R. H. (1996) 'The effectiveness of inpatient and outpatient alcohol abuse: the need to focus on mediators and moderators of setting effects'. *Addiction*, 91, 1773–96.

Government of Ireland (1982) *Planning for the Future.* Dublin: Stationery Office.

Haemmig, R. B. (2003) 'Re: What would constitute failure then?' *British Medical Journal*, http://bmj.com/cgi/eletters/327/7407/122-a.

King, M. (1986) 'At risk drinking among general practice attenders: validation of the cage questionnaire'. *Psychological Medicine*, 16, 213–17.

Marsden, J., Gossop, M., Stewart, D., Best, D., Farrell, M., Lehman, P., Edwards, C. and Strang, J.(1998) 'The Maudsley Addiction Profile (MAP): A brief instrument for assessing treatment outcomes'. *Addiction*, 93, 1857–67.

McLellan, T., Luborsky, L., Cacciola, J., and Fuerman, I. (1992) 'The fifth edition of the Addiction Severity Index: cautions additions and normative data'. *Journal of Substance Abuse Treatment*, 9, 461–80.

Miller, W. R. and Rollnick, S. (2002) *Motivational Interviewing: Preparing People to Change Addictive Behaviour* (2nd edn). New York: Guilford Press.

Moore, G., McCarthy, P., MacNeela, P., MacGabhann, L., Philbin, M. and Proudfoot, D. (2004) *A Review of Harm Reduction Approaches in Ireland and Evidence from the International Literature.* Dublin: Stationery

Office/National Advisory Committee on Drugs.

Moore, P. (2007) *An Exploratory Study of Young Offenders' Views Concerning Drugs, Crime and Drug Policy.* Lisbon: European Monitoring Centre for Drugs and Drug Addiction.

O'Malley, S. S. (1996). 'Opioid antagonists in the treatment of alcohol dependence: clinical efficacy and prevention of relapse'. *Alcohol Supplement,* 1, 77–81.

Prochaska, J. O., Di Clemente, C. C. and Norcross, J. C. (1992) 'In search of how people change: applications to addictive behaviours'. *American Psychologist,* 47(9), 1102–14.

Project MATCH (1997) 'Secondary a priori hypotheses. Project MATCH Research Group'. *Addiction,* 92, 1671–98.

Qureshi, N. A., Al-Ghamdy, Y. S., and Al-Habeeb, T. A. (2000) 'Drug addiction: a general review of new concepts and future challenges'. *Eastern Mediterranean Health Journal,* 6(4), 273–733.

Riastrick, D., Bradshaw, J., Tober, G., Weiner, J., Allison, J. and Healey, C. (1994) 'Development of the Leeds Dependency Questionnaire (LDQ): a questionnaire to measure alcohol and opiate dependence in the context of a treatment evaluation package'. *Addiction,* 89, 563–72.

Sass, H., Soyka, M., Mann, K. and Zieglgansberger, W. (1996) 'Relapse prevention by acamprosate. Results from a placebo-controlled study on alcohol dependence'. *Archives of General Psychiatry,* 53, 673–80.

Selzer, M. (1971) 'The Michigan alcoholism screening test'. *American Journal of Psychiatry,* 127, 1653–8.

Simini, B. (1998). 'Naloxone supplied to Italian heroin addicts'. *Lancet,* 352, 967.

Sporer, K. A. (2003) 'Strategies for preventing heroin overdose'. *British Medical Journal,* 326, 442–4.

Stockwell, T., Murphy, D., and Hodgson, R. (1983) 'The severity of alcohol dependency questionnaire: its uses, reliability and validity'. *British Journal of Addiction,* 78, 145–55.

World Health Organisation (WHO) (1992) *The ICD-10 Classification of Mental and Behavioural Disorders. Clinical Descriptions and Diagnostic Guidelines.* Geneva: WHO.

World Health Organisation (2007), www.who.int/substance_abuse/terminology/who_lexicon/en/, downloaded 8 June 2007.

20

Aggression and Violence in Mental Health/Psychiatric Services

Seamus Cowman

The increased concern among employees, employers and professional organisations over the escalation in violence and aggression has created an urgent requirement for all nurses and other employees to be aware of hospital policy and procedures for safety and security and the management of violence across mental health services.

In mental health services, violence and assaultive behaviour is manifested in many different directions including: patient violence and assault on staff; patient violence and assault on other more vulnerable patients; violence and assault from outsiders; patient violence towards visitors and the public generally. Prevention of violence through adequate measures in safety and security serve as the root of nursing practice in the management of patients with violent and aggressive behaviour in mental health care settings. An Irish-based study by Cowman and Walsh (2004) reported on less than favourable conditions, the prevailing situation being that psychiatric nurses must continue to provide nursing services in the absence of standardised approaches to safety and security policy and procedure on wards.

This chapter will present the widest possible view of mental health workplace violence and its management. Specifically, the aims of the chapter are to review and define violence and related concepts. Matters related to safety and security in psychiatric services will be explored, with some broad direction given to nurses. Organisational culture and other issues of direct importance to nursing in the mental healthcare setting will also be discussed. Finally, the chapter will discuss principles, procedures and care in the management of violent incidents.

VIOLENCE AS A PROBLEM IN MENTAL HEALTH SERVICES

The extensive range of international literature and data from health service bodies has described the exposure of healthcare staff to patient violence in the workplace. The United States Department of Labor (1998) reported that more assaults occur among healthcare and social services workers than in any other sector. A great concern expressed in many reports, including the Department of Labor (1998) and the North Eastern Health Board (NEHB 2004), is the likely under-reporting of violence and a persistent perception within the health sector that assaults are part of the job for employees of mental health services.

In the UK, as far back as 1987 the Health Services Advisory Committee reported that 11 per cent of National Health Service (NHS) staff had been assaulted resulting in major injury. The NHS Health and Safety Executive described nursing as Britain's most dangerous profession (Gould 2000). In Ireland, the Advisory Committee on Health Services highlighted that the number of assaults against staff in the health and social work category had more than trebled between 1994 and 1999 (HSA 2001). Assaults as a percentage of all accidents and injuries had increased from eight per cent in 1994 to 17 per cent in 1999.

In Ireland a large-scale interdisciplinary study conducted by the North Eastern Health Board described the extent of work-related violence (NEHB 2004). The study reported that work-related violence is a highly complex and serious problem for health services and has a significant impact on many functional aspects of the organisation. The study indicated that a violent episode impacts heavily on the life of an individual at many levels. At a professional level it damages the therapeutic milieu and at an organisational level the cost of staff sickness due to violence impacts heavily on the health service finances. A significant finding was the lack of a unified and agreed approach to the management of violence and the inadequate and inappropriate provision of training.

DEFINITION OF VIOLENCE AND RELATED CONCEPTS

One of the major limitations encountered in the literature on work-related violence is the lack of a universally agreed definition of violence and aggression. It has been suggested that in the UK health services more than twenty different definitions of work-related violence are currently used (National Audit Office 2003). Definitions of a violent act also vary, with some studies concentrating exclusively on physical acts of violence (Walker and Seifert 1994) and others including verbal abuse and threats (Graydon *et al.* 1994).

Generally, dictionary definitions describe aggression as a forceful action or procedure, especially when intended to dominate or master, and as hostile, injurious or destructive behaviour or outlook. Violence is described in stronger terms as the exercise of physical force so as to inflict injury on, or cause damage to, persons or property, treatment or usage tending to cause bodily injury or forcibly interfering with personal freedom. It may be concluded that by definition violence is synonymous with aggression and they will be treated as synonymous in this chapter.

Perhaps the most significant and important definition to note is that of the Health and Safety Authority (1992). The HSA broadly discussed violence in terms of physical assault, threat and verbal abuse and this provides a useful baseline for considering violence and aggression in mental health services (Figure 20.1).

Figure 20.1 Categorisation of violence and aggression

Category	Example
Physical assault	Use of weapon, kicking, pushing, slapping, pinching
Threat	Warning of intent to injure, physical intimidation
Verbal abuse	Abusive/offensive language, obscene comments

Source: HSA (1992)

Safety and security is inextricably linked to the study of violence. Safe and secure environments are the first step in combating the problem of violence in healthcare and very much support the old adage that prevention is better than cure. In the aftermath and review of a violent incident it is often identified that safety and security measures were inappropriate, ineffective or not commensurate with the likely threats posed in caring for patients in the acute phase of a mental illness.

The approach to safety and security measures that is adopted is most likely determined by the type of mental health services provided. The strictest measures in safety and security are to be found in the forensic and acute mental health settings, with more relaxed approaches outside these settings. This means that standards in safety and security and best practice approaches across mental health services are ill defined. There is wide variation across mental health services regarding levels of physical security, inappropriate placement and patient mix. Kennedy (2002) discussed safety and security and defined it in three main contexts: environmental; relational; and procedural (Figure 20.2).

Figure 20.2 Definitions and concepts in safety and security

Environmental Safety and Security	Design and maintenance of estate and fittings Building access CCTV, alarms, mobile phones
Relational Safety and Security	Quantitative: staff–patient ratios Qualitative: quality of care, therapeutic regimes
Procedural Safety and Security	Policy and procedure Patient level: systems and routines for checking and searching System levels: arrangements for risk management, professional governance, audit, training

Source: Kennedy (2002)

In Ireland, the HSA (2001) has suggested that organisations in the health sector:
- review work practices and procedures and what precautions are in place
- evaluate the type of security presence to provide a deterrent and protection for staff

- evaluate the requirements for devices such as alarms (personal and general), surveillance (CCTV), mobile phones, two-way radios and panic buttons.

CATEGORISING PATIENT VIOLENCE

There is general agreement in the literature that there are certain factors associated with violent behaviour. A useful classification is provided by Jansen (2005), who categorises the factors associated with patient violence into three main areas: patient issues; staff issues; and environmental issues.

Patient Issues

Many diverse issues have been reported, including biological issues, gender, age, social and economic status and psychopathology. The biological issues highlighted chiefly include heredity, hormonal effects (testosterone) and the limbic system and cerebral cortex. Research on the neurobiology of aggression has shown that different types of aggression are controlled by different subsets of brain structures within the limbic system, for example the septum and the hypothalamus. Anger was also shown to be associated with activation of the left orbit frontal cortex (Dougherty et al. 1999). It is noted that gender studies are inconclusive, with some studies reporting no differences between men and women (Lam et al. 2000). Some studies show that younger in-patients commit more assaults (Whittington et al. 1996).

The potential for psychotic patients to exhibit violent behaviour is greatest during the acute phase of the illness (Daffern and Howells 2002). Steinert et al. (1999), in a study of patients with a first episode of schizophrenia or schizo-affective disorder reported that 75 per cent of men and 53 per cent of women exhibited some type of aggressive behaviour. More recently a review study by Walsh et al. (2002) reported a significant association between violence and schizophrenia.

Staff issues

A lack of training or inappropriate training and low staff to patient ratios are the main staff issues that increase the threat of violent behaviour. There has been a plethora of studies over many years highlighting the positive effects of staff training in violence management, e.g. Paterson et al. (1992), and Whittington and Wykes (1996). Over fifteen years ago it was reported that skilful clinical management training will reduce the number of assaults on staff and diminish the severity of any injuries resulting from such assaults (Carmel and Hunter 1990). More recently, authoritative bodies such as the UK's National Audit Office (2003) recommended that each employer conduct a training needs analysis and that training should be relevant to the risk management and clinical concerns of those being trained. Similarly in Ireland the HSA (2001), in promoting staff safety and security, concluded that there is a clear need for the availability of authoritative advice on best practice in training staff to deal with aggression and violence.

Environmental Issues

Studies show that most violent incidents occur during the day, with most assaults occurring at mealtimes and early in the afternoon (Bradley *et al.* 2001). It has also been shown that most assaults take place during the first three days after admission to hospital (Barlow *et al.* 2000). Most violent incidents on acute admission wards were reported as occurring on a Monday and the fewest on a Friday, and the most common locations were the ward corridor and day room, the nurses' station and outside the locked door where interaction between patients and staff takes place (Nijman 1999). Overcrowding and occupancy levels have positively correlated with violent incidents (Bradley *et al.* 2001; Kumar and Bradley 2001), with the explanation being density, lack of privacy and control over work environment and related social environment.

COMBATING THE PROBLEM OF VIOLENCE

The Department of Health (UK) (2000) produced a report on safety in high-security hospitals and suggested that patients be locked in their rooms at night because of lapses in security and the wide availability of pornography and illicit drugs. The USA has initiated very specific proactive measures to combat violence and promote safety and security. In some states of the US mental health security technicians are employed to promote safer environments for care. The duties and responsibilities of the security technician encompass elements of safety and security including: behaviour management; observing patients for potential violence or socially destructive behaviour, with intervention as required; security monitoring and control; emergency response co-ordination; and transportation of patients.

In contrast to the USA, in many EU countries (including Ireland) mental health professionals are required to take more confrontational approaches with patients and clients. The responsibility for security monitoring and control also lies with mental health care staff.

In the UK the National Institute of Clinical Excellence has produced guidelines for effective prevention and short-term management of violence in adult psychiatric inpatient settings and emergency departments (NICE 2005). The recommendations contained in the NICE guidelines as best practice are based on the best available evidence and can make a significant contribution towards ensuring safe and secure environments in mental health services.

RISK ASSESSMENT

The assessment of risk is a vital element in the cycle of violence management in mental health settings. The process of risk assessment must be ongoing and requires frequent review and upgrading. The availability of actuarial data enriches the process of risk assessment. For example, sometimes in the clinical setting a patient may be a cause of anxiety and concern to staff who may estimate a potential for violent behaviour. Actuarial measures and their data refer to instruments or statistics based on what is known about violent or harmful behaviour. Therefore, using previous case examples, we can examine the distribution, characteristics, influencing variables and outcomes of previous violent behaviours (Monaghan *et al.* 2001). The HRC-20 (Webster *et al.* 1997) is an example of a good multidisciplinary risk assessment framework that guides the collection of information pertinent to the risk of violence.

Jones and Plowman (2005) highlight the importance of a full and detailed history of the individual being assessed and suggest a minimum amount of information on which to begin to base a risk assessment. Such information includes:

- Family history — quality of relationship with parents and other significant childhood experiences.
- Educational history — adaptation to his/her educational environment.
- Occupational history — experience of employment.
- Relationship history — experience of intimate relationships through adolescence and adulthood.
- Psychiatric history — contacts with mental health services.
- Substance abuse history — the relationship between substance abuse and violence should be established.
- Forensic history — any previous arrests, charges or convictions.

Prediction and, at the very least, anticipation of psychiatric patients who are likely to be violent must be a central working philosophy of any acute psychiatric service (Blumenthal and Lavender 2000). Risk assessment is therefore an essential activity in ensuring safe environments for staff and patients. The creation of safe and secure environments is heavily dependent upon mental health professionals having well-developed skills in clinical reasoning and decision-making. In mental health the process of decision-making is determined as being enormously complex, and decisions sometimes have to be made rapidly in stressful clinical circumstances. It is important to note that expert nurses rely extensively on their personal knowledge and experience and it has been reported that the better that nurses felt they knew the patient, the lower the level of subjective risk reported (Trenoweth 2003).

PROSECUTION OF PATIENTS

Zero tolerance to workplace violence and aggression has emerged in contemporary health services policy and mental health discourse. It has gained widespread support because its emphasis and stance is acceptable. Whittington (2002) reviews the concept of zero tolerance and identifies a number of inherent problems. There is a lack of clarity in defining the problem behaviour of violence. It may also be the case that implementing a zero tolerance approach in mental health services may disturb the subtle balance that needs to be struck in deciding what is acceptable staff and patient behaviour in any healthcare interaction. In mental health services a sudden move from what has traditionally been a lax attitude (violence accepted as part of the job) to one of zero tolerance may raise serious tensions and hostilities that leads to further confrontation.

The amount of interest and number of publications on the prediction and management of violence is not matched by a similar emphasis on systematically reporting assaults to the police or assault being followed by prosecution of the assailant (Coyne 2002). In recent years the involvement of the police and law enforcement agencies has played an increasingly important role in the management of people with mental illness. This in the major part has arisen from a policy of deinstitutionalisation in the care and management of persons with a mental illness and a policy of normalisation, integration and community care. The primary purpose of police intervention in the lives of persons with a mental illness most often arises from the power and authority of the police to protect the safety and welfare of the community. The initial role of the police can be to transport persons for psychiatric evaluation and treatment when the individual may be a danger to themselves or others. A violent act or the likelihood of violence underlines the majority of psychiatric emergencies involving the police.

It has been suggested (Turnbull 1999) that the public have learned that assaulting doctors, nurses and other healthcare staff brings few punishments or sanctions, unlike, for example, assaulting a member of the police. Therefore safety and security in mental health services is further undermined by creating the false impression that if patients' crimes are ignored these patients are justified in believing that their conduct is acceptable. It has also been reported that a small proportion of patients are responsible for a large percentage of the violence that occurs (Convit *et al.* 1990). Unfortunately the strongly held view among healthcare professionals that violence is an occupational hazard in mental healthcare and that staff in this field should expect to be assaulted tends to exclude the notion of police prosecution in more situations of violence.

CLINICAL NURSING ENVIRONMENTS

Changing health policy has also impacted on the role of mental healthcare professionals. With the change of emphasis from institutional care to community care the traditional role of the psychiatric nurse is moving from one of custodian to therapist (Cowman *et al.* 2001). However, it is also the case that the culture of admission wards has changed. Sanders *et al.* (2000) investigated aggression among psychiatric admissions (n = 199) and identified that almost a quarter of patients admitted reported thoughts of violence directed at specific individuals. Nearly one in ten patients owned a weapon and one in twenty admitted to carrying one. Ryrie and McGowan (1998) highlighted the illicit use of drugs among psychiatric in-patients as a major security issue.

Staff safety and security must be a key concern of all mental health service providers. Bowers *et al.* (2002) demonstrated wide-scale variation in safety measures and security features across acute admission wards in a London survey. Cowman and Walsh (2004) undertook a study of all acute admission psychiatric wards in the Republic of Ireland and identified great variation between hospitals, with no overall policy or agreement on best practice in terms of safety and security. This study also reported on a lack of standardised security measures at the entrance to hospital wards and the limited access to security guards suggested that nurses were expected to adopt more confrontational roles during episodes of violence.

The Royal College of Psychiatrists (UK) (2000) published guidelines on appropriate general layout and structure of the clinical environment. The guidelines proposed that in managing and providing care to psychiatric patients the following areas should be considered:

- Access to privacy — telephones, toilets, showers, privacy for conversations with visitors and friends.
- Access to spacious facilities — confrontations may result from cramped conditions.
- Access to open spaces and fresh air — patients being able to leave the ward.
- Making the clinical setting more 'homely' — access to television, having a wardrobe/locker, access to private telephones.

Other important clinical environmental factors to be considered in combating patient violence were boredom, lack of therapy and social groups. The infrastructure was highly significant in ensuring a safe environment, e.g. entrances and exits in sight of staff, accessible exit doors, moveable objects being of a safe weight, size and construction.

The National Patient Safety Agency (NPSA) which was established in the UK in 2001 has introduced a national reporting and learning system for adverse events across the National Health Service in England and Wales. The reporting system, which is electronic, collects structured and unstructured data about patient safety incidents and has now been incorporated into local risk management systems. There are positive reports on the introduction of the reporting system, in particular its effects in reducing a culture of blame that has permeated mental health services.

The Royal College of Psychiatrists (1999) provided advice and guidelines to individual medical staff and trainees on establishing a culture of personal safety in clinical practice. The advice and guidelines included a number of useful practical suggestions such as:

- Preserving personal privacy through not divulging home address, telephone number or personal information to patients.
- Personal appearance that engenders confidence and trust: expensive, flamboyant or sexually provocative clothing may be misinterpreted by a patient.
- Clothing should not be tight in case the staff member has to move quickly.
- Scarves, long hair and loose items of clothing should be avoided.
- Isolation should always be avoided; familiarity with the emergency alarm system is also essential.
- At night staff should avoid walking in poorly lit, isolated areas either inside or outside buildings.
- Staff should not be expected to make assessments alone in an emergency situation or at night.

- Always assess the level of security and avoid situations that compromise safety.
- A personal alarm should be worn and care should also be taken when conducting an interview — where possible other members of staff should be present.
- If the staff cannot control a disturbance the police should be called without delay.

KEY PRINCIPLES IN MANAGING VIOLENCE AND AGGRESSION

Aggressive and violent behaviour may develop gradually or occur suddenly in a patient who is psychotic or intoxicated. Some signs that a client may become violent include restlessness, increasing tension, agitation, making threats and verbal abuse. In managing such a situation safety is paramount. The basic aim of care in such a situation is to protect the client and others from harm and to provide a safe and non-threatening environment. Helping the client to express feelings in a non-violent way is also a very important therapeutic aim.

There is little agreement on best practice in the management of patients who exhibit violent behaviour. International practice is wide and varied and includes tranquillisation medication, physical restraints and seclusion. Seclusion is a long-standing practice, used since the foundation of psychiatry as a branch of medicine. Nursing has played a central role in seclusion and this is well documented by Maguire (2002). Preventing episodes of violence and the de-escalation and management of potentially violent situations is a fundamentally important nursing role that can impact positively on reducing episodes of violence and aggression in the clinical area.

De-escalation is constantly used by nurses in daily practice and all nurses should know how to perform de-escalation. Cowin *et al.* (2003) describe de-escalation as a gradual resolution of a potentially violent/aggressive situation through the use of verbal and physical expression, empathy, alliance and non-confrontational limit-setting that is based on respect.

The key principles of care in the management of violence and aggression may be considered in terms of pre-incident, peri-incident and post-incident perspectives.

Pre-incident Perspective
- Building a trusting relationship with the patient well in advance of any outbursts of violence. This can help communication and allay patient anxieties.
- Being aware of factors that increase the likelihood of agitation or violent behaviour. Identify signs of impending violence (A, B, C).
  A = antecedents — what is happening in the environment prior to the incident. Factors such as patient agitation, pacing, verbal abuse, threatening behaviour, mistrust of staff, withdrawal.
  B = behaviour — changed behaviour often indicates a period of rising tension.
  C = consequences — awareness of the consequences for the individual client, staff and organisation. Actions may include possible physical interventions, restraint, seclusion, medication and police involvement.

Peri-incident Perspective

- Remain calm and reassure the patient that support is available and that you can provide control if he/she cannot control themselves. The patient may fear loss of control and may be afraid of what he/she may do if they begin to express anger. Give personal space and allow expression of feeling in an emphatic way.
- Avoid arguing or contradicting the patient's comments and do not take verbal abuse personally.
- Assess the risk of personal safety, assess the environment and identify escape routes. Do not confine the patient to a narrow space. Be aware of the patient's territory and within safe limits allow them to move around.
- Always maintain control of yourself and the situation and remain calm. If you do not feel competent seek assistance and do not attempt to use physical techniques unless you have received the appropriate training.
- Be aware and familiar with PRN medications and policies for seclusion and control/restraint. In an emergency situation of violence you may have to act quickly.
- Always speak in a low, calm voice, addressing the patient by name, and keep them informed of your actions at all times. Use simple and direct speech, display confidence and if necessary state limits and expectations. Assertive and directive statements can be effective when used by skilled and appropriately trained staff.
- Decrease stimulation by turning the television or radio off and lowering the lights if possible. Reduce the numbers of people in the vicinity; if a patient feels threatened he/she may perceive any stimulus as a threat.
- When a decision to restrain or sedate the patient has been made, act quickly, work in accordance with the agreed policy and procedure and co-ordinate the process to which people have been trained.
- At all times talk to the patient. Never strike or subdue the patient as punishment.
- Be aware that de-escalation does not work in all cases, especially those complicated by alcohol or drugs, hallucinations and delusions.
- An experienced qualified member of staff should take control of a potentially escalating situation.
- If restraining the patient or placing him/her in seclusion, explain to the patient what you are doing and the reason and reassure him/her that they will be safe and that they will be checked regularly.
- If placed in seclusion the patient should be nursed in accordance with institutional policy. Regularly reassess the patient's needs for continued seclusion or restraint and release the client as soon as it is safe and therapeutic.

Post-incident Perspective

- Principles of personal safety and security are combined with debriefing after the incident. Stress reduction, reporting documentation and resumption of normal therapeutic activities with the patient are important post-incident considerations.

- Victims of aggression/violence must talk about their experience with a suitably qualified person, other staff and colleagues.
- Reflect on the event — what happened? Who was involved? What feeling/emotions, strengths/weaknesses were associated with the event and what was learned?
- Documentation and reporting post-incident:
  1. Be aware of local clinical reporting system. Under-reporting puts people at risk.
  2. The protocol usually requires the recording of information relating to: who was involved; where it happened; what action was taken to de-escalate the situation; if anybody was injured; what was the outcome.
- Assess requirements and options for further training/support.
- Be aware of how one's own actions/attitudes/values influenced the patient.
- Do not reject the patient as a person and re-engage with the patient in normal activity programmes as soon as possible.

CONCLUSION

Given the increased concerns among employers, employees and professional organisations over the escalation in workplace violence there is an urgent requirement for strong direction on the management of violence and aggression in mental health services. The consolidation and regularisation of safety and security procedures is essential to the creation of stable mental health care settings that are safe and secure for patients and staff and that espouse a therapeutic milieu.

The publication of position papers and guidelines on the management of violence and aggression, including safety and security measures, will inform and direct employers and appropriate professional bodies. The establishment of national directives on risk assessment and violence management is essential to workplace violence. Psychiatric nursing is now practised in more open environments than was traditionally the case when the majority of psychiatric nurses worked in large mental hospitals. The education and training of psychiatric nurses must ensure appropriate preparation to maximise the competence of nurses in dealing with potentially violent patients in the new environments of care. Nurses must be knowledgeable about policy and procedure and the importance of adherence to policy and procedure in managing episodes of violence cannot be over-emphasised.

Reflective Questions
1. Discuss the importance of safety and security in the prevention of violence.
2. What is the key role of the nurse in the management of a violent episode?
3. What are the measures available to mental health professionals in combating the escalating level of violence in mental health services?

4. What are the factors associated with violent and aggressive behaviour in mental health? Make particular reference to:
- patient issues
- staff issues
- environmental issues.

References

Barlow, K., Grenyer B. and Ilkia-Lavalle, O. (2000) 'Prevalence and precipitants of aggression in psychiatric inpatient units'. *Australian and New Zealand Journal of Psychiatry*, 34, 967–74.

Blumenthel, S. and Lavender T. (2000) *Violence and Mental Disorder: A Critical Aid to the Assessment and Management of Risk*, New York: Jessica Kingsley.

Bowers, L., Crowhurst, N., Alexander, J., Callaghan, P., Eales, S., Guy, S., McCann, E. and Ryan, C. (2002) 'Safety and security policies on psychiatric acute admission wards: results from a London-wide survey'. *Journal of Psychiatric and Mental Health Nursing*, 9, 427–33.

Bradley, N., Kumar, S., Ranclaud, M. and Robinson, E. (2001) 'Ward crowding and incidents of violence on an acute psychiatric inpatient unit'. *Psychiatric Services*, 52, 521–5.

Carmel, H. and Hunter, M. (1990) 'Compliance with training in managing assaultive behaviour and injuries from inpatient violence'. *Hospital and Community Psychiatry*, 41(5), 558–60.

Convit, A., Isay, D., Otis, D. and Volavka, J. (1990) 'Characteristics of repeatedly assaultive psychiatric inpatients'. *Hospital and Community Psychiatry*, 41: 1112–15.

Cowin, L., Davies, R., Estall, G., Berlin, T., Fitzgerald, M. and Hoot, S. (2003) 'De-escalating aggression and violence in the mental health setting'. *International Journal of Mental Health Nursing*, 12(1), 64–73.

Cowman S., Farrelly, M. and Gilheaney, P. (2001) 'An examination of the role and function of the psychiatric nurse in clinical practice'. *Journal of Advanced Nursing*, 34(6).

Cowman, S. and Walsh, J. (2004) 'Safety and security procedures in psychiatric acute admission wards'. *Nursing Times Research*, 9(3), 185–93.

Coyne, A. (2002) 'Should patients who assault staff be prosecuted?' *Journal of Psychiatric and Mental Health Nursing*, 9, 139–45.

Daffern, M. and Howells, K. (2002) 'Psychiatric inpatient aggression: A review of structural and functional assessment approaches'. *Aggression and Violent Behaviour*, 7, 477–97.

Department of Health (UK) (2000) *Report of the Review of Security at the High Security Hospital*. London: HMSO.

Department of Labor (USA) (1998). 'Guidelines for preventing workplace violence for healthcare service workers'. Washington DC: OSHA 348.

Dougherty, D., Shin, L., Alpert, N., Pitman, R., Orr, S., Lasko, M., Macklin, M., Fishman, A. and Rauch, S. (1999) 'Anger in health men: a PET study using script driven imagery'. *Biological Psychiatry*, 46 (4), 466–72.

Gould, D. (2000) 'Security alert'. *Nursing Times*, 96, 26–8.

Graydon, J., Kasta, W. and Khan, P. (1994) 'Verbal and physical abuse of nurses'. *Canadian Journal of Nursing Administration*, 7, 89.

Health and Safety Authority (HSA) (1992) *Report of the Advisory Committee on Health Services Sector to the Health and Safety Authority*. Dublin: Health and Safety Authority.

Health and Safety Authority (HSA) (2001) *Report of the Advisory Committee on Health Services Sector to the Health and Safety Authority*. Dublin: Health and Safety Authority.

Jansen, G. (2005) 'The attitudes of nurses towards inpatient aggression in psychiatric care' (PhD dissertation). University of Groningen.

Jones, J. and Plowman, C. (2005) 'Risk assessment: a multidisciplinary approach to estimating harmful behaviour in mentally disordered offenders', in S. Wix and M. Humphries, *Multidisciplinary Working in Forensic Mental Health Care*. Oxford: Elsevier Churchill Livingstone.

Kennedy, H. G. (2002) 'Therapeutic uses of security: mapping forensic mental health services by stratifying risk'. *Advances in Psychiatric Treatment*, 8, 433–43.

Kumar, S. and Bradley, Ng (2001) 'Overcrowding and violence on psychiatric wards. Explanatory models'. *Canadian Journal of Psychiatry*, 46, 437.

Lam, J., McNeil, D. and Blinder, R. (2000) 'The relationship between patients and gender and violence leading to staff injuries'. *Psychiatric Services*, 51, 1167–70.

Maguire, J. (2002) 'Seclusion usage in psychiatric institutions in the Republic of Ireland and an analysis of nursing attitudes, knowledge and experiences regarding seclusion' (unpublished MSc dissertation). Royal College of Surgeons in Ireland, Dublin.

Monaghan, J., Steadman, H., Silver, E., Appelbaum, P., Clark Robbins, P., Mulvey, E., Roth, L., Grisso, T. and Banks, S. (2001) *Rethinking Risk Assessment: The McArthur Study of Mental Disorder and Violence*, Oxford: Oxford University Press.

National Audit Office (UK) (2003) *A Safer Place to Work: Protecting NHS Hospital and Ambulance Staff from Violent Aggression*. London: National Audit Office.

National Institute of Clinical Excellence (NICE) (UK) (2005) *Violence: The Short-term Management of Disturbed/Violent Behaviour in In-patient Psychiatric Settings and Emergency Departments*, Clinical Guideline 25. London: NICE.

Nijman, H. (1999) 'Aggressive behaviour of psychiatric inpatients: measurement, prevalence and determinants'. University of Maastricht.

North Eastern Health Board (NEHB) (2004). *Study of Work Related Violence. Committee on Workplace Violence*, Kells: North Eastern Health Board.

Paterson, B., Turnbull, J. and Aitken, L. (1992) 'An evaluation of a training course in the short-term management of violence'. *Nurse Education Today*, 12, 368–75.

Royal College of Psychiatrists (UK) (1999) *Report of the Collegiate Trainees Committee Working Party on the Safety of Trainees*, Council Report CR78. London: Royal College of Psychiatrists.

Royal College of Psychiatrists (UK) (2000) *National Audit of Management of Violence in Mental Health Setting*. London: Royal College of Psychiatrists.

Ryrie, I. and McGowan, J. (1998) Staff perceptions of substance use among psychiatric in-patients. *Journal of Psychiatric and Mental Health Nursing*, 5, 137–42.

Sanders, J., Milner, S., Brown, P. and Bell, A. J. (2000) 'Assessment of aggression in psychiatric admissions: semi-structured interview and case note survey'. *British Medical Journal*, 320 (72420), 1112.

Steinert, T., Wiebe, C. and Gebhardt, R. (1999) 'Aggressive behaviour against self and others among first admission patients with schizophrenia'. *Psychiatric Services*, 50, 85–90.

Trenoweth, S. (2003) 'Perceiving risk in dangerous situations: risks of violence among mental health inpatients'. *Journal of Advanced Nursing*, 42(3), 278–87.

Turnbull, J. (1999). 'Theoretical approaches to violence and aggression', in J. Turnbull and B. Paterson (eds), *Aggression and Violence: Approaches to Effective Management*. London: Macmillan.

Walker, Z. and Seifert, R. (1994) 'Violent incidents in a psychiatric intensive care unit'. *British Journal of Psychiatry*, 826–8.

Walsh, E., Buchanan A. and Fahey, T. (2002) 'Violence and schizophrenia: examining the evidence'. *British Journal of Psychiatry*, 180, 490–5.

Webster, C., Douglas, K., Eaves, D. and Hart S. (1997) *HCR-20: Assessing Risk of Violence (Version 2)*. Vancouver: Vancouver Mental Health Law and Policy Institute, Simon Fraser University.

Whittington, R. (2002) 'Attitudes towards patient aggression amongst mental health nurses in the "zero tolerance" era: associations with burnout and length of experience'. *Journal of Clinical Nursing*, 11, 819–25.

Whittington, R., Shuttleworth, S. and Hill, L. (1996) 'Violence to staff in a general hospital setting'. *Journal of Advanced Nursing*, 24, 326–33.

Whittington, R. and Wykes, T. (1996) 'An evaluation of staff training in psychological techniques for the management of patient aggression'. *Journal of Clinical Nursing*, 5, 257–61.

21
Dual Diagnosis
Gerard Moore

Dual diagnosis is a relatively new phenomenon that has become an issue for mental health services since the 1980s, alongside the move from hospital to community-based care. Patients who present with a dual diagnosis can be understood as having multiple complex needs associated with both mental health and substance abuse issues. While understanding the complexity of the human condition would alert mental health workers to the reality that all cases have some level of complexity, this does not always indicate that a dual diagnosis is present, which underlines the need for considered and careful diagnosis. This chapter will examine the concept of dual diagnosis and its clinical implications alongside a discussion on treatment and management issues.

PREVALENCE OF DUAL DIAGNOSIS

The number of people with a dual diagnosis in Ireland is unknown. Studies conducted in other jurisdictions suggest various prevalence rates ranging from fifteen to sixty-five per cent of patients with a serious mental illness. Estimates of prevalence rates change over time, reflecting differences in how research is conducted and the lack of consensus on a definition. More research is required before an accurate rate can be suggested. Hein *et al.* (1997) estimate up to two-thirds of outpatient populations meet the dual diagnosis criteria. A study conducted the previous year suggested a much lower rate of 15 per cent (Menezes *et al.* 1996).

Kamali (2000) found that 39 per cent of Irish patients with a diagnosis of schizophrenia fulfilled diagnostic criteria for a lifetime history of substance abuse. A study conducted the following year with outpatients in Dublin broadly supports this finding, indicating that 45 per cent of people with schizophrenia meet dual diagnosis criteria (Condren *et al.* 2001). Earlier studies conducted outside Ireland report rates of substance abuse among individuals with schizophrenia as rising at a significantly higher rate than in non-psychiatric populations (Cuffel 1992; LeDuc and Mittleman 1995).

DEFINING DUAL DIAGNOSIS

The relationship between diagnoses in an individual with dual diagnosis is more complex than simply having two conditions. The associated difficulties and implications for healthcare interventions and provision of appropriate and timely healthcare are significant. However, the lack of consensus on an agreed definition of dual diagnosis remains problematic. The first published study on the management of dual diagnosis by the addiction and mental health services in Ireland offers a definition that will be utilised for this chapter. Dual diagnosis can be understood as 'the co-existence of both mental health and substance misuse problems for an individual' (McGabhann *et al.* 2004:25) An earlier definition, 'the concurrent existence of both substance abuse or dependency and one or more psychiatric disorders' (Gafoor and Rassool 1998:497) provides a similar understanding of the patient presenting with a dual diagnosis.

CONCEPT OF DUAL DIAGNOSIS

Use of the term *dual diagnosis* is not confined to patients who present with mental health and addiction problems, which often leads to confusion among service providers about how to diagnose, treat and manage patients. The term is applied to the co-existence of mental health and physical problems, intellectual disabilities and addiction or even the co-existence of two mental health diagnoses in an individual, e.g. psychosis and mood disorder. In many ways the complex nature of any mental health problem can be understood as potentially becoming a dual diagnosis.

To address this multiple use of the term the Expert Group on Mental Health opted to use the term 'co-morbid' in its 2006 policy document *A Vision for Change*. The failure of service providers at policy, research and clinical levels to agree a term to describe dual diagnosis is indicative of the overall failure of services to agree on treatment structures. Terms such as co-morbidity do not describe the degree or nature of drug abuse or whether a causal relationship exists between two or more conditions. An individual's health status can become co-morbid in many different ways, depending on the time sequence and interactions between the two primary conditions (Fischer and Akram 2001). However, the term co-morbid can be viewed as being equally incomplete in its ability to describe the complexities of the co-existence of mental health and substance abuse in one individual.

Without an adequate agreed concept of dual diagnosis individuals needing treatment are at risk from the competing paradigms prevalent in substance abuse or mental healthcare systems. Mental healthcare providers often find it difficult to engage patients with a history of substance abuse, as they do not respond well to a typical mental health service. Services that embrace an abstinence model have difficulty engaging clients who have opted for a harm reduction approach. Some addiction services fully endorse an abstinence-based approach up to and including the use of prescribed psychotropic drugs, making it difficult for people in receipt of mental health care to access services. Mental health services occasionally refuse to dispense methadone, creating difficulties when patients on maintenance programmes need to avail of in-patient treatment.

CAUSES OF DUAL DIAGNOSIS

Attempting to understand why a person has developed a dual diagnosis is a useful tool that has a clinical value, allowing the individual to explore the impact of their past on their current life experience. Life-story work, in which people review their past and present it to others in a treatment context, is an established part of many treatment programmes in addiction services. Mental health workers need to be conservative in their attribution of causative factors in individual cases as many people with a dual diagnosis use legal and illicit substances for the very same reasons that others in society engage in their use: for social and recreational purposes.

The Expert Group on Mental Health (2006) stated that co-morbidity contributes to greater severity of addiction and mental disorder. For patients this increases the likelihood of a relapse of their condition. Patients with a vulnerability to psychosis may find substance misuse worsening or altering the course of psychiatric illness. Substance misuse may often lead to an exacerbation of symptoms and relapse in major illness (Gournay *et al.* 1997). Patients may be using multiple substances or experiencing addiction on different levels, for instance alcohol and gambling. For example the use of cocaine is linked to mood swings, general restlessness, irritability, hallucinations and the development of paranoid psychosis, highlighting the complexity of making an accurate diagnosis. Cocaine use may exacerbate a current condition or be the causative factor for the production of symptoms of mood disorder, psychosis or both.

Research into the link between mental illness and substance abuse has led to a number of different beliefs in the field including the impact of stress, the process of deinstitutionalisation, attempts to self-medicate for symptom management and the direct impact of substance abuse. It is not always viewed as the person having two distinct mental health problems. According to Evans and Sullivan (1990) mental health symptoms are sometimes seen as illness and substance abuse is often considered bad behaviour. This supports the belief that if relief for the mental health symptoms can be found the individual will cease or reduce their substance abuse. Similarly, providers of substance abuse services have been found to believe that symptoms of mental ill health are the result of substance abuse. Both these positions are problematic as the individual is at risk of remaining undiagnosed and consequently finding it difficult to access timely appropriate interventions.

Some research supports the stress vulnerability model. Intoxication and/or substance dependence is linked to the development or exacerbation of psychological problems such as poor self-esteem, mood changes and difficulties with self-image. This model hypothesises that drug abuse may precipitate schizophrenia or increase the likelihood of its expression in an already vulnerable person (Dixon *et al.* 1991). During the past thirty years researchers such as Richard *et al.* (1985) have recognised a link between substance use in adolescence and the development of psychotic illness. Specific substances have been linked to the development of psychiatric symptoms, for example amphetamine use is associated with the development of psychotic symptoms (McLellan *et al.* 1979). Studies on the use of cannabis have suggested a similar link (Andreasson *et al.* 1987). Cannabis use in particular is linked to depression, anxiety, memory loss, learning, social functioning and the onset of psychosis.

The deinstitutionalisation of the mental health system can be seen as a contributing factor in the rise in prevalence of dual diagnosis. The seemingly new patient group, 'young adult chronic patients' who do not experience the prolonged hospitalisation of previous eras, are particularly vulnerable to the development of a dual diagnosis (Pratt *et al.* 2007). Possibly, the mental health services are a victim of their own success as a reduction in the provision of long-term care in hospital settings has resulted in more patients living in the community and more exposure of this group of people to substance abuse. Consequently there is an increase in the rate of patients with a dual diagnosis.

The high rate of substance abuse in individuals with a psychotic illness has been linked to attempts at self-medication (Khantzian 1985; Kasten 1999). Mental health disorders are almost three times as common among those with alcohol dependence compared to the general population, and forty per cent of service users managed by community mental health teams report drug or alcohol misuse problems (McGabhann *et al.* 2004). A primary psychiatric illness may precipitate or lead to substance misuse (Expert Group on Mental Health 2006). A patient with depression may drink in order to cope with or manage his or her feelings. This exacerbates the problem, as alcohol is a depressant leading to a lowering of the mood and the necessity to drink increasing amounts to effect any change. Prolonged substance misuse or the withdrawal from a substance can lead to development of psychiatric symptoms or illness. Prolonged alcohol use is linked to early onset dementia.

SUBSTANCE USE CHOICE IN DUAL DIAGNOSIS

The nature and type of substance abuse most common in patients with a dual diagnosis will generally mirror that of the society in which they live, so mental health workers can expect to see patterns of abuse similar to those with a single diagnosis of substance abuse disorder. However, an early study on psychoactive substances used by people with a diagnosis of schizophrenia found that they used more stimulants than the general population (Schneier and Siris 1987). This is not supported by later work by Lehman *et al.* (1994), who found that cannabis and alcohol are more common substances of abuse.

RELATIONSHIP BETWEEN MENTAL ILLNESS AND SUBSTANCE ABUSE

There are a number of possible issues surrounding the relationship that develops between mental health and substance abuse to be taken into account when assessing the individual and planning care.

• Substance use (even one dose) may lead to psychiatric syndromes or symptoms.

- Harmful use may produce psychiatric syndromes.
- Dependence may produce psychological symptoms.
- Intoxication from a substance may produce psychological symptoms.
- Withdrawal from substances may produce psychological symptoms.
- Withdrawal from substances may lead to psychiatric symptoms.
- Substance use may exacerbate pre-existing psychiatric disorders.
- Psychological morbidity not amounting to a disorder may precipitate substance use.
- Primary psychiatric disorder may lead to substance use disorder.
- Primary psychiatric disorder may precipitate substance use disorder which, in turn, may lead to psychiatric syndromes (Crome 1999).

It is evident that substance use or misuse may alter the course of a primary mental health problem, or the reverse may occur. However, individuals with a dual diagnosis are mostly likely to come from four particular categories:
- A primary psychiatric disorder with a secondary substance misuse disorder.
- A primary substance misuse disorder with psychiatric complications.
- Concurrent substance misuse and psychiatric disorders, for example alcohol dependence and depression.
- An underlying traumatic experience, for example post-traumatic stress disorder, resulting in both substance abuse and mood disorders (Gafoor and Rassool 1998).

MANAGEMENT OF DUAL DIAGNOSIS

Recognising whether the substance abuse or the mental health problem is primary, secondary or concurrent is essential to diagnosis and the instigation of an appropriate treatment regime. Careful and timely management of dual diagnosis is essential as rates of relapse are higher, service utilisation is increased, in-patient treatment is more common and treatment outcomes are poor for both conditions (Expert Group on Mental Health 2006).
Clinical implications include:
- exacerbation of psychiatric symptoms
- increased use of institutional services
- poor medication adherence
- homelessness
- increased risk of HIV infection
- poor social outcomes, including impact on carers and families
- contact with criminal justice system (DoH 2002).

Assessment of Dual Diagnosis
In an increasingly complex care system, nurses working in mental health, substance abuse and general health services all need to have the skills and tools available for accurate diagnosis and appropriate intervention. According to

Gournay *et al.* (1997) due to their increased susceptibility to accidents and to being victims of assault dual diagnosis patients will often be found in Emergency Departments. Furthermore, the increasing separation of substance abuse from the field of mental health indicates that the first presentation of a percentage of patients with a dual diagnosis will not be to either the general or mental health services but to a separate substance abuse service. The site of the person's first presentation may be a factor in the diagnostic process as staff with a particular set of skills centred around a specialist area may be prone to valuing the onset of one set of symptoms over another and/or arriving at a clinical judgement about which symptom set, dual diagnosis or mental illness, is primary.

Assessment should serve a number of different purposes, screening the patient, a tool to aid diagnosis, a guide to creating a treatment plan and provision of a baseline from which to measure outcomes of any interventions. A number of tools have been developed to assess drug use in an individual and to assess their mental state. Because of the complexities associated with dual diagnosis there are limitations to how current assessment tools can be applied. The mental health worker could consider using an established mental health assessment tool in combination with a tool designed to measure substance abuse and combine both results in order to screen a patient for dual diagnosis. However, this rather crude application of assessment tools is often inaccurate, as the course of the individual's mental illness and substance abuse may not follow a regular pattern and indeed each is most likely to impact on the other. The complexity of the case could be lost if standard tools are applied. The individual may deliberately misreport symptoms and behaviours in order to disguise their drug use or mental illness as a means of accessing a treatment centre.

Few assessment tools have been developed in relation to dual diagnosis, and reliability and validity of those that do exist are still being established (McGabhann *et al.* 2004). The difficulty of establishing an accurate assessment tool for dual diagnosis is well reported by Wolford *et al.* (1999), who found that many of the available tools used to measure substance abuse were insensitive when used in a population with a mental illness. As patients with severe mental illness differ in their patterns of substance misuse (e.g. they tend to use lower quantities of substances), norms established for the general population may not be applicable to psychiatric patients (McGabhann *et al.* 2004).

Service Model Approaches

Mental health and substance abuse services often come from different educational and philosophical traditions; consequently the service providers for these different conditions occasionally have conflicting and contradictory approaches to care. Traditionally Irish addiction services dealt primarily with alcohol misuse and developed in conjunction with the mental health services. These services offered an abstinence-based programme often closely adhering to a twelve-step model. In contrast, the substance abuse services targeting illicit drug use developed separately from mental health services and they tend to take a more pragmatic approach towards addiction, utilising a harm reduction approach such as methadone maintenance to treat heroin addiction. As a result, substance abusers who require in-patient mental health services may experience difficulty in having their methadone prescription continued when in receipt of care in a service with an abstinence-based philosophy.

The Expert Group on Mental Health (2006) advocate that local community mental health teams should manage individuals with co-morbid conditions and that mental health services are responsible for providing a service only to those who have co-morbid substance abuse and mental health problems. However, if the primary problem is addiction it is not the responsibility of the community mental health team to manage the patient. Patients who present without co-morbidity (e.g. with a primary substance abuse problem and no mental health problems) clearly do not fall into the remit of the mental health services. There are positive and negative aspects to this approach. Services for people with alcohol problems in Ireland are clearly linked to and frequently managed by the mental health services. Services for other substances of abuse such as opiates are not managed by the mental health services. The rate of service development has not kept pace and it may be difficult, if not impossible, for opiate users to find primary addiction services in their community that meet their needs. Interventions are therefore delayed, allowing problems to become more complex and increasing the possibility of co-morbidity occurring. There are issues around diagnosis and identifying which problem occurs first, mental health or addiction. This can be a matter of clinical opinion subject to the skill of the diagnostician. The increased specialisation of both mental health and addiction services include an inherent risk that practitioners become deskilled and symptoms go undetected or unaddressed. In other jurisdictions three distinct models for addressing dual diagnosis have emerged: serial services; parallel services; and an integrated model.

Serial Services
In serial or sequential services the person initially receives treatment for one condition. Once initial treatment has succeeded in stabilising the condition the person is then referred for treatment of the second or dual disorder. There are clear problems with this approach: the disorder that is not being treated can impact negatively on the disorder being addressed, exacerbating the condition. A patient who experiences paranoid delusions and is in receipt of serial services initially for substance abuse may discontinue attending services because they have developed paranoid ideation about the service providers. Treatment for the mental health disorder in the absence of treatment for the substance abuse disorder is ineffective for both disorders (Pratt et al. 2007).

Parallel Services
Both disorders are treated simultaneously. Different staff, who may be working for different agencies, carry out this treatment. It appears to be a more desirable approach as both disorders are given equal priority and addressed simultaneously.

This reduces the possibility of the symptoms of one disorder impairing the treatment outcomes of the other. This model is not without its critics; for example Drake *et al.* (1993) argue that parallel services can lead to fragmented, contradictory and inadequate care.

Issues include differences in treatment approaches and treatment goals, differences about which service should advocate for the person in relation to accessing other agencies such as social services. Misunderstanding or poor communication between organisations can lead to needs not being met in a timely and appropriate manner. Contradictory advice may be delivered from both services, leading to confusion. All these problems can be overcome but not without careful co-ordination of services and mutual understanding of problems.

Integrated Services

With integrated services the person receives treatment in the same place at the same time by the same practitioners (Pratt *et al.* 2007) and this is the favoured approach for dual diagnosis. This is a better option for the person, provided the service providers are knowledgeable about both disorders and the complications that occur with a dual diagnosis. Within an integrated service nine principles are identified by Drake *et al.* (2004) that have been shown to be critical for effective treatment.

1. *The same clinical team*, who are knowledgeable in both disorders and their interaction, provide integrated treatment; mental health and substance abuse treatment occurs concurrently and services are individualised and address the specific characteristics of dual diagnosis.
2. *Stage-wise approach*. Services are alert to the person's specific stage of change as outlined by Prochaska *et al.* (1994) (see Chapter 19).
3. *Engagement interventions*. Motivational counselling is used to increase the likelihood of individuals engaging in treatment. This includes active outreach, flexibility in approach, practical as well as psychological support and culturally sensitive services models.
4. *Motivational counselling interventions*. Services use counselling techniques that develop readiness for a shift towards individualised goals.
5. *Active treatment interventions*. Services include interventions, such as motivational counselling, cognitive behavioural approaches and family interventions, that allow individuals to manage their own illness.
6. *Relapse prevention interventions*. Services assist the individual in planning towards relapse interventions as they recognise that those with a dual diagnosis are at greater risk of relapse.
7. *Long-term perspective*. Services are designed to support people not just through crisis but also for the longer term as they recognise both the increased risk of relapse and that recovery is a long-term process.
8. *Comprehensive service*. Services address all the person's needs and liaise closely with other agencies, particularly in the areas of housing, employment and justice.

9. *Interventions for treatment of non respondents.* Here again the individual's needs are considered in terms of addressing social issues in relation to money management, family intervention and occasionally the need for residential treatment.

Treatment Maintenance and Change

The initial step in the treatment of any person should be the process of conducting a clear and thorough assessment. Assessment can act as a baseline from which to measure the person's progress as well as a guide to the development of a collaborative care plan. Assessment is difficult and clinicians need to be cautious about attributing symptoms to either a mental health or a substance abuse disorder in the initial stages of engagement. Establishing an accurate history of the person's life is a useful first step in an integrated approach towards care.

Pharmacological interventions may change when a person has a dual diagnosis. Maremmani *et al.* (1998) reported that the average methadone dosage required to stabilise heroin addicts with a dual diagnosis of anxiety disorder was 80mg/day, compared to 100mg/day for patients with a single diagnosis of substance abuse disorder. This has implications for clinicians in their assessment and prescription of treatment regimes for complex cases, particularly when drug regimes such as methadone stabilisation programmes are frequently instituted by agreed protocols which dictate the dosage and duration of treatment.

Developing a therapeutic alliance should be given special consideration as the establishment of a good working relationship between the individual and the service providers will be invaluable should any slips or relapses occur. The complexity of dual diagnosis often requires staff to engage with the patient on a long-term basis and to work towards achievable goals as well as actively engaging in the psychosocial aspects of care.

CONCLUSION

Dual diagnosis refers to the co-existence of a mental health and substance abuse problem in an individual. There is disagreement at the level of service planners and service providers about how to categorise and treat people who present with a dual diagnosis. Some of these differences have their bases in beliefs about mental health and substance abuse. People who present with a dual diagnosis are complex and have multiple needs in terms of achieving short-, medium- and long-term goals. They provide a real challenge to service providers. More work is required to develop accurate assessment tools for dual diagnosis. Early appropriate interventions can reduce the exacerbation of symptoms.

Reflective Questions

1. What are the mostly likely reasons that dual diagnosis has emerged as a problem during the past two decades?
2. What role could a mental health team play in the treatment of people newly diagnosed with schizophrenia in relation to alcohol and drug use?

3. In relation to your own practice structure and location, can you identify difficulties people with a mental health issue may experience if they needed to access substance abuse services?
4. How could you phrase questions when assessing a patient to uncover the motivating factors for the substance use?

Useful Websites
Some useful Irish and international website addresses:
www.nacd.ie
www.hrb.ie
www.drugsalcohol.info
www.dancesafe.org
www.nida.nih.gov

References
Andreasson, S., Engstom, A. and Allebeck, P. (1987) 'Cannabis and schizophrenia longitudinal study of Swedish conscripts'. *Lancet*, 2, 1483–6.

Condren, R. M., O'Connor, J. and Brown, R. (2001) 'Prevalence and patterns of substance misuse in schizophrenia: a catchment area case-control study'. *Psychiatric Bulletin*, 25, 17–20.

Crome, I. B. (1999) 'Substance misuse and psychiatric co-morbidity: towards improved service provision. *Drugs: Education, Prevention and Policy*, 6, 151–73.

Cuffel, B. J. (1992) 'Prevalence estimates of substance abuse in schizophrenia and their correlates'. *Journal of Nervous and Mental Disease*, 180, 589–96.

Department of Health (DoH) (UK) (2002) *Mental Health Policy Implementation Guide: Dual Diagnosis Good Practice Guide*. London: Department of Health Publications.

Dixon, L., Haas, G., Eider, P. J. and Sweeney, J. (1991). 'Drug abuse in schizophrenic patients: clinical correlates and reasons for use'. *American Journal of Psychiatry*, 148, 224–30.

Drake, R. E., Bartels, S. J., Teague, G. B., Noordsy, D. L., and Clarke, R. E. (1993) 'Treatment of substance abuse in severely mentally ill patients'. *Journal of Nervous and Mental Disease*, 181 (10), 606–11.

Drake, R. E., Mueser, K. T., Brunette, M. F., and McHugo, G. J. (2004) 'A review of treatment for peoples with severe mental illness and co-occurring substance use disorders'. *Psychiatric Rehabilitation Journal*, 27 (4), 360–74.

Evans, K., and Sullivan, J. M. (1990) *Dual Diagnosis: Counselling the Mentally Ill Substance Abuser*. New York: Guilford Press.

Expert Group on Mental Health (2006) *A Vision for Change*. Dublin: Stationery Office.

Fischer, M. and Akram, G. (2001) 'Prevalence of co-morbid mental illness and drug use recorded in general practice: preliminary findings from the general practice research database'. *Drugs: Education, Prevention and Policy*, 8, 275–80.

Gafoor, M. and Rassool, G. H. (1998) 'The co-existence of psychiatric disorders and substance misuse: working with dual diagnosis patients'. *Journal of Advanced Nursing*, 27, 497–502.

Gournay, K., Sandford, T., Johnson, G. and Thornicroft, G. (1997) 'Dual diagnosis of severe mental health problems and substance abuse/dependence: a major priority for mental health nursing'. *Journal of Psychiatric and Mental Health Nursing*, 4, 89–95.

Hein, D., Zimberg, S. and Weisman, S. (1997) 'Dual diagnosis sub types in urban substance abuse and mental health clinicians'. *Psychiatric Services*, 48.

Kamali, M., Kelly, L. and Gervin, M. (2000) 'The prevalence of co-morbid substance misuse and its influence on suicidal ideation amongst inpatients with schizophrenia'. *Acta Psychiatrica Scandinavia*, 101, 452–6.

Kasten, B. P. (1999) 'Self-medication with alcohol and drugs by persons with severe mental illness'. *Journal of the American Psychiatric Nursing Association*, 5, 80–7.

Khantzian, E. J. (1985) 'The self-medication hypothesis of addictive disorders. Focus on heroin and cocaine dependence'. *American Journal of Psychiatry*, 142, 1259–64.

LeDuc, P. A. and Mittleman, G. (1995) 'Schizophrenia and psycho-stimulant abuse: A review and re-analysis of clinical evidence'. *Psychopharmacology*, 121, 407–27.

Lehman, A., Myres, C., Dickson, L. and Johnson, J. (1994) 'Defining sub-groups of dual diagnosis patients: for service planning'. *Hospital and Community Psychiatry*, 45, 556–61.

Maremmani, I., Marini, G., and Fornai, F. (1998) 'Naloxone induced panic attacks'. *American Journal of Psychiatry*, 155, 447.

McGabhann, L., Scheele, A., Dunne, T., Gallagher, P., MacNeela, P., Moore, G. and Philbin, M. (2004) *Mental Health and Addiction Services and the Management of Dual Diagnosis in Ireland*. NACD: Dublin Stationery Office.

McLellan, A. T., Woody, G. E., and O Brien, C. P. (1979) 'Development of psychiatric illness in drug abusers: possible role of drug preference'. *New England Journal of Medicine*, 301, 1310–14.

Menezes, P. R., Johnson, S. and Thornicroft, G. (1996) 'Drug and alcohol problems among people with severe mental illness in south London'. *British Journal of Psychiatry*, 168, 612–19.

Pratt, C. W., Gill, K. J., Barrett, N. M. and Roberts, M. M. (2007) *Psychiatric Rehabilitation* (2nd edn). London: Elsevier Academic Press.

Prochaska, J. O., Norcross, J. C. and DiClemente, C. C. (1994) *Changing for the Good*. New York: Harper Collins.

Richard, M. L., Liskow, B. L. and Perry, P. J. (1985) 'Recent psychostimulant use in hospitalised schizophrenics'. *Journal of Clinical Psychiatry*, 46, 79–83.

Schneier, F. and Siris, S. (1987) 'A review of psychoactive substance use and abuse in schizophrenia patterns of drug choice'. *Journal of Nervous and Mental Disease*, 175, 641–52.

Wolford, G. L., Rosenburg, S. D. and Drake, R. E. (1999) 'Evaluation of methods for detecting substance use disorder in persons with severe mental illness'. *Psychology of Addictive Behaviours*, 13 (4), 313–26.

22
Physical Health and Mental Health Nursing

Frances Ryan, Brian Keogh and Louise Doyle

This chapter considers the physical aspects of mental health problems and is divided into two sections. First the assessment of the physical health of clients with mental illness in the clinical setting will be discussed. Second, severe adverse events caused by the administration of certain psychotropic drugs (lithium toxicity, agranulocytosis, neuroleptic malignant syndrome and serotonin syndrome) will be described. The medical interventions and the nursing management of these events will also be outlined.

GUIDELINES TO PHYSICAL ASSESSMENT

People with severe mental health problems have the propensity to be overweight, physically inactive and smoke heavily. It is noted that as a group, they have higher levels of morbidity and mortality than other people (NIMHE/Mentality 2004). Similarly, certain antipsychotic medications have the potential to lead to weight gain and metabolic disorders, thus increasing the risk of cardiovascular complications and the incidence of diabetes. Physical health issues may exacerbate existing mental health problems, thereby delaying recovery and acting as a deterrent to the achievement of holistic well-being for the client. Consequently, the assessment and management of physical health problems among people with mental illness has become an important and pressing issue for mental health nurses. The report of the Chief Nursing Officer in the United Kingdom (Department of Health (UK) 2006) emphasises the need for mental health nurses to develop physical assessment skills and engage in health promotion in order to ensure that clients with mental illness receive regular assessment of their physical needs and appropriate physical healthcare. This chapter does not use a head-to-toe approach to assessment; rather the key areas relating to physical assessment will be examined from a broad perspective. In practice, more detailed assessment may ensue from the interpretation of the initial clinical findings. A systematic approach to the collection of information will assist the mental health nurse in conducting a physical assessment in the clinical area. Vital signs and baseline interventions will be outlined and discussed. Lifestyle behaviours, nutritional assessment, mobility and personal hygiene issues will also be included. Documentation and appropriate referral will be an integral component of each section.

A physical assessment is usually performed after obtaining the client's overall medical history. The initial health history usually provides the nurse with an individual profile that will guide certain aspects of the physical examination and will act as a baseline against which all other information can be used.

While physical assessment is usually sequential in nature, incorporating all the main body systems, it is pertinent to note that it is also individualistic and the sequence of inspection and examination will depend on the circumstances and the client's presenting mental health problem. Therefore, a complete examination may not always be routine. Many of the body's systems may be selectively assessed on the basis of the individual's presenting problem and an accurate assessment requires trust and co-operation from the client, coupled with adept and competent interpersonal skills on the part of the nurse.

Special care must also be taken in obtaining a complete history of medications used by the client. Oftentimes including a family member, with the client's permission, in the overall assessment may provide missing information, enhance the assessment and validate information received.

Central to any assessment is observation, inspection and obtaining specific baseline information. Baid (2006) asserts that inspection is the first part of the physical examination and commences the moment the nurse makes initial contact with the client. Inspection includes acquiring an initial impression of how the client appears. Specific descriptions need to be based on careful observation and inspection. Does the client appear sick? What specific physical manifestations indicate that the client is physically sick? What is the client's posture and gait like? Does the client appear to be in pain, distressed or confused? This preliminary impression gained by the nurse will provide a focus for more detailed specific information to follow. It is a vital part of the initial physical assessment and a precursor to the attainment of more specific information relating to vital signs and lifestyle behaviours.

THE ASSESSMENT OF VITAL SIGNS

The recording of vital signs is an important part of every physical examination. Baseline readings for temperature, pulse, blood pressure and respiration need to be obtained and documented accurately.

Temperature
Body temperature may change according to diurnal variations and individual variation is normal. Fever is an indicator of possible infection; therefore baseline temperature recordings are necessary to monitor any deviations from the norm. In addition, hyperthermia is also an indicator of possible neuroleptic malignant syndrome or agranulocytosis, which are discussed later in this chapter.

Cardiovascular Function
Cardiovascular function may be assessed by measuring blood pressure and pulse rate. An alteration in blood pressure is a key physiological change in many

psychiatric conditions (e.g. anxiety) and is also a common side effect of many psychotropic medications. The nurse is required to make an accurate recording of blood pressure, noting whether there are any postural blood pressure changes, usually accompanied by dizziness or light-headedness once the client assumes an upright position. It is also necessary to obtain data regarding any cardiac medications the client may be taking, in conjunction with carrying out a risk factor assessment. Factors such as familial history of hypertension or hyperlipidaemia, diabetes, obesity, physical inactivity and cigarette smoking are all essential elements of the cardiovascular assessment and such information needs to be documented in the appropriate nursing records. For the initial cardiac assessment the radial pulse rate should be counted for one minute, paying attention to the rate, rhythm and volume of the pulse (Smeltzer and Bare 2000). Minor variations in rate and rhythm are normal and both may vary according to whether the patient is anxious or otherwise, hence it may be appropriate to reassess at the end of the examination if the rate is higher than expected.

General inspection of the skin is also an indicator of cardiovascular function. Pallor, most evident around the nails, lips and mouth, may be caused by anaemia or decreased arterial perfusion. Cyanosis, indicating decreased blood flow to a particular area, is usually apparent on the skin of the nose, lips and earlobes and may be associated with conditions such as congestive heart failure. Similarly, peripheral oedema in dependant areas such as the feet and legs is usually observed in patients with congestive heart failure and peripheral vascular disease. Lower extremity ulcers are also an indication of arterial or venous insufficiency (Smeltzer and Bare 2000). During the assessment of vital signs it is imperative that the nurse details any abnormalities. Such deviations from normal are required to be documented and reported to the general physician to enable the client's physical condition to be monitored, and followed up if necessary, during the period of hospitalisation.

Respiratory Function

Detailed respiratory assessment is a sound indicator of both cardiac and lung function. Clients with underlying cardiac disease may exhibit the following symptoms in varying degrees: tachypnoea or rapid shallow breathing may be noted in clients who have heart failure; haemoptysis or pink frothy sputum may also be a manifestation of pulmonary oedema associated with heart failure. A dry hacking cough may be a symptom of pulmonary congestion. Crackles or a wheeze heard on examination of the lungs may be due to fluid accumulation and certain cardiac drugs such as beta blockers may precipitate airway narrowing, also leading to wheezing (Smeltzer and Bare 2000).

Smoking is a contributor to respiratory impairment and lung disease. Smoking prevalence is significantly higher among people with mental health problems than in the general population. Meltzer et al. (1996) suggest that between 70 and 74 per cent of psychiatric in-patients smoke. When assessing respiratory function the nurse needs to be cognisant of the impact of smoking, and any obvious respiratory impairment, on the client's ability to perform the activities of daily living. This information can then be used to formulate a care plan where necessary. Some of the major signs of respiratory compromise are dyspnoea, cough, sputum production, wheezing and cyanosis. A preliminary test of the client's ability is performed by measuring the respiratory rate for one minute, paying attention to the rate, depth and rhythm of respirations.

Additional nursing interventions include observation of the client's colour, use of accessory muscles of respiration such as the sternomastoid and intercostal muscles, as well as lung examination and physical inspection of the thorax, to rule out any structural abnormalities such as barrel chest, kyphosis or scoliosis (both curvatures of the spine) that may restrict the client's ability to breathe. Oxygen saturation levels may also be performed to give baseline information, if indicated. During the assessment the nurse collects information about any underlying respiratory problems, their duration and severity and any precipitating risk factors, such as smoking, that may contribute to the patient's condition.

Once baseline temperature, pulse and respiratory observations are taken and recorded, the next part of the assessment should include an evaluation of the client's renal and endocrine function.

Renal Function

Urinalysis is an important test in providing clinical information on renal function and a routine urinalysis done on admission is a useful baseline assessment procedure. Urine testing for glucose and ketones is particularly useful in the detection of early onset diabetes. In addition, a raised level of ketones may be indicative of fasting (e.g. anorexia nervosa). In conjunction with performing a dipstick test, assessment of urine colour, clarity and odour are important to note and document. The client should also be assessed for any dependant oedema such as in the feet or sacral areas, which may be indicative of fluid retention.

Endocrine Function

Unhealthy lifestyles, weight gain and substance abuse, coupled with some of the side effects of antipsychotic medications, leave clients with mental illness at risk of developing physical health problems such as cardiovascular disease and diabetes (Ohlsen *et al.* 2005). The risk of developing non-insulin dependant diabetes may occur as a result of weight gained on antipsychotic medication but also as a direct drug effect (Mir and Taylor 2001). An initial physical assessment should include such blood tests as urea and electrolyte levels (U & Es), liver function tests (LFTs), thyroid function tests (TFTs) and a baseline blood glucose reading. Any abnormalities should be documented and reported and prompt referral made to suitable specialist sources where appropriate. Hypothyroidism or hyperthyroidism may produce symptoms which mimic depression or mania respectively.

While underlying physical health problems can impact on the general well-being of the person with mental illness, so too can lifestyle behaviours, so this is another essential factor in the overall assessment process.

The Assessment of Lifestyle Behaviours

A comprehensive and focused physical assessment will consider how factors such as nutrition, obesity, physical activity and alcohol and nicotine intake can impact on physical wellness. Cormac *et al.* (2004) suggest that mortality and morbidity rates are higher in long-term psychiatric patients than in the general population. The attributed causes in increased mortality may be linked to the client's mental disorder and altered lifestyle behaviours. For example, there is a high prevalence of substance abuse among those with mental health problems. Therefore it would seem pertinent to include an assessment of smoking habits, physical activity and diet and weight management in the overall plan of care for the client with mental illness.

Nutritional Assessment

A person's state of nutrition is often reflected in their physical appearance. Nursing assessment should include an initial appraisal of the client's weight, height and other indicators such as hair, teeth, gums and skin. Oral examination is important as poor oral hygiene may be an indication of malnutrition and a result of long-term medication. Oral health also affects comfort, eating, speech and general well-being. Signs and symptoms of poor oral hygiene include a smooth, swollen or coated tongue with red, receding, bleeding gums and dental caries. Nursing assessment should include documentation of the problem and formulation of a plan of care for any problems identified.

Assessment of the musculoskeletal system provides information about muscle wasting and weakness. Poor posture with flaccid, wasted muscles may present as physical signs that the client's nutritional status is poor. Similarly, dry flaky skin with diminished elasticity and turgor, and poorly healing wounds, are indications of poor nutrition and dehydration.

Dietary habits are an important aspect of the nutritional assessment. The appraisal of food intake should consider the type and quantity of food consumed. The history should also include the frequency with which some foods are consumed as well as information about cigarette, alcohol and illicit drug use. Obesity may be a problem in clients with severe and enduring mental illness and can be exacerbated by physical inactivity and the side effects of certain medications. Weight gain due to antipsychotic medication should be noted and detailed in the nursing documentation and appropriate nursing interventions, such as promotion of physical activity, possible dietary restriction and psychological support included in the care plan. Certain clients may have specific dietary requirements, such as the need for texture-modified meals due to swallowing difficulties. This should also be included in the plan of care and referral made to the dietician to assess dietary needs and advise on the management of those who are under- or overweight. The role of the nurse in nutritional assessment is to formulate a care plan based on dietary assessment and the client's profile. This should be carried out in liaison with specialist sources such as the dietician and should meet the client's needs for a balanced diet and to maintain or control weight.

Assessment of Mobility and Physical Activity

Comprehensive assessment of the client's mobility and functional capacity provides baseline information on the ability to perform the activities of daily living. These include basic needs such as personal cleansing and dressing, eating, moving and toileting. As functional ability will be influenced by joint movement and co-ordination, cardiovascular and respiratory reserve and an intact neurological system, these factors will also need to be included in the evaluation. The nurse is required to assess and determine the client's level of independence in self-care and the need for nursing interventions. Possible reasons for restricted mobility include pain, systemic disease, loss of muscle strength, the presence of an immobilising device such as a cast, poor activity tolerance, or dementia. Many clients with enduring mental illness may have been inactive for years and it is important to assess not only the physical ability of the client to mobilise but also their views on activity and exercise so that any interventions for physical activity may be incorporated into care plans.

Physical activity has many beneficial effects on health, and while there is widespread acknowledgement of the benefits of exercise for people with mental illness (Daley 2002), it is necessary to undertake a detailed physical assessment before including an exercise regimen in a plan of care. Assessment of the client's mobility involves noting the ability to move, muscle strength and tone, joint function, balance, impaired walking and risk of injury. Conditions such as underlying postural hypotension may cause the client to be dizzy, nauseous and tachycardic on assuming a vertical position and thus limit tolerance to certain activities. People with respiratory impairment secondary to cardiac disease may not be able to tolerate standing for prolonged periods or lying flat. Similarly, people with emphysema may assume a forward position with arms thrust outwards in order to maximise their breathing capacity.

Abnormalities of body movements should also be observed for. Involuntary movements such as tremors may exist in people with Parkinson's disease or alcohol withdrawal delirium. Assessment should not only include the client's baseline activity and rest patterns, but also identify barriers and facilitators to exercise, and promote self-care where possible. The nurse may need to collaborate with the physical and occupational therapist in the overall assessment and plan of care for clients with alterations in mobility and physical activity.

Assessment of Personal Hygiene

Immobility and prolonged inactivity, poor nutritional status and impaired sensory perception and cognition may all contribute to impaired skin integrity, thereby necessitating an assessment of the client's skin and personal hygiene. In addition, clients with obsessive compulsive disorder may have obsessions concerning cleanliness and clients with schizophrenia or depression may neglect their personal hygiene needs. In assessing the skin and potential risk for pressure ulcer development, factors such as mobility, cognitive function, nutrition, age and tissue perfusion need to be included in the assessment. The overall condition of the skin needs to be taken into account, along with more specific factors such as: the presence of erythema or redness; breaks in the skin; circulatory status; temperature, pallor, oedema; compromised mobility; advanced age; and the presence of incontinence. Appropriate nursing interventions for any problems identified need to be documented in the care plan.

Urinary and bowel incontinence are problems that may exacerbate existing skin disorders as well as causing embarrassment and curtailing a person's independence. The physical assessment should be used to investigate bladder and bowel function and symptoms associated with dysfunction such as stress incontinence or functional incontinence. The history should include information on fluid intake; episodes of incontinence and any associated physical activity such as coughing, sneezing, etc., functional factors such as the ability to get to the toilet; normal bowel and bladder patterns; underlying medical conditions such as colitis; medication history (for example, a person on diuretics will have an increased volume of urine produced); and the use of laxatives. This record can be used to determine the relationship of episodes of incontinence to other activities and factors.

Assessment and prevention of constipation is equally important when evaluating a client's elimination patterns. Food and fluid intake and levels of activity need to be reviewed. Furthermore, psychotropic medications may cause altered bowel and/or urinary function in some people. Based on the assessment data a nursing care plan may be developed to include appropriate nurse-led interventions suited to the individual client's needs. The client may need to be referred to specialist sources such as the physical therapist or dietician where appropriate.

The aim of assessment is to gather information about the client that can be useful in developing a plan of care for that person. It involves a systematic appraisal of the individual from a biopsychosocial perspective. The purpose of such an assessment is to provide individualistic, holistic, competent nursing care. The physical assessment of the client with mental illness is crucial to the monitoring of the ongoing care that the client requires and is central to ensuring both the physical and mental well-being of the person. The principles of assessment outlined in this chapter are largely relevant to clients with mental illness in the hospital setting, however, whatever the setting, it has become incumbent on mental health nurses to acknowledge their responsibility to ensure that their clients receive adequate physical health care and to do so requires developing competencies in physical assessment skills.

The next section of this chapter is related to severe adverse reactions to prescribed psychopharmacology.

LITHIUM TOXICITY

Lithium is a commonly used drug in the treatment and prophylaxis of the affective disorders. It has many side effects and contraindications (a detailed list is available in the *British National Formulary*) but its most worrying is lithium toxicity, which can be fatal and should be treated urgently. Lithium is well known for its narrow therapeutic/toxic range and doses are adjusted to a serum lithium level of 0.4–1mmol/litre (BNF 2007). Toxic symptoms can occur at serum levels of 1.5mmol/litre and require emergency treatment if levels are 2mmol/litre or above. Patients can become toxic for a number of reasons — overdose (accidental or intentional), dehydration or infections — although in certain instances the cause is unclear (Healy 2005).

Recognising Lithium Toxicity

The symptoms associated with lithium toxicity are:
• nausea
• vomiting
• diarrhoea
• tremor (Healy 2005).

However, in more serious cases symptoms include:
• hyperflexia
• hyperextension of limbs
• convulsions
• toxic psychoses
• syncope
• renal failure
• circulatory failure
• coma (BNF 2007).

Treatment is dependent on the seriousness of the toxicity and careful observation is required by the nurse and the client to recognise symptoms early and to act accordingly. A medical practitioner should review the client immediately and blood serum levels should be taken to ascertain the client's condition. No further lithium should be administered to the client and large volumes of intravenous isotonic saline are usually prescribed (Healy 2005). In more severe cases, the client will need to be treated as an emergency and may require haemodialysis (BNF 2007).

Prevention

Clients prescribed lithium need information about the drug's actions, the side effects and other specific information required to assist them to remain within their therapeutic index (Downie *et al.* 2004). Clients must be assessed for their motivation to take the drug and to attend for regular serum lithium levels and thyroid and renal function tests (Prosser *et al.* 2000). Clients receiving lithium should be encouraged to carry a lithium card which will explain how to take the drug, what to do if they miss a dose, side effects (including lithium toxicity) and what medications and illnesses alter serum levels. Other information on the lithium card includes:

- only drink alcohol in small quantities
- avoid some medications such as diuretics and non-steroid anti-inflammatory drugs such as Brufen
- remain hydrated (especially when hot or during exercise) and do not fluctuate daily salt intake
- if the client is a female, they should consult their medical practitioner if considering pregnancy (Downie *et al*. 2004).

Clients taking lithium should be advised to contact their community mental health nurse, pharmacist or general practitioner if they have any queries about lithium. They should also be aware of the symptoms of lithium toxicity and advised to get medical help if they are feeling unwell, regardless of the cause.

BLOOD DISORDERS

Rosenfeld and Loose-Mitchell (1998) suggest that blood disorders (dyscrasias) are relatively rare for clients taking antipsychotic drugs, except in the case of clozapine, which may induce agranulocytosis in up to three per cent of clients taking the drug. Agranulocytosis is a blood disorder characterised by a selective reduction in white blood cells, particularly neutrophils, which make the client more susceptible to infections (Downie *et al*. 2004). In the case of clozapine, clients prescribed the drug must have a blood test to eliminate agranulocytosis weekly for the first 18 weeks, fortnightly for up to a year after this initial period and then monthly thereafter (Healy 2005).

Agranulocytosis in itself is difficult to detect and is usually identified when symptoms of infection appear. These symptoms include fever, sore throat and mucosal ulcers. Psychiatric nurses should also be aware that agranulocytosis, although rare, may occur in patients taking other neuroleptic drugs such as Chlorpromazine. Nurses should be vigilant of the symptoms and intervene accordingly. Clients who continue on antipsychotic medication after discharge should also be aware of this side effect and what to do if it occurs. Early detection is essential and interventions should only require cessation of the drug in question; treatment for the infection may be indicated. There is spontaneous recovery for most people within about two weeks (Downie *et al*. 2004).

NEUROLEPTIC MALIGNANT SYNDROME

Neuroleptic malignant syndrome (NMS) is a rare but potentially life-threatening idiosyncratic reaction to neuroleptic medications. It can occur in response to any neuroleptic medication but occurs most often in response to low-dose/high-potency typical antipsychotics, e.g. Haloperidol. It also occurs more frequently in those who are on higher doses of antipsychotic medications and where polypharmacy occurs (Healy 2005). Many clients will experience NMS shortly after initial exposure to antipsychotic medications, and almost all clients who develop it do so within two weeks of commencing antipsychotic medications. However, it may also develop in clients who have taken antipsychotics for many years. Diagnosis of NMS can be complicated as it initially presents in a similar way to serotonin syndrome.

The symptoms associated with NMS include:

- muscular rigidity ('lead pipe rigidity')
- tremor
- hyperthermia
- urinary incontinence
- hypo- or hypertension
- tachycardia
- altered mental status
- elevated serum creatinine phosphokinase secondary to muscle breakdown
- elevated white blood cell count.

Prevention

Prevention of NMS can be difficult as it is rarely possible to predict accurately who will develop the syndrome. Early detection is essential to the prevention of severe NMS, however early diagnosis can be made difficult if the cardinal symptom of muscle rigidity is not clearly evident. It is imperative that nurses are familiar with other key symptoms such as altered mental status, fever and altered autonomic function. However, these symptoms could be indicative of changes to the client's mental health or could have an alternative medical cause. Pelonero *et al.* (1998) identify that agitation, dehydration and a prior history of NMS are risk factors in the development of the syndrome. Therefore it is important that nurses are familiar with a client's previous reaction to antipsychotic medication and are aware and respond to deficits in fluid balance in clients taking antipsychotic medications.

Treatment

Immediate discontinuation of the antipsychotic is essential. Pharmacological interventions include the possible use of a dopamine agonist such as Bromocriptine to increase the production of dopamine, and/or a muscle relaxant such as Dantrolene (BNF 2007). In conjunction with this, antipyretics can be given to reduce fever. Electroconvulsive therapy (ECT) may produce a rapid response to NMS and may also be beneficial for the underlying psychiatric condition (Pelonero *et al.* 1998; Healy 2005).

Apart from pharmacological interventions, the main course of treatment for NMS is symptomatic management. A cooling blanket and/or a fan may be required to help reduce pyrexia. Intravenous fluids may also be necessitated to correct dehydration and electrolyte abnormalities. Attention to nutritional support is required as many clients may not be able to eat/drink due to altered mental status.

The syndrome, which usually lasts for five to seven days after drug discontinuation, may be unduly prolonged if depot antipsychotics have been used.

Where possible, clients with a history of NMS should not be recommenced on antipsychotic therapy and should instead be prescribed alternative medications such as lithium, carbamazepine or benzodiazepines. However, this may not always be possible and in these cases the client should be switched to an antipsychotic in a different class and with a lower D2 affinity (e.g. atypical antipsychotics) than the one which produced the NMS.

SEROTONIN SYNDROME

Serotonin Syndrome (SS) is a rare but life-threatening drug reaction caused by an excess of serotonin. It is most often caused when drugs which act on the serotonergic system are prescribed with other drugs that also work on this system (e.g. SSRIs with tricyclic medications). Serotonin syndrome is more likely to occur within the first 24 hours after taking the medication or after an increase/overdose in medication. With the increased incidence of serotonin syndrome since the introduction of the SSRIs and its potentially life-threatening effects, nurses need to know how to recognise and manage this condition.

The symptoms associated with SS include:
- myoclonus (jerks and twitches)
- tremors of the tongue or fingers
- shivering
- hyperthermia
- sweating
- confusion, agitation or restlessness
- tachycardia
- hyperreflexia
- diarrhoea.

At least three major symptoms should be present before a diagnosis is made and the client must be taking a medication that affects the serotonergic system. The main differential diagnosis is NMS and both conditions share many features, however the more rapid onset of SS, the presence of diarrhoea and the absence of 'lead pipe' rigidity can help to establish a diagnosis of SS (Birmes *et al.* 2003).

In most cases, serotonin syndrome is a self-limiting condition and will resolve once the offending agent(s) have been stopped. Supportive care is essential in the management of SS. Intravenous fluids may be required and the nurse should monitor vital signs and urine output regularly. As with NMS, hyperthermia can be managed by introducing measures to reduce the high temperature (e.g. cooling blankets, fans, etc.). In more severe cases, a serotonin antagonist such as cyproheptadine may be used to reduce serotonin levels, although the beneficial effects of such medications are not firmly established.

CONCLUSION

Clients with mental illness are, for a variety of reasons, often more vulnerable to physical illness. Psychiatric nurses are in a key position to use their skills to detect early warning signs of disease and instigate appropriate responses. Therefore the importance of conducting a physical assessment in conjunction with a mental state assessment cannot be underestimated. The treatment regimes for people with mental illness often include psychopharmacology and nurses have a key role in ensuring that adverse effects such as those mentioned in this chapter are recognised and appropriate treatment regimes are implemented immediately.

Reflective Questions
1. What are the important factors to consider when carrying out a physical health assessment for clients with mental illness?
2. Think about how certain lifestyle behaviours can affect the physical well-being of clients with mental health problems. How can these be addressed during a physical health assessment?
3. How would you recognise whether a client were exhibiting signs of neuroleptic malignant syndrome?
4. You have been asked to talk to a group of clients about lithium therapy. What factors would you consider before meeting with the group?

References
Baid, H. (2006) 'The process of conducting a physical assessment: a nursing perspective'. *British Journal of Nursing*, 15 (13), 710–14.
Birmes, P., Coppin, D., Schmitt, L. and Lauque, D. (2003) 'Serotonin syndrome: a brief review'. *CMAJ*, 168(11), 1439–42.
British National Formulary (BNF) (2007). London: British Medical Formulary and Royal Pharmaceutical Society of Great Britain.
Cormac, I., Martin, D. and Ferriter, M. (2004) 'Improving the physical health of long-stay psychiatric in-patients'. *Advances in Psychiatric Treatment*, 10, 107–15.
Daley, A. J. (2002) 'Exercise therapy and mental health in clinical populations: is exercise therapy a worthwhile intervention?' *Advances in Psychiatric Treatment*, 8, 262–70.
Department of Health (UK) (2006) *From Values to Action: The Chief Nursing Officer's Review of Mental Health Nursing*. London: Department of Health.
Downie, G., MacKenzie, J. and Williams, A. (2004) *Pharmacology and Medicines Management for Nurses*. Edinburgh: Churchill Livingstone.
Healy, D. (2005) *Psychiatric Drugs Explained*. Edinburgh: Churchill Livingstone.
Meltzer, H., Gill, B., Hinds, R. and Petticrew, M. (1996) 'Economic activity and social functioning of residents with psychiatric disorders (OCPS surveys of psychiatric morbidity in Great Britain)', Report 6. London: HMSO.

Mir, S. and Taylor, D. M. (2001) 'Antipsychotics and hyperglycaemia'. *International Clinical Psychopharmacology*, 16, 63–73.

NIMHE/Mentality (2004) *Healthy Body and Mind: Promoting Healthy Living for People Who Experience Mental Distress*. London: Mentality/NIMHE.

Ohlsen, R. I., Peacock, G. and Smith, S. (2005) 'Developing a service to monitor and improve physical health in people with serious mental illness'. *Journal of Psychiatric and Mental Health Nursing*, 12, 614–19.

Pelonero, A. L., Levenson, J. L. and Pandurangi, A. K. (1998) 'Neuroleptic malignant syndrome: a review'. *Psychiatric Services*, 49(9), 1163–72.

Prosser, S., Worster, B., MacGregor, J., Dewar, K., Runyard, P. and Fegan, J. (2000) *Applied Pharmacology*. London: Harcourt.

Rosenfeld, G. and Loose-Mitchell, S. (1998) *Pharmacology* (3rd edn). Philadelphia: Lippincott Williams and Wilkins.

Smeltzer, S., Bare, B. (eds), (2000) *Brunner and Suddarth's Textbook of Medical-Surgical Nursing*. Philadelphia: Lippincott.

SECTION 4

Contemporary Issues and Challenges in Psychiatric/Mental Health Nursing

23
Helping People make a Recovery in the Community

Mike Watts

This chapter seeks to explore the processes of mental breakdown and recovery through the lens of personal experience and through my work with GROW. It seeks to place the service user at the very heart of the mental health system and to begin to explore the vital role in recovery of helping relationships, the psychiatric nurse, other professionals and the community in general. As such it is very much in line with the aims laid down in *Vision for Change* (DoHC 2006).

A PERSONAL EXPERIENCE OF BEING MENTALLY ILL

I first became conscious that I had 'problems' when I left school. I had been struggling for a couple of years and had failed my final exams. In the world outside I found it quite difficult to cope with simple things like meeting people. I soon discovered that the anxiety lessened, at least temporarily, if I had a drink. Over the next few years I spiralled into increased difficulties. I would stick at things for about a year and then 'let go'. I worked on a farm and I went to college before dropping out. I travelled in the East where soft drugs were readily available. I began to hear menacing voices. I developed very peculiar ideas such as 'people with blue eyes come from the sky'. I read in the Bible that you can't trust someone whose eyebrows meet in the middle and on examining my own found to my dismay that I had hair between them. I can remember telling my best friend he could no longer trust me. It was a very frightening conclusion because it also meant I couldn't trust myself (GROW 1996).

On my return home I reluctantly agreed to seek help and attended an outpatient psychiatric clinic in a well-known teaching hospital. Here I was asked if I would mind if a group of students were present at my first interview. I did, but didn't have the courage to say so. I was diagnosed as being 'pathologically shy'. I don't know whether that diagnosis had anything to do with the fact that I had a head injury at the age of 12. After my diagnosis and a prescription of Librium, I decided the hospital couldn't help so I continued on under my own direction, finding it increasingly difficult to cope and increasingly contemplating suicide.

I then met a young woman who was to become my wife. Being in love is a great motivator! I started to try to look after myself and I took a series of manual jobs, which helped me gain stability. I also stopped taking all drugs. We went to India together, this time to a yoga school.

We eventually married and came to Ireland. We were going to create the perfect alternative lifestyle. I had inherited some money and we were able to buy a small farm. When our first son was born, Fran, my wife, had a classic psychotic breakdown. The doctor met me at the door of the maternity hospital on the third day after the birth and said she needed to be transferred to the local psychiatric hospital. I was absolutely horrified and promptly discharged my wife and baby son. After a truly terrifying night at home when Fran sat up in bed and screamed, tearing at her hair and banging her head against the wall, I had no option but to sign her in to hospital. A big part of Fran had completely lost touch with reality. She thought our son was Jesus, and that she had to give him to an old man down the lane, because he had a picture of the Virgin Mary on the kitchen wall. After the trauma of Fran's psychosis her admission was a relief. I remember being so grateful that all the staff were kind and friendly.

Over the next three years we battled against a recurring nightmare of hospital admissions, a growing cocktail of drugs and diagnoses that went from post-puerperal depression to schizoaffective disorder to manic depression. One of the most peculiar phenomena was the fact that because Fran was sicker than I was, I was treated as though I was completely well, even though my own life continued to be a nightmare of anxiety that often crossed over into terror. During this time we were continually trying to find a way out. We both expected that one day we would wake up and everything would be all right.

One of the main difficulties of that period was not knowing what to do to help ourselves. No one seemed to know. In fact, quite often we would get conflicting advice from different doctors. The prevailing feeling was that we wouldn't in fact get better (GROW 1996). The message was, 'the tablets have made you better, go and behave as if you were better'. However, the tablets presented many side effects that became problems in themselves. Fran put on a large amount of weight. Her tongue was as dry and hard as a piece of wood and she would often sit for days by the fire rocking backwards and forwards, before exploding again into a rage that would lead to further hospitalisation and further medication.

The experience of mental illness is an isolating one. While it is a different experience for each person, whatever form your illness takes you become increasingly isolated in your own thoughts and feelings. In this way you may progressively lose touch with a commonly accepted reality. The whole process of recovery can be viewed as a process of re-involvement, first with other friendly minds, then with your own strengths and finally with participation within the community and a common-sense set of values that in themselves maintain your mental health.

The Start of Recovery

What helped us both recover was stumbling on to an organisation called GROW. GROW is a self-help organisation which was started by people in Australia in

1957 on their release from psychiatric hospital. It is a twelve-step programme that offers its members direction and a practical programme of recovery or personal growth. It also has a highly structured and effective weekly meeting and, most important, a hopeful and encouraging community of people who will patiently and consistently nurture your spirit and give you affirmation, reassurance and sound advice.

GROW's programme has over the years expanded into a complete practical psychology of mental health based on the experience of thousands of people. It is a main player in what has become known as the recovery movement. It differs significantly from most philosophies used in the mental health system in that it is a philosophy of mental health that is required for recovery from mental illness. When people are ill they need their distress alleviated, they need to gain insight into reasons for their condition, but, most important, they need help to become mentally healthy.

What GROW did for us initially

1. It gave us real **hope**. Here were people who were talking about mental illness in a constructive way as something that happens, but that can be overcome.
2. It helped us **accept** what had happened and reduced the awful sense of stigma. It helped us accept ourselves.
3. It **encouraged** us to take very small but worthwhile risks.
4. It gave us **direction** and as we progressed we gained a **sense of control**. As we became familiar with the meetings the group helped us identify a starting point for recovery. I was given a piece from the book *The Program of Growth to Maturity*, which said quite simply, 'Don't be shy about being shy' (GROW 2004). It was incredible the power those words had in releasing me from the crippling idea of being pathologically shy, which for me had connotations of liar, thief and psychopath.
5. It made our struggles **meaningful** because we realised any progress we made helped others in the group. This idea of being useful and valuable was extremely important. Having a leadership role has been identified as a key factor in recovery (Rappaport *et al.* 1985).
6. It enabled us to learn to meet what GROW calls our **three vital needs** (GROW 2004):
   • To be someone ... to have a sense of personal value and unique identity.
   • To be at home ... to have a sense of security and loving harmony.
   • To be going somewhere ... to have a sense of purpose and progress.

TOWARDS A NEW MODEL OF MENTAL HEALTH CARE

Prior to the publication of the Green Paper on Mental Health (Government of Ireland 1992), GROW presented a view that recognised and traced a naturally occurring evolutionary process at work in mental health care. This evolution has seen a movement in the care of people with mental illness from mainly custodial care prior to the 1950s to one that embraces community care and the inclusion of service users in the development and planning of the mental health services in Ireland. Perhaps now we are on the verge of a major breakthrough in mental health care. Two recent documents, *A Vision for Change* (DoHC 2006) and *A Vision for a Recovery Model in Irish Mental Health Services Discussion Paper* (Mental Health Commission 2006a) indicate a belief in the value of a new way forward. There is a general recognition among all players that we need a multi-disciplinary approach and the possibility of a real two-stranded system is emerging.

A Two-stranded Mental Health System

The first strand of a mental health system consists of diagnosis and treatment; the second, and by far the most important, is concerned with rehabilitation and education. This is where the nurse's role could become vitally important. Jan Foudraine, a Dutch psychiatrist working in the USA, noted that, of all his team of professionals, nurses were the people who got to know their patients best. It is this knowledge of each person's uniqueness that is vital to a person-centred system (Foudraine 1974).

Figure 23.1 A two-stranded mental health system

Strand One	Strand Two
Diagnosis and Treatment	Rehabilitation and Recovery
	Education and Prevention
↓	↓
Psychiatrists and psychiatric nurses	• a whole range of experts
	• service users' own feedback
	• the voluntary sector in mental health
	• key players in the community
	• the general public

DIAGNOSIS

Diagnosis can be valuable if it is used as a means to let a person know what they need to do to overcome their difficulties. What tends to happen is that it becomes a life sentence when used to label a person at the very worst time of their crisis (Crepaz–Keay 2006). It also tends to ignore the 'well part' of the person and exclude that person from creating a recovery plan. In GROW we have found that people who experience schizophrenia have become terribly isolated. If a diagnosis of schizophrenia could be understood as a need to become increasingly involved with people it would provide an acceptable way forward. If, however, diagnosis becomes a fancy way of saying to a person, 'you have a terrible lifelong disease, which is a mystery to us and from which you will not recover', it becomes a cruel and self-fulfilling prophecy.

TREATMENT

Obviously psychiatric drugs can be extremely valuable. Anyone who has experienced deep depression or acute mania and its damaging consequences will know how medication can provide a level of stability that just about allows you to function. However, the aim of good treatment should be the end of that treatment (GROW 1997) and this can only come about if intense work is put in on rehabilitation and recovery.

RECOVERY

There is a body of knowledge that has built up from what is known as the recovery movement. The recovery movement consists of a loose amalgam of people and organisations composed of people who have experienced mental illness and recovered. For example, GROW, the National Empowerment Centre, Irish Advocacy Network, Steer (Support Training Education Employment Research) are all composed of people in this category. GROW has published two volumes of a book called *Soul Survivors* (GROW 1996, 2003), which give personal accounts of the two journeys into and out of mental illness. The National Empowerment Centre has put together some core principles of recovery (Ahern and Fisher 1999). These include:

1. the need for hope
2. the need to have people who believe in you
3. the need to have dreams
4. the need to take small risks
5. the need for direction and to take small steps.

The European Commission recently published a document on mental health in which they target education and prevention as the most important priority for a community mental health system (Jane–Llopis and Anderson 2005).

INTEGRATING THE MEDICAL MODEL INTO A RECOVERY MODEL

Roberts and Wolfson (2004) illustrate the differences between the recovery model and the medical model (see Figure 23.2). While many commentators see these two views as diametrically opposed, they can actually complement each other. However, we need to find a way to integrate the medical model into one that allows and encourages recovery. In other words we need a system that identifies the type of illness or distress, provides the minimum amount of drugs needed and sees this as a starting point on a road to recovery. This road provides professional help of many kinds and leads a person into personal support systems that promote positive mental health. Integral to the success of this is a gradual and appropriate reduction in medication and professional help as the person recovers. A longitudinal study undertaken by Salem *et al.* (1988), which followed the progress of matched groups of people with mental illness engaged in the recovery process, found evidence of all this happening over a nine-month period.

Figure 23.2 The recovery model versus the medical model

Recovery Model	Medical Model
Distressing experience	Psychopathology
Biography	Pathography
Interest centred on the person	Interest centred on the disorder
Pro-health	Anti-disease
Strengths-based	Treatment-based
Experts by experience	Doctors and patients
Personal meaning	Diagnosis
Understanding	Recognition
Value-centred	Apparently value-free
Humanistic	Scientific
Growth and discovery	Treatment
Choice	Compliance
Modelled on heroes	Underpinned by meta analysis
Guiding narratives	Randomised control trials
Transformation	Return to normal
Self-management	Expert care co-ordinators
Self-control	Bringing under control
Personal responsibility	Professional accountability
Within a social context	Decontextualised

Mental Health Commission (2006)

The idea of a slow progression from hospitalisation and medication to more personal relationships is cleverly expanded in a page from GROW's Programme of Recovery and Personal Growth entitled 'Which tranquillisers do you use?' (GROW 2004). The following are some 'tranquillisers' that could be utilised by the individual with mental health difficulties:

1. God
2. your own personal resources: habitually, or in a crisis
3. friendly help, individual and group
4. professional guidance: nurse; social worker; marriage guidance counsellor; pastoral counsellor; psychologist; psychiatrist
5. medical intervention: physical or chemical means (ECT, drugs)
6. compulsory help: restraint by the state authority in hospital or prison.

The nurse is crucially placed at the top of the list of professionals. His or her job is to provide friendly yet professional help which will aim to involve the individual in their local community and to help him/her nurture friendships and develop personal resources in the way that all of us need to in order to deal with life successfully.

As a nurse:
1. Be friendly and interested.
2. Get to know the person you are trying to help.
3. Encourage them to get involved in mutual help and realise that their experience is valuable to others; they have a leadership role (GROW 1996).
4. Set up a GROW group for a group of your clients (GROW 1996)
5. Instead of developing a care plan, work with your clients to make a recovery map.
6. Apply the principles of recovery to your relationship with your patient.
7. Get beyond the labels of nurse and mental patient and dare to share your own humanity and struggles (in an appropriate way).
8. Give positive feedback on all efforts to recover.
9. As a member of a multidisciplinary team, be your patients' advocate for enabling rather than disabling forms of help.

We live in a world that increasingly recognises that mental health, like physical health, is something we all have to work at. Mental illness can and does happen to all of us. When we are very well there is still a vulnerable and *shadow side*. When we are terribly sick, there is still a strong, healthy part.

CARE PLAN OR RECOVERY MAP?

Ultimately the success of a recovery approach will depend on a change of mindset and a change of practice by those 'in power' in the health system. Language becomes a very important tool in effecting that change. At present mental illness is seen as a lifelong condition. Care plans, where they exist, tend to be cautious affairs couched in medical language. They give the impression of dependence on the professional and often on medication instead of growing independence. An idea that has developed through GROW is the creation of a recovery map (Watts 2005). The words themselves are much more dynamic and proactive. To illustrate this I will return to my own and Fran's stories.

A Personal Experience of Recovery from Mental Illness

When we were mentally sick we were in several different types of places. As well as having a geographical location, which contained many resources, we were in an emotional or spiritual place as well. The pain of these places represented our needs. We were both in isolation. Fran was in despair and rage, and I was in despair and fear, bordering on terror. The question was how we could find resources locally that would help us move from this position to one of security, personal value and purpose. Once we started looking we found them in the most unlikely places.

I found my way out of fear slowly and progressively, by allowing others to show me the way. This included many ordinary people. An old neighbour of ours would bang his fist on the table while playing cards and shout out 'Up sticks and wallop Carthy'. To me this was inspirational and attractive. I was so over-controlled I had lost the ability to be spontaneous and to express joy.

I eventually got a job in a factory when we decided to leave the farm, and the warmth of other people, playing football at lunchtime, and even throwing food round the canteen, all assisted my recovery. I also went back to third-level education, studied for a degree in psychology and subsequently a master's in family therapy. During my recovery, creative writing, tin whistle classes, Toast Masters, hill walking and badminton classes all played their part.

Meanwhile Fran was finding her way through a very different set of relationships and people. Someone suggested that she might teach reading and writing to Traveller women, as she spoke four languages. The women warmed to her and taught her how to sew! She became involved in the Irish Countrywomen's Association and won best actress in a drama competition. A back-to-work course, language exams and teaching, plus a horticultural course, all played their part. Along the way we have had help from experts, including spiritual direction, marriage guidance, some family therapy and small pieces of professional counselling.

In 1987 we discovered we were expecting our fourth child after a gap of 11 years. Fran's doctor advised her to cease taking lithium during the pregnancy. This was the only medication she was still on. After a complicated birth, she found she was enjoying being a mother and persuaded her doctor to again stop the lithium, which she had been advised to resume taking. This was twenty years ago.

CONCLUSION

Salem *et al.* (1988:408) wrote the following conclusion at the end of five years of research into the recovery process through GROW:

Ultimately, the success or failure of efforts in community care will depend less on mental health professionals' ability to create supportive environments or to teach specific skills and more on the ability to find and encourage naturally occurring niches. These niches are where people find meaning in life; mutual rather than uni-directional relationships; and consistent ongoing structures on which to depend. These are the settings that those who experience serious psychopathology often are unable to find. Mutual help organisations may provide naturally occurring settings (that is, not professionally developed), that are available to people who are left to maintain themselves in the world when the professionals, the aftercare workers, and the volunteers have gone home.

If you would like to experience one of GROW's mutual help groups and see for yourself recovery in action we have a network of groups throughout the country and you can get further information by visiting www.grow.ie.

Reflective Questions
1. How can you as a psychiatric nurse assist the person who is being discharged from hospital on their road to recovery?
2. What challenges might you face when adopting a recovery-based model in clinical practice?
3. Reflecting on the author's experience of mental illness and the mental health care system, how can this help you to understand the experiences of people who use the service?
4. What steps can you take to be more inclusive to the needs of the people who use mental health services in Ireland?

References

Ahern, L. and Fisher, D. (1999) *Personal Assistance in Community Existence: A Recovery Guide.* Lawrence, MA: National Empowerment Centre. Available at www.power2u.org/pace_manual.pdf. Accessed 28 November 2006.

Allott, P. and Loganathan, L. (2003) 'Discovering hope for recovery from a British perspective — a review of a sample of recovery literature, implications for sample and practice change' (West Midlands Partnerships for Mental Health, Birmingham), in Mental Health Commission (2006a).

Crepaz-Keay, D. (2006) *Lecture to Mental Health Commission*, Galway.

Department of Health and Children (DoHC) (2006) *A Vision for Change: Report of the Expert Group on Mental Health Policy.* Dublin: Stationery Office.

Foudraine, J. (1974) *Not Made of Wood: A Psychiatrist Discovers his own Profession.* USA: Macmillan.

Government of Ireland (1984) *The Psychiatric Services: Planning for the Future.* Dublin: Stationery Office.

Government of Ireland (1992) *Green Paper on Mental Health.* Dublin: Stationery Office.

GROW (1996) *Soul Survivors*, Vol. 1. Kilkenny: GROW in Ireland.

GROW (1997) *Summary Introduction to GROW.* Kilkenny: GROW Publications.

GROW (2003) *Soul Survivors*, Vol. 2. Kilkenny: GROW in Ireland.

GROW (2004) *The Programme of Growth to Maturity* (17th edn). Australia: Aussie Press.

Jane-Llopis, E. and Anderson, P. (2005) *Mental Health Promotion and Mental Disorder Prevention. A Policy for Europe.* Nijmegen: Radboud University.

Mental Health Commission (2006a) *A Vision for a Recovery Model in Irish Mental Health Services Discussion Paper*. Dublin: Mental Health Commission.

Mental Health Commission (2006b) *The Views of Adult Users of the Public Sector Mental Health Services*. Dublin: Mental Health Commission.

Ralph, R., Lambert, D. and Kidder, K. (2002) 'The recovery perspective and evidence based practice for people with serious mental illness: a guideline developed for the behavioural health recovery management project' (University of Chicago: Centre for Psychiatric Rehabilitation), in Mental Health Commission (2006a).

Rappaport, J., Seidman, E., Toro, P., McFadden, L., Reischl, T., Roberts, L., Salem, D., Stein, C. and Zimmerman, M. (1985) 'Collaborative research with a mutual help organisation'. *Social Policy*, 15, 12–24.

Roberts, G. and Wolfson, P. (2004) 'The rediscovery of recovery: open to all. Advances in psychiatric treatment', in Mental Health Commission (2006a).

Salem, D., Seidman, E. and Rappaport, J. (1988) 'Community treatment of the mentally ill: the promise of mutual-help organisations'. *Social Work*, 33, (5), 403–8.

Watts, M. (2005) *Growing*. Kilkenny: GROW Publications.

24
Sexuality and Mental Health

Agnes Higgins

Sexuality is both a core dimension of personhood and an important aspect of health and well-being. Psychiatric nurses are in a unique position to provide sexual health care to people with mental health problems. The aim of this chapter is to commence a discussion on sexuality in the context of people who are experiencing mental distress, and the role of the psychiatric nurse. Although some might consider the paraphilias and gender identity disorders as important aspects of sexuality, the focus of this chapter is not on 'pathological' sexuality. Instead, emphasis is placed on core issues that impact on the vast majority of people attending psychiatric services and the implications of research in these areas for best nursing practice.

THE CONCEPT OF SEXUALITY

Sexuality is a difficult concept to define. It is a complex and elusive phenomenon that has multiple interlinkages with all aspects of our lives. Sexuality is much more than anatomy and physiology and more than sexual intercourse. Sexuality is a symbol for a complex attribute that goes beyond the confines of copulation and gender designation. Each person's sexuality is as unique to the person as their fingerprint and is an integral part of their being human, being alive and being real. The Pan American Health Organisation and World Health Organisation (PAHO/WHO) (2002:6) state that:

> Sexuality refers to a core dimension of being human which includes sex, gender, sexual and gender identity, sexual orientation, eroticism, emotional attachment/love and reproduction. It is experienced or expressed in thoughts, fantasies, desires, beliefs, attitudes, values, activities, practices, roles, [and] relationships. Sexuality is a result of the interplay of biological, psychological, socio-economic, cultural, ethical and religious/spiritual factors. While sexuality can include all of these aspects, not all of these dimensions need to be experienced or expressed.

From this definition, it is evident that sexuality is about who we are, our identity, our relationship with the self and with others. It is intimately bound up with our self-concept, self-esteem, body image and total self-image. Sexuality or expression of sexuality is not a fixed and static state, but a dynamic, evolving and fluctuating potential. It is an aspect of one's humanness, which exists in the young, middle-aged and old, whether single or coupled; in opposite- and/or same-sex partnerships; it is part of the person living with a mental health problem in the community or an environment of long-term care.

Figure 24.1 Definitions of other concepts related to sexuality

Biological sex	Sex refers to the sum of biological characteristics that define the spectrum of humans as female, male and intersex.
Transsexual	Transsexuals are people who see themselves as 'really being the other gender' — e.g. a woman who feels she is a man, locked in a woman's body.
Gender	Gender relates to the cultural values, attitudes and roles associated with a particular biological sex.
Gender identity	The term given to the way an individual's identity is gendered — the way of being a man or woman.
Sexual orientation	Refers to the gender to whom the person is attracted sexually. Many people think of sexual orientation in an essentialist way (you are either heterosexual or homosexual), but it should be viewed as a spectrum rather than a dichotomy.
Sexual activity	The behavioural expression of one's sexuality. It is through sexual activity that the erotic component of one's sexuality is most evident.
Sexual identity	An internal framework that is constructed over time and enables the person to organise her/his self-concept based upon biological sex, gender identity and sexual orientation and to perform socially in regard to her/his perceived sexual capabilities.
Sexual health	Not merely the absence of disease or dysfunction, but includes a positive and respectful approach to sexuality and sexual relationships, as well as the possibility of having pleasurable and safe sexual experiences, free from coercion, discrimination and violence.
Heterosexism	An automatic assumption that everyone is heterosexual and that heterosexuality is superior to, and preferable to, other sexualities.

As the person grows and changes, the recognition, acceptance and expression of the self as a sexual being continues as a lifelong process. How a person views and expresses her/his sexuality is influenced by their stage of development, beliefs, attitudes and values, which are shaped and influenced by cultural, societal and religious norms. Hence what it means to be a girl or boy, man or woman, will vary from culture to culture and will change with time as societal values change. Equally, how people choose to express their sexuality may also change.

Figure 24.2 An overview of how the various dimensions of sexuality might be integrated into one's sexual identity

Biological sex	Gender identity	Sexual orientation/ attraction	Sexual expression/ activity
Man	Feminine	Attracted to members	Sexual thoughts
Woman	Masculine	of the same sex	Sexual fantasies
Intersex	Gay	Attracted to members	Sexual touch/caressing
	Lesbian	of the opposite sex	Kissing
	Bisexual	Attracted to both,	Masturbation (self/other)
	Transsexual	or neither	Vaginal sex
	Heterosexual		Oral sex
	Concept of body image		Anal sex
	(sexual attractiveness)		Sexual fetishes
			Celibacy
			Illegal sexual activity
			(e.g. child pornography,
			sexual violence)

Sexuality is a force that has the potential to promote intimacy, pleasure, self-esteem and support the deepest longing for human connection, while paradoxically being a force that can diminish, hurt and exploit the vulnerabilities of others. As psychiatric nurses, instead of seeing sexuality as a unified whole, it is necessary to recognise that there are many sexualities and that this emotionally charged issue is best defined by both the service user and caregiver within the context of factors such as age, gender, personal attributes, religious and cultural norms.

SEXUAL RIGHTS AND PEOPLE WITH MENTAL HEALTH PROBLEMS

The history of sexuality and people with mental health problems has largely been a history of misunderstanding, misconception, stigma and myth. Historically, the expression of sexuality was viewed as either a cause or a symptom of mental illness, thus linking the expression of sexuality to people with mental health problems in a negative way. The genetic and degenerative theory of inheritance also fuelled the idea that people with mental health problems were hypersexual, immoral, governed by animalistic sexual urges and a danger to the human race (Deegan 1999). Consequently, psychiatric services took on a control and regulator function in relation to sexual behaviour. People with any disability are still frequently treated as asexual beings and are denied their sexual rights and needs for intimacy and sexual expression (Shakespeare *et al.* 1996).

Holistic, person-centred care, the core of psychiatric nursing, is predicated on the value of personhood. Central to this is a valuing of the person as a biological, psychological, social, spiritual and sexual being, with rights as a sexual citizen.

Sexual rights include: the right to express one's full sexual potential; the right to sexual autonomy, privacy, equity and pleasure; the right to make free and responsible reproductive choices; the right to comprehensive sexual health education; and the right to sexual health care (PAHO/WHO 2002). The UN's principles for the protection of persons with mental illness and for the improvement of mental health care (the MI principles) states that people 'shall have the right to exercise all civil, political, economic, social and cultural rights' (Office of the High Commissioner for Human Rights 1991:2). Although not explicitly stated, the term 'civil rights' does include the right to sexual expression. The UN Convention (to which Ireland is a signatory) also assigns people with mental health problems the right to be sexually active and the right to knowledge.

The *Report of the Commission on the Status of People with Disabilities* in Ireland in 1996 marked a watershed in Irish disability policy. It set out a legislative policy and service framework for people with disabilities and the realisation of their economic, social and cultural rights, including their sexual rights (Government of Ireland 1996). Discrimination on the grounds of sexual orientation or disability are also included within the nine grounds covered by the Irish equality legislation (Government of Ireland 1998). In addition, the promotion of sexual health has also been identified by policy makers as a central component of the health strategy (DoHC 2000).

For sexual health to be attained and maintained, the sexual rights of people must be recognised, acknowledged and upheld by psychiatric nurses. In order to do this, nurses must challenge the assumptions that act as barriers to the inclusion of sexuality within the domain of psychiatric nursing practice and create a context for discussion of sexual health issues with service users and their families.

INCLUDING SEXUALITY IN NURSING ASSESSMENT AND CARE

Needs assessment is important both for individual care planning and service provision for people experiencing mental health problems. McCann (2000) suggested that if psychiatric nurses wanted to be truly responsive to people they needed to include sexuality as a dimension of assessment and to explore sexual and relationship issues. However, psychiatric nurses often fear discussing sexual issues and passively wait for service users to tell them of any concerns or worries in this aspect of their lives. In defending their actions, nurses frequently put forward a number of rationalisations such as lack of time, fear of upsetting or offending the person, assuming that service users will volunteer concerns or that service users lack the ability to talk about sexuality. Underpinning some of these views is a belief that people with mental health problems are not capable of handling their sexuality responsibly. In other cases these rationalisations reflect a projection of personal and social anxieties onto service users and families. Talking about sexuality should begin at the initial stages of care; in this way, nurses can act as role models, educating service users that sexuality and sexual relationships can be openly discussed without shame or guilt.

Suggestions for commencing a discussion on sexuality with a service user:
- Has your mental health problem changed the way you see yourself (feel about yourself) as a man/woman?
- Has your mental health problem affected your relationship with your family/partner or changed the way you get close to your partner/friends/family?
- Is there someone you are involved with sexually right now?
- Other people in similar situations have said the physical part of their relationship has been affected by the drugs. Would you like to talk ...
- Some people have questions regarding (...). If you would like to talk ...
- Many people undergoing this type of treatment have concerns about what will happen to their sex lives, and I would be happy to answer any questions you may have.

SEXUAL VIOLENCE

Research suggests that sexual violence among men and women is a pervasive dimension of contemporary Irish society that is both under-reported and under-acknowledged (McGee *et al.* 2002). Although not all people who have been sexually abused will attend a mental health service, a history of sexual violence significantly increases the person's chances of experiencing a mental health problem. While exact figures are unknown, some estimate that approximately thirty per cent of the people attending mental health services in Ireland will have experienced some form of sexual violence and require focused therapeutic interventions (National Counselling Service 2003).

Research into the long-term impact of child sexual abuse on both men and women has repeatedly demonstrated that people who have been sexually abused experience low self-esteem, decreased self-worth, shame, stigma and powerlessness; they have difficulty forming relationships, trusting people in intimate and sexual relationships and maintaining sexual boundaries. Survivors of abuse frequently develop negative attitudes towards their own sexuality, and either avoid all sexual contact or unconsciously enact aspects of early sexual abuse in subsequent sexual relationships. Although it is not possible to say conclusively that childhood abuse 'causes' adult re-victimisation, there is evidence that people who have experienced sexual abuse in childhood are frequently left vulnerable to sexual re-victimisation (McGee *et al.* 2002).

Survivors of sexual abuse are also found to be at risk of long-term psychological effects, which will bring them into contact with the mental health services and psychiatric nurses. High rates of sexual abuse have been reported among people who experienced depression, anxiety, self-harm, post-traumatic stress disorder, personality disorders, eating disorders and alcohol problems (McGee *et al.* 2002). A significant correlation has been found between depression, post-traumatic stress disorder and the more severe forms of sexual violence, such as penetration or attempted penetration. A link between childhood sexual abuse and subsequent psychosis, especially hallucinations, has been reported in people diagnosed with schizophrenia and bipolar affective disorder. Read and Argyle (1999) suggest that there is a relationship between the content of the hallucination and sexual abuse, e.g. the voice telling the person to kill themselves being the voice of the abuser.

Revealing a history of abuse could be the first step in dealing with a psychological burden that may have been kept secret for years and ensuring that service users get focused therapeutic support. However, stigma, self-hatred, shame, perceiving what happened to them as 'too trivial' to tell others, blaming themselves, and fearing that nobody will believe them often leads to service users not disclosing sexual violence (McGee *et al.* 2002). Therefore, avoiding talking about sexual violence or not giving permission to service users to talk about their experiences may reinforce the person's belief that their experience is 'too bad' or 'too unpleasant' to discuss with anyone, or may be perceived as a further collusion with society's denial of the prevalence of sexual abuse. Even if adult sexual violence or childhood sexual abuse did occur but is denied by the person, the fact that the subject is mentioned signals to the person that the nurse is willing to explore the issues at some future time when the person is ready.

PRESCRIBED DRUGS AND SEXUALITY

Although contested, the use of prescribed drugs is considered by some an essential part of the treatment of many people with mental health problems. Currently, in the Republic of Ireland, the focus of mental health services is on drug treatment, with a significant number of service users being prescribed three or more drugs (Schizophrenia Ireland 2002).

However, antipsychotic, antidepressant and anticholinergic drugs can have many adverse side effects, which severely impact directly and indirectly on sexuality and sexual function (see Figure 24.3). In most cases, side effects that impact on sexual function are idiosyncratic and unpredictable, with no apparent relationship between the type of drug used, dose and the incidence of a specific sexual dysfunction. However, it is thought that drugs that enhance serotonin or decrease dopamine tend to diminish sexual function and desire. In addition drugs that block the cholinergic and alpha-adrenergic receptors may have 'asexual properties' (Higgins *et al.* 2005).

There is a commonly held view that people with a mental health problem suffer from reduced libido or sex drive as a result of their 'mental illness'. Thus their experience of drug-induced iatrogenic sexual dysfunction is often minimised or ignored. All conventional (typical) neuroleptics (phenothiazines, butrophenones, thioxantines) can lead to some form of sexual dysfunction. The reported rates of sexual dysfunction in people treated with conventional neuroleptics range from 45–60 per cent in men to 30–93 per cent in women (Higgins *et al.* 2005).

The last decade has seen the introduction of the so-called atypical antipsychotics (olanzapine, risperidone, clozapine, etc). These drugs, when compared to the older antipsychotics, are considered to be more effective in the treatment of symptoms such as withdrawal and lack of energy, and thus have favourable effects on interpersonal relationships, sexual interest and activity. However, there are an increasing number of case reports of sexual dysfunction with these drugs. Treatment emergent sexual dysfunction has also been reported with virtually all antidepressant medication. Reported rates of sexual problems as a result of antidepressant drugs range from 40 to 62 per cent. Anticholinergic drugs are frequently used to treat acute Parkinsonism, dystonia and akathesia, all of which have been found to respond to this group of drugs. While anticholinergic drugs do diminish some side effects, they can cause erectile dysfunction in men and a failure of vaginal lubrication in women (Higgins *et al.* 2005). In addition, some drugs are unsafe to take during pregnancy, hence the need for discussion and advice on options available, such as contraception.

Gregoire and Pearson (2002) reported on four cases of unplanned pregnancy in women who had been changed from older, typical oral or depot antipsychotics to atypical drugs. They suggest that this can be explained by the loss of the contraceptive side effect produced by drug-induced hyperprolactinaemia in these women. Therefore, nurses need to explain this risk to women and provide advice on contraception.

Registered nurses have various roles in relation to medication, including the functions of administration, education and monitoring of both the benefit and side effects of drugs. However, research from service users' perspectives suggests that they are dissatisfied with the information they receive on drugs and would like more education; in particular, on the side effects of medication that impact on sexual function. In a survey of over 2,000 service users, 39 per cent reported that they experienced sexual side effects from drugs. In comparison with the other side effects, such as fatigue, weight gain and tremors, the sexual side effects were rated as the most troublesome by those experiencing them (National Schizophrenia Foundation 2000).

In many cases, nurses may be reluctant to inform service users about side effects that impact on sexuality, or to enquire about sexual issues, for a number of reasons, such as fear that service users will discontinue taking their drugs, lack of knowledge about side effects, and embarrassment. In addition, there is often an erroneous assumption that these side effects will diminish with time as the person's body adjusts to the drug. Failure on the part of nurses to educate service users may result in them blaming themselves for their sexual dysfunction, feeling too ashamed to talk or disclose the facts to healthcare professionals, or becoming fearful of engaging in intimate relationships (Deegan 1999).

To prevent service users feeling isolated and confused, nurses need to provide oral and written information to service users about the impact of drugs on sexual function and include sexual issues in assessment tools used to assess side effects. It is no longer ethical for psychiatric nurses to continue with the paternalistic attitude that views the withholding of information as being in the best interest of service users (Higgins *et al.* 2006). In situations where service users are embarrassed or reluctant to inform their doctor about these side effects, psychiatric nurses need to take personal action and inform the medical practitioner, so that available options may be discussed with the service user and an alternative treatment plan jointly designed.

Figure 24.3 Impact of prescribed drugs on sexuality and sexual function

Drug groups	Men	Women
Conventional neuroleptics (e.g. phenothiazines, butrophenones, thioxantines)	Erection difficulties (difficulty in achieving or maintaining an erection, including morning erections)	Desire and arousal problems Poor vaginal lubrication Diminished orgasm or anorgasmia
Atypical antipsychotics (e.g. olanzapine, risperidone and clozapine)	Ejaculatory difficulties (reduced ejaculatory volume, retrograde ejaculation, delayed ejaculation or total inhibition of ejaculation) Gynecomastica Galactorrhea Breast discomfort Weight gain Fatigue Sedation Priapism (engorgement of the penis – must be treated as a medical emergency)	Menstruation changes (irregular menses, amenorrhea, or menorrhagia) Gynecomastica Galactorrhea Breast discomfort Weight gain Fatigue Sedation
Antidepressants	Erection and delayed ejaculation problems, painful ejaculation Decreased nocturnal erections Galactorrhoea Loss of sensation in the penis (mainly associated with Fluoxetine)	Decreased sexual desire Decreased sexual excitement Diminished or delayed orgasm Loss of sensation in the vagina and nipples (mainly associated with Fluoxetine)
Anticholinergic	Erectile dysfunction	Decreased vaginal lubrication

SEXUAL DIVERSITY AND MENTAL HEALTH

Being gay/lesbian/bisexual/transgender (GLBT) is not in itself a mental health problem and GLBT people are not inherently any more prone to mental health problems than anybody else. However, coping with the effects of discrimination can be detrimental to GLBT mental health. Like many other minorities in society, they face many forms of prejudice, harassment and discrimination, which are rooted within the heterosexist structures of society and societal homophobic attitudes (Wilton 2000). While most gay, lesbian and bisexual young people develop positive coping strategies to manage the ensuing stress and become healthy, productive adults, psychiatric nurses need to understand the relationship between sexual orientation and mental distress in order to be in a position to identify vulnerable individuals and promote mental health among this group of people.

The invisibility of GLBT identity in mainstream culture can damage people's self-esteem and make it hard for people to feel a sense of belonging to a society that seems not to recognise they exist (Wilton 2000). The negative internalisation of society's attitudes and the constant monitoring and censoring of one's thoughts and actions in social situations can result in feelings of social alienation, anxiety, loss of self-esteem and an inability to express the 'true self'. The possible consequence of ostracism, stigma and reprisal in a homophobic culture makes 'coming out' extremely difficult. These feelings are exacerbated during adolescence and early adulthood, when many GLBT men and women remain isolated from the adult gay and lesbian movements. For those people who come out, the experience of being perceived as deviant and rejected by either family or society can have a profound effect on identity and sense of worth. In addition, GLBT people with mental health problems often suffer a combined stigma, the stigma of their mental health problem and their sexual orientation (National Disability Authority 2005).

Research studies focusing on the mental health and social well-being of gay men, lesbians, and bisexuals suggested levels of alcohol and drug abuse and depression are high among this group of people (Robertson 1998; King and McKeown 2003). Reasons suggested for this included using alcohol and drugs as a means of coping with depression and societal oppression. Although statistical data for completed suicides among the homosexual population are skewed, as sexual orientation is not recorded as part of mortality data, there is a growing body of international research suggesting that lesbian, gay and bisexual people are at increased risk of mental health problems, particularly self-harm and suicidal behaviour. As the exact relationship between social prejudices and mental health problems has yet to be firmly established, the extent to which this vulnerability is dependent on the prevailing negative social attitudes is difficult to say, but probably accounts for a large part.

Homosexuality was declassified as a mental disorder by the American Psychiatric Association in 1973 and the World Health Organisation in 1992. However, a number of research studies exploring lesbian, gay and bisexual people's experience of the mental health services suggested they experience the same discrimination in the mental health service as they do in wider society (McFarlane 1998; Robertson 1998; King and McKeown 2003). Many participants in these studies did not feel safe to be 'out' in the mental health service and reported experiencing insensitivity, prejudice and discriminatory practices from staff in the form of homophobia, biphobia and heterosexism. Although participants did identify sensitive practices, a number cited examples of overt homophobia and subtle forms of discrimination, including lack of empathy, the presumption of heterosexuality and an unwillingness to discuss sexuality.

Participants who reported discussing their sexuality with staff often received 'clumsy and ill informed responses' (King and McKeown 2003:44).

Psychiatric nurses need to be aware of their own assumptions and prejudices that may marginalise GLBT service users and ensure that they are not reinforcing the heterosexual assumptions of society, thus exacerbating isolation. They need to create an environment where disclosure can take place by avoiding heterosexual language in assessment discussions or in sexual education offered to service users. In addition, psychiatric nurses need to ensure that they include information and advice on resourses that are relevant to gay, lesbian and bisexual people.

SEXUAL RISK BEHAVIOUR AND PEOPLE WITH SEVERE MENTAL HEALTH PROBLEMS

The growing spread of the human immunodeficiency virus (HIV) and other sexually transmitted diseases has led to an increased interest in the study of at-risk populations and the development of prevention programmes. The first studies addressing cognitive and behavioural factors that placed people with severe mental health problems at risk of sexually transmitted infections did not emerge in the literature until the beginning of the 1990s. This was possibly due to prevailing stereotypes that people with 'severe' mental health problems, such as those diagnosed with schizophrenia, were asexual or not interested in sex. The belief that people with mental health problems had diminished sex drive was fuelled by studies in the early 1980s, which reported decreased incidence of sexual activity among people with mental health problems living in institutions (Buckley *et al.* 1999). This decreased incidence was possibly due to low reporting and institutional segregation rather than an aspect of the illness.

Although sexual activity does not in itself pose a risk of infection, evidence suggested that people with severe mental health problems engage in sexual risk behaviour, such as having multiple partners, engaging in sex with high-risk groups, trading sex for some material gain, and using condoms infrequently (Kelly *et al.* 1997; Grassi *et al.* 1999). While many of the behaviours identified are important risk factors for people who do not experience mental health problems, the sequelae of severe mental illness, including cognitive and social skills and problem-solving deficits, and the coexistence of substance abuse problems, contribute to the risk of sexually transmitted infections. By impairing judgement and disinhibiting behaviour, substance abuse increases the risks of inconsistent condom use and engaging in sex with a high-risk partner. People with severe mental health problems may lack the assertiveness needed to negotiate safer sexual relationships. The presence of delusions, hallucinations and social dysfunction may negatively affect the person's ability to sustain long-term relationships; consequently they may engage in sexual behaviour in the context of unstable and transient relationships.

A disadvantaged social and economic status often leaves people with transient living arrangements, placing them in contact with high-risk populations, subject to 'survival sex pressures' and vulnerable to sexual abuse, exploitation and victimisation (Kelly *et al.* 1997:295). In addition, many researchers reported a lack of knowledge around sexually transmitted diseases, the reproductive system and safe sexual practices among people with severe mental health problems.

Although many of the research studies were conducted with people outside Ireland, given the lack of knowledge around issues of sexuality and the incidence of sexual risk behaviour among the general public in Ireland (Layte *et al.* 2006), it is reasonable to propose that similar deficits in knowledge and risk behaviour in people with mental health problems in Ireland are possible and quite probable. Psychiatric nurses therefore have a key role to play in educating service users around areas such as relationship development, courtship, prevention of pregnancy, sexually transmitted diseases and negotiating safe sexual practices. By developing programmes that assist people to develop intimacy skills and sexual health relationships, psychiatric nurses may assist service users to overcome some of the social isolation and loneliness they experience. Consideration also needs to be given to developing programmes that encompass diversity in sexual behaviour as opposed to basing education programmes on the normative assumption of heterosexuality.

CONCLUSION

This chapter has addressed issues such as the concept of sexuality, barriers in talking to service users about sexual issues, sexual violence, prescribed drugs and sexuality, sexual diversity and sexual risk behaviour.

What is evident is the growing body of evidence that suggests that people experiencing mental health problems have problems in relation to sexuality. A high number of clients attending psychiatric services have experienced sexual violence prior to coming to the service and an equally high number of clients experience side effects of drugs, which impact on sexuality. Some client groups, such as people who experience 'severe' mental health problems, have poor knowledge of sex-related issues, lack the necessary skills to negotiate safe sexual relationships and are vulnerable to exploitation and sexually transmitted diseases. Therefore, the main message of this chapter is that sexuality is an aspect of service users' lives that nurses should no longer ignore. If nurses are to be truly holistic in their approach to care they need to acknowledge service users as sexual beings and provide support, advice and education in this area of life and living. In conclusion, I will leave the final word to Patricia Deegan (1999:21), who described herself as a mental health consumer and reminds us that people:

> ... who have been diagnosed with major mental illness do not cease to be human beings by virtue of that diagnosis. Like all people we experience the need for love, companionship, solitude and intimacy. Like all people we want to feel loved, valued and desired by others.

Reflective Questions

1. What type of messages did you receive about sexuality and how have these messages influenced your perceptions of sexuality and the care you offer service users?
2. What possible barriers (cultural, personal, professional, organisational) might you face when talking to service users about their sexuality, and how might you overcome these barriers?
3. List the prescribed drugs you have seen administered. Now imagine yourself in the position of the person receiving the medication and how you would feel if you experienced the sexual side effects for that group of drugs (see Figure 24.3). What help or advice would you like from the team and to whom would you like to talk about your experiences, and why?
4. You have been allocated to care for a service user who has been sexually abused as a child. What challenges would caring for this person raise for you and how might you meet these challenges?

References

Buckley, P., Robben, T., Friedman, L. and Hyde, J. (1999) 'Sexual behaviour in people with serious mental illness: patterns and clinical correlates', in P. Buckley (ed.) *Sexuality and Serious Mental Illness*. Amsterdam: Harwood.

Deegan, P. (1999) 'Human sexuality and mental illness: consumer viewpoints and recovery principles', in P. Buckley (ed.) *Sexuality and Serious Mental Illness*. Amsterdam: Harwood.

Department of Health and Children (DoHC) (2000) *The National Health Promotion Strategy 2000–2005*. Dublin: Stationery Office.

Government of Ireland (1996) *Report of the Commission on the Status of People with Disabilities: A Strategy for Equality*. Dublin: Stationery Office.

Government of Ireland (1998) *Employment Equality Act*. Dublin: Government of Ireland.

Grassi, L., Peron, L., Ferri, S. and Pavanati, M. (1999) 'Human immunodeficiency virus-related risk behaviours among Italian psychiatric inpatients'. *Comprehensive Psychiatry*, 40(2), 126–30.

Gregorie, A. and Pearson, S. (2002) 'Risk of pregnancy when changing to atypical antipsychotics'. *British Journal of Psychiatry*, 180, 83–4.

Higgins, A., Barker, P. and Begley, C. (2005) 'Neuroleptic medication and sexuality: the forgotten aspect of education and care'. *Journal of Psychiatric and Mental Health Nursing*, 12(4), 439–46.

Higgins, A., Barker, P. and Begley, C. (2006) 'Iatrogenic sexual dysfunction and the protective withholding of information: in whose best interest?' *Journal of Psychiatric and Mental Health Nursing*, 13(4), 437–46.

Kelly, J., McAuliffe, T., Sikkema, K., Murphy, D., Somlai, A., Mulry, G., Mill, J., Stevenson, L. and Fernandez, M. (1997) 'Reduction in risk behaviour among adults with severe mental illness who learned to advocate for HIV prevention'. *Psychiatric Services*, 48(10), 1283–8.

King, M. and McKeown, E. (2003) *Mental Health and Social Wellbeing of Gay Men, Lesbians, and Bisexuals in England and Wales*. London: Mind.

Layte, R., McGee, H., Quail, A., Rundle, K., Cousins, G., Donnelly, C., Mulcahy, F. and Conroy, R. (2006) *The Irish Study of Sexual Health and Relationships*. Dublin: Crisis Pregnancy Agency and Department of Health and Children.

McCann, E. (2000) 'The expression of sexuality in people with psychosis: breaking the taboos'. *Journal of Advanced Nursing*, 32(1), 132–8.

McFarlane, L. (1998) *Diagnosis Homophobic – The Experience of Lesbians, Gay Men and Bisexuals in Mental Health Services*. London: PACE.

McGee, H., Garavan, R., de Barra, M., Byrne, J. and Conroy, R. (2002) *The SAVI report: Sexual Abuse and Violence in Ireland. A National Study of Irish Experiences, Beliefs and Attitudes Concerning Sexual Violence*. Dublin: Liffey Press in association with Dublin Rape Crisis Centre.

National Counselling Service (2003) *SENCS: Survivors' Experiences of the National Counselling Service for Adults who Experienced Childhood Abuse*. Dublin: Health Board Executive.

National Disability Authority (2005) *Disability and Sexual Orientation: A Discussion Paper*. Dublin: National Disability Authority.

National Schizophrenia Foundation (UK) (2000) *A Question of Choice*. London: National Schizophrenia Foundation.

Office of the High Commissioner for Human Rights (1991) *Principles for the Protection of Persons with Mental Illness and the Improvement of Mental Health Care*. Geneva: Office of the High Commissioner for Human Rights.

Pan American Health Organisation (PAHO)/World Health Organisation (WHO) (2002) *Promotion of Sexual Health: Recommendations for Action*. Proceedings of a regional consultation convened by Pan American Health Organisation (PAHO), World Health Organisation (WHO) in collaboration with the World Association of Sexology. Antigua/Guatemala: PAHO/WHO.

Read, J. and Argyle, N. (1999) 'Hallucinations, delusions and thought disorder among adult psychiatric inpatients with a history of sexual abuse'. *Psychiatric Services*, 50(11), 1467–72.

Robertson, A. (1998) 'The mental health experiences of gay men: a research study exploring gay men's health needs'. *Journal of Psychiatric and Mental Health Nursing*, 5(1), 33–40.

Schizophrenia Ireland (2002) *A Question of Choice – Ireland Service Users' Experience of Medication and Treatment*. Dublin: Schizophrenia Ireland.

Shakespeare, T., Gillespie-Sells, K. and Davies, D. (1996) *The Sexual Politics of Disability*. London: Cassell.

Wilton, T. (2000) *Sexualities in Health and Social Care: A Textbook*. Buckingham: Open University Press.

25

Clinical Supervision and Mental Health Nursing

Jean Morrissey

Clinical supervision (CS) has received increasing attention in mental health nursing during the last two decades, mainly in the United Kingdom and Australia. Its value in developing high-quality nursing care and in supporting nurses who often work in difficult and challenging situations has been recognised and supported. However, while CS is gaining momentum in Ireland its implementation is at an embryonic stage. This chapter aims to introduce the reader to the concept of CS and examine some of the key issues that need to be addressed if CS is to be implemented effectively in the workplace. Although the chapter focuses primarily on CS for registered nurses, the ideas and application will be of relevance to students either in their current role as learners or as potential supervisees, supervisors, or both, in the future.

UNDERSTANDING CLINICAL SUPERVISION

Issues relating to the practice of CS are complex and the subject of much debate among academics and practitioners. These issues are further compounded by the fact that the term *clinical supervision* is often used in different contexts as though there was a shared agreed meaning of the terminology used. It is essential therefore to be explicit about what is meant by the term CS and, more important, how it is translated into practice. Throughout the literature there are many definitions of CS. At its simplest, it is essentially a formal learning alliance whereby a supervisee meets regularly with an experienced practitioner — a supervisor — to reflect on clinical and professional issues relating to the supervisee's ongoing professional learning and clinical practice. It is a formal process of professional support and learning which enables practitioners to develop knowledge and competence, assume responsibility for their own practice and enhance consumer protection and the safety of care in complex clinical situations. Cutcliffe *et al.* (2001:3) view CS as 'supportive, safe, centred on developing best practice for service users, an invitation to be self-monitoring and self-accountable and an activity that continues throughout one's working life'. Ultimately, its purpose is twofold: to promote and protect 'the welfare of the client and the development of the supervisee' (Carroll 1996:45) or as Barker (1992:66) asserts, 'to protect people in care from nurses and to protect nurses from themselves'. These overarching goals are sometimes placed chronologically with the emphasis on enhancing client care through reflective practice and the ongoing professional development of the supervisee within the context of the supervisory relationship.

In nursing, CS embraces a range of strategies such as preceptorship and peer support, which adds to the blurring and confusion of terminology between the different teaching and supportive aspects of these roles. (See Figure 25.1 for comparisons.) There is also an increasing connection being made between CS and the activity of reflective practice. In nursing, reflective practice has adopted ideas from CS and attempted to make the connection more formal by providing practitioners with a space in which reflection can take place with a more experienced and skilled practitioner (Driscoll 2000). However, Faugier (1994) argues that much of what is described as 'reflective practice' remains ill-defined and usually involves practitioners reflecting alone or with their peer group without adequate guidance and/or formal structures. While the practice of self-reflection is generally promoted, Casement (1985:63) argues that the capacity for self-reflection, which he terms 'the internal supervisor', can only be developed and maintained against a background of continuing CS with a skilled supervisor. As such, it could be argued that self-reflection should be considered as a preparation for CS, rather than a substitute for it.

Figure 25.1 Structured support systems in nursing: similarities and differences

	Preceptorship	Supervised Practice	Peer Support	Clinical Supervision
Supervisee	Student nurse	Student nurse on final clinical placement	Any nurse	Qualified nurse
Period of time	Throughout training especially on clinical placements	Final stages of student's course	Varies; support groups have a reputation of petering out	Intended to be throughout career
How widespread	Integral part of course	Integral part of course	Patchy; not widely accepted	Patchy, rapidly accelerating
Assessment function	Preceptor often has part to play in assessment of practical work	Supervisor has a defined assessment role: nurse cannot qualify without passing this part of the course	None: colleagues do not report to anyone unless there is evidence of unsafe or unethical practice	None: clinical supervisor does not report to anyone unless there is evidence of unsafe or unethical practice

Source: Adapted from Bond and Holland (1998) to fit Irish context

MANAGERIAL SUPERVISION

While CS focuses exclusively on the supervisee's reflections on his/her clinical work with their supervisor, managerial supervision is usually between the line manager and employee and focuses primarily on the tasks and general performance of the employee, which at times may extend to discussion and reflection of the employee's clinical work. Other pertinent issues within this relationship may also include:

- fitness to practice issues
- professional development and lifelong learning
- organisation and prioritisation of work
- monitoring and reviewing performance (appraisal)
- career development.

CS and managerial supervision should not be amalgamated. Occupying and managing the dual relationship of manager and clinical supervisor undoubtedly presents several professional and ethical challenges for both participants of the supervisory dyad, particularly given the power differential that exists between the manager/clinical supervisor and supervisee. In order for the most effective CS to take place, the role of manager and clinical supervisor should be separate and distinct from one another. Failure to separate the roles may give rise to misunderstanding and mistrust about the purpose and function of CS and may lead to resistance to its successful implementation.

CLINICAL SUPERVISION AND THERAPY

In nursing there is often conceptual confusion between what is understood as personal support and therapy (Yegdich 1999), which is not surprising given that there are often elements of personal therapy in CS; for example, both are helping processes, comprise an authority–dependency relationship and use, albeit differently, similar skills (Page and Wosket 2001). However, they are not the same: each is a separate activity with different aims. 'The aim of CS is to help supervisees become better therapeutic workers whereas the aim in counselling stresses becoming a better person' (Carroll 1996:59).

THE DEVELOPMENT OF CLINICAL SUPERVISION IN MENTAL HEALTH NURSING

Early accounts of CS can be traced back to the process of training in psychoanalysis. In the early days of Freud, CS comprised small informal groups in which trainees discussed and reviewed each other's clinical work. Since then and with the emergence of other counselling therapies (e.g. cognitive behaviour therapy, among others), CS has been employed in psychotherapy and other associated disciplines such as psychology, counselling and social work. However, while CS has been performed over the years, its development as a distinct profession in its own right — i.e. with its own concepts and techniques — is relatively new, at least in the mental heath professions (Bernard and Goodyear 1998).

In the UK, CS in mental health nursing did not emerge until the 1990s. In 1993 the Department of Health (DoH (UK) 1993) issued a strategy document which placed CS as an important agenda item for the profession. This paper provided key statements broadly defining the purpose of CS and approved its establishment in the interests of maintaining and improving standards of care. The Department of Health's definition included reference to a formal process of professional support and learning and defined professional skills explicitly as knowledge, competence, assuming responsibility and enhancing consumer satisfaction.

Two years later, the profession's statutory body, the United Kingdom Central Council for Nursing, Midwifery and Health Visiting, set out its initial position on CS and published definitive guidance for the nursing and health visiting professions the following year (UKCC 1996). More recently the Nursing Midwifery Council (NMC) (formerly the UKCC) (2001), described CS as an integral part of lifelong learning, enabling the nurse to constantly evaluate and improve their contribution to patient/client care. Currently implementation of CS is advancing in many parts of the UK and is increasingly being used as part of clinical governance (Winstanley and White 2003).

In Ireland, mental health nursing has undergone several changes in the provision and delivery of services since the introduction of the government's policies for mental health *Planning for the Future* (DoH 1984) and more recently *A Vision for Change* (DoHC 2006). Such changes have added to the demands on psychiatric nurses' expertise. The *Scope of Nursing and Midwifery Practice Framework* (An Bord Altranais 2000) outlines the need for accountability and autonomy in nursing and identifies continuing professional development (CPD) as a means of achieving these objectives. CS is one of a number of examples of CPD strategies identified by An Bord Altranais which nurses should embrace in their scope of practice to meet the changing needs of society and mental health services. However, only nurses seeking to be registered as Advanced Nurse Practitioners are required by the National Council for the Development of Nursing and Midwifery to have undergone CS (NCNM 2003).

Interest in CS in mental health nursing has also been influenced by the practices of other professions, e.g. psychology and social work, which have generally accepted CS as standard practice. Lyth (2000) suggests that clinical supervision has become an important concept in nursing because of the benefits it can bring to both patient care and nurses. However, while there is interest in the development of CS, the majority of mental health nurses in Ireland are not exposed to it. Furthermore, given the dearth of published research on mental health nurses' experience of CS from an Irish context, it is difficult to assess how it is being implemented and/or to determine its future role in mental health nursing.

MODELS OF CLINICAL SUPERVISION

Numerous models of CS have been described throughout the literature, e.g.:
- developmental model of supervision (Stoltenberg and Delworth 1987)
- double matrix model (Hawkins and Shohet 2005)
- tasks of supervision (Carroll 1996).

These theoretical concepts inform and guide how supervision is understood and implemented. Also, the supervisor's own theoretical background and the nature of his/her practical experience (i.e. whether s/he subscribes to the humanistic, psychoanalytical or behavioural school of psychotherapy) will influence the model of supervision. For example, CS using a psychoanalytical framework will differ from CS using a different theoretical orientation, for example a humanistic approach. Given the extent and range of models, relationships and styles of CS, it is not surprising that different supervisors have different approaches/methods to monitor supervisees' clinical work and professional development. However, Jubb Shanley and Stevenson (2006:588) point out that as an emergent profession 'the discipline of nursing is not as well established in its use of other therapies as other disciplines e.g. psychology and the employment of a system of CS is also not yet as well established'.

Proctor's Model of Clinical Supervision

Within nursing, Proctor's (1986) model of clinical supervision is the most widely adapted and commonly used (Winstanley and White 2003). Proctor (1986) outlines the three tasks and categories of responsibilities of the supervisor and supervisee as follows.
- **Normative task (managerial)**: monitoring the various contexts in which the supervisee works. Involves all aspects of the work that involve accountability and responsibility of the supervisee and the welfare of the client, e.g. promoting and complying with policies and procedures, developing standards and contributing to clinical audit.
- **Formative task (educative)**: understanding how people learn, and facilitating these processes, underpins this task of clinical supervision. The supervisor joins and facilitates the supervisee in a process of enquiry and mutual challenge, rather than as an expert transmitter of knowledge. The supervisor's role is to help the practitioner enhance and fully utilise his/her knowledge, skills and competence as they are presented in relation to work with particular clients.
- **Restorative task (supportive)** involves offering supervisees a forum to reflect on their personal reactions arising from working with clients, or indeed with supervisors, e.g. enabling practitioners to understand and manage the emotional distress of nursing practice.

The prominence of these tasks will vary depending on the context of the CS and the different aspects will overlap. However, it is the degree to which one particular task is more prominent than another that may fuel tensions, uncertainties and conceptual complexities within the practice of CS.

Clinical Supervision Formats

Regardless of the particular model being used, all CS models use a specific format, e.g. one-to-one (individual) or group supervision. While one-to-one CS is the most frequently used format in nursing, group supervision is a close second. Each format has its advantages and disadvantages and presents different learning opportunities and challenges that are often interchangeable and context-dependent (Carroll 1996) (see Figures 25.2 and 25.3).

Figure 25.2 Advantages and disadvantages of one-to-one clinical supervision

Advantages	Disadvantages
More time for supervisee	Full focus on the individual supervisee
Opportunity to create clearer and more focused learning objectives	Input from only one person (supervisor)
Highly personalised	Becomes difficult if supervisory relationship breaks down
Allows for strong mentoring	Can become collusive with very little challenge
Allows supervisee to concentrate on a number of clients	Can create dependency in supervisees
Supervisee can work at his/her own pace	No comparisons for supervisee on other ways of working
Development of the supervisee can be monitored more easily	
Non-competitive environment (no sibling rivalry)	
Development of supervisee can be monitored more easily	

For the supervisee, what is important is the ability to know which format might best meet his/her learning needs at that particular stage of professional development. Having experience of both formats can provide a good learning opportunity for supervisees: the supervisee can experience both the intensive attention of individual supervision and the opportunity to contribute to and learn with and from others in a group. Equally, it is important for supervisors to be aware of their preferred format and competence in the different formats of supervision. However, in practice, compromises often occur and supervisees and/or supervisors may find themselves in one or other of these supervisory formats not from choice but because alternatives are not feasible (e.g. because of time or financial constraints) or available, which can influence the quality of both the supervisory experience and the learning process. Where possible, group or individual supervision should start from a positive choice for all participants.

Figure 25.3 Advantages and disadvantages of group clinical supervision

Advantages	Disadvantages
Input from a number of people — supervisor is not the only person with knowledge and experience	Scapegoating can take place
Supportive atmosphere from peers, especially for novice	Individual can get lost/hide in the group
Value of listening to others describe how they work and the problems they face	May be less time for experimenting with other supervisory interventions
Cost-effective in terms of time and economics	Supervisees who carry heavy case loads may not have enough time
Risk-taking can be higher in a group setting	Not all individuals are suited to group work
Emotional support from peers who are in a similar learning situations	Group dynamics can interfere with individual earning
Someone of the same age, gender, race	Pressure to conform to group norms
Evaluation and feedback from a number of people	Difficulty of entering an already established group as a new member
Dilutes power of supervisor	Time spent on areas not of interest to other group members
	Confidentiality is less secure
	More experienced supervisees tend to lose out in group supervision

Source: Adapted from Carroll (1996)

THE FREQUENCY OF CLINICAL SUPERVISION

Guidance about the frequency of CS will vary and depend on the practitioner's case load, area of practice and supervisor's availability. As a guideline, Butterworth *et al.* (1997) recommend that CS should be of a significant length to be effective, i.e. not less than 45 minutes per session every four weeks. Winstanley's (2001) study found that CS sessions should be a maximum of one hour for hospital nursing staff to be of use, whereas community-based staff might benefit from extending CS to last longer than one hour.

THE SUPERVISORY RELATIONSHIP

CS is uniformly regarded as a professional relationship characterised by certain boundaries. The importance of the supervisory relationship, whether it comprises a dyad or a group, cannot be over-estimated if effective supervisory practice is to take place. The knowledge, skills and modelling that a supervisor conveys are important aspects of helping the supervisee assist the client by promoting best practice in both the therapeutic and the supervisory relationship. However, the supervisory relationship is a complex interpersonal process and comprises a combination of different elements, such as personalities, functions, roles, models, strategies, tasks, and process issues (Carroll 1996).

Furthermore, each supervisory dyad is different, so the skill of establishing the supervisory relationship cannot be prescribed and, like everything else in the supervisory experience, it is context-dependent and grounded in supervisory judgement and skill rather than a product of chronology. Despite this, there is a scarcity of empirical research in the nursing literature on this issue. However, several writers have outlined the core features of the role of supervisor (e.g. Butterworth and Faugier 1992; Rolfe *et al.* 2001). One fundamental feature of the role of supervisor is a willingness to facilitate learning in others while being open to learning about themselves.

Not all good clinicians make good supervisors. Carroll (1996) asserts that good supervisors are good teachers and have access to a wide range of teaching/learning methods that can be adapted to individual supervisees. In addition, supervisors are flexible in their relationships with supervisees, moving easily across roles of teacher, evaluator, role model, mentor, counsellor (Hawkins and Shohet 2005). This shift involves a change in role, an increased field of responsibility, the acquisition of a different range of skills and personal demands of another order (Clarkson and Gilbert 1991).

Fowler's (1995) study of post-registration students' perceptions of a 'good' supervisor identified the following characteristics:
- is capable of forming a relaxed and supportive relationship
- has relevant knowledge and clinical skills
- can assess learning needs, supervise and evaluate learning
- is aware of the pressures and demands of the course
- demonstrates effort in putting themselves out to help the student.

Other characteristics seen as important were 'being approachable', 'willing to negotiate' and 'showing interest'. While some of the above qualities may specifically apply to student nurses, many are likely to be of equal importance whether the supervisee is a student or a qualified nurse.

As a multi-faceted activity, the supervisee expects and respects the supervisor's ability to evaluate and insure the quality of both the therapeutic and supervisory process. However, certain elements of the supervisory relationship are conducive to the development of anxieties for both participants. For the supervisor, the responsibility to provide constructive feedback is anxiety-provoking for both members of the supervisory dyad. Also, the supervisor's status and prestige in the organisation may further complicate the anxieties in the supervisory process. No matter what efforts are made to minimise it, both are aware that the supervisor's judgement may affect the supervisory relationship. For the supervisee, sharing anxieties and doubts about one's clinical practice can be a threatening experience, often making them feel under scrutiny and giving them the uncomfortable sensation of not feeling *good enough*. Thus, in a similar way to the therapeutic situation, change may be both desired and simultaneously feared by the supervisee and in seeking help they may defend the ways in which they have previously learned. Essential to this experience is the supervisor's ability to assist the supervisee to overcome his/her fears of learning. However, as Bishop (1998:16) points out, 'to be challenging while maintaining a positive approach is not always easy, yet good supervisors must achieve this if supervisees are to benefit from supervision and be open to feedback, willing to question their practices and explore new interventions'. This process is more likely to be achieved if the supervisee has had some choice in choosing his/her supervisor.

CLINICAL RESPONSIBILITY AND CONFIDENTIALITY IN CLINICAL SUPERVISION

Given the nature of CS, there is no line of responsibility between the client and the clinical supervisor. Nevertheless, clinical supervisors cannot abdicate their responsibility: they have a professional and ethical duty to anticipate (within reason) and minimise the possibility of negligence to the client, supervisee or both. The fiduciary role of the supervisor therefore not only carries a responsibility for taking an ethical approach to conducting CS but also the responsibility to ensure that the supervisee's practice is both safe and ethical (Scaife 2001).

The duty of confidentiality in CS is twofold: it applies to both clients and supervisees. Essentially, the supervisory relationship must be confidential; however, given the different circumstances of each case it is difficult, if not impossible, to provide absolutes. If the clinical supervisor believes that the client's welfare may be compromised this may require informing either the CNM II or the CNM III.

Clearly any breach of confidentiality by the clinical supervisor is never an easy decision and requires careful consideration about the needs of the client and supervisee, although fundamentally the client's welfare must take precedence. Such decisions also require collegial and supervisory support and discussion about the presenting professional, ethical and legal issues of the specific issues, along with the consequences of taking action (or not) rather than simply responding to a code of ethics. As such, it is essential that the parameters of confidentiality are clarified and agreed upon by the supervisee(s) and supervisor when establishing the supervisory contract at the outset.

ESTABLISHING A CLINICAL SUPERVISION CONTRACT

In implementing CS, it is essential that clear boundaries are clarified and agreed upon by all parties — supervisees, supervisors and the organisation — at the outset, in the form of best practice guidelines and organisation policy/protocol documents. Issues to be addressed include:

- Understanding of CS in mental health nursing — aims and functions.
- Involvement in CS — recommended or required attendance; frequency.
- Role of supervisor — allocated or chosen; internal/external; nurse or other related discipline.
- Operational arrangements for carrying out CS — model of supervision; format (i.e. individual or group); location.
- Training for supervisors and supervisees.
- Resource commitment — protected time for CS; cover for staff to be involved in CS.
- Record keeping and documentation by supervisors and supervisees.
- Understanding — of confidentiality; accountability; and responsibility in CS.
- Evaluating and auditing implementation of CS.

ORGANISATIONAL FACTORS AND CLINICAL SUPERVISION

For many nurses, CS is located at the interface between the supervisee and the organisation. The organisational setting provides the fundamental backdrop for understanding the roles in the supervisory relationship. Additionally, the hierarchical structure of the organisation and the organisational role of the supervisor can also dictate the nature of the supervisory relationship. Moreover, there may be all sorts of pressures on either the supervisor or supervisee or both, from the profession, organisation or society in which they both work. So, as well as dealing with the client in question (in CS) the supervisor and supervisee have to pay attention to their supervisory relationship and the wider system in which they both operate.

Furthermore, these elements contain a number of assumptions within which the multidimensional process of supervision may be applied. Therefore, the need for a shared understanding and agreement between all participants involved in the supervisory process (i.e. supervisor, supervisee and organisation) via a mutually negotiated contract is essential before implementing CS in the workplace (Rolfe et al. 2001). Failure to do so may result in the potential efficacy of CS being undermined and undervalued.

EVALUATING AND AUDITING THE IMPLEMENTATION OF CLINICAL SUPERVISION

It is unlikely that organisations will invest in the process of CS supervision without being satisfied that there will be tangible improvements to the service. Therefore if CS is to be implemented more widely, measurable evidence will be required to confirm that CS improves client care.

In the UK a number of evaluative studies have addressed issues of effectiveness and CS over the last decade. Several studies have reported that nurses find the provision of support through CS a positive and worthwhile experience and have identified better client outcomes when recalling the benefits of CS (Butterworth *et al.* 1997; Scanlon and Weir 1997; Green 1999). However, there is still a lack of knowledge about what makes clinical supervision effective, particularly in terms of its benefits to client care. Clearly, there are methodological challenges in this area, i.e. the variation and permutation of the variables involved along with the challenge of identifying what and how to measure in terms of the outcomes of CS. To address this issue the Manchester Clinical Supervision Scale (MCSS) (Winstanley 2000) was developed and has been recommended as a robust tool for assessing the effectiveness of CS. More recent studies have utilised this tool in their research, e.g. Edwards *et al.* 2005.

Notwithstanding this, the research to date has highlighted a number of issues concerning the organisation and application of systems of CS which influence the quality of the practice of CS that supervisees receive. These include: the length and frequency of CS; choice of supervisor; barriers to the uptake of clinical supervision; training of supervisors; record keeping; and confusion about the amalgamation of clinical and managerial supervision (Green 1999; Kelly *et al.* 2001; Edwards *et al.* 2005). Such issues require serious attention in terms of their impact on the welfare of the client and the process of learning.

Example of Clinical Supervision

Rachel, a staff nurse of six months' experience, has attended monthly group supervision since qualifying. The group comprises John and Anne (staff nurses), who have been qualified for three years and who recently started working in the home care team, along with their supervisor Joan, an experienced nurse of many years' standing.

On commencing CS, Rachel was very anxious joining the group, believing that she would be perceived as 'incompetent' in front of her fellow supervisees and supervisor. As a result, during the initial months of CS Rachel was hesitant to disclose her uncertainties about her lack of confidence and skills in certain areas of her clinical practice. However, having the opportunity to listen to John and Anne discuss how they work and the problems they face working for the first time in the community, she slowly began to gain more confidence and contributed more actively, by asking questions and offering her opinions.

Being sensitive to the fact that Rachel might feel anxious joining an established CS group, her supervisor Joan encouraged and validated her contribution. Since attending CS, Rachel has presented the following issues:

- Finding it difficult to delegate duties to colleagues, resulting in her feeling stressed and overworked.
- Feeling sad and helpless following the death (suicide) of a client while Rachel was off duty.

Having a regular space in her working environment which provides a safe, supportive and encouraging atmosphere has enabled Rachel to reflect on these issues, gain support and to learn possible approaches/strategies in managing them.

CONCLUSION

The concept of CS and its implementation can be a valuable component of continuous professional development and learning in mental health nursing. However, there can be problems in its implementation — it can be underused, undervalued and/or used ineffectively, which can distort the supervisory experience and learning outcomes for both the supervisor and supervisee and indeed possibly the client. Caution is therefore advised in implementing CS so that it enhances both the supervisory process and the task of teaching and learning for supervisees. Furthermore, it is necessary to consider the broader organisation and cultural context within which the supervisory dyad or group takes place. While several studies provide support for its use as an effective supervisory intervention, there is a need for more empirical research to explain and support its effectiveness further.

Reflective Questions
1. How does clinical supervision differ from therapy?
2. Which format of clinical supervision — i.e. individual or group — would you prefer, and for what reasons?
3. Reflecting on your current clinical practice, what issues might you take to discuss with your clinical supervisor?
4. What factors might encourage and/or discourage you in availing of clinical supervision in your practice area?

References
An Bord Altranais (2000) *Scope of Nursing and Midwifery Practice Framework.* Dublin: An Bord Altranais.
Barker, P. (1992) 'Psychiatric nursing', in T. Butterworth and J. Faugier (eds), *Clinical Supervision and Mentorship in Nursing.* Cheltenham: Stanley Thorne.
Bernard, J. M. and Goodyear, R. K. (1998) *Fundamentals of Clinical Supervision.* Boston, MA: Allyn and Bacon.
Bishop, V. (1998) (ed.) *Clinical Supervision in Practice.* London: Macmillan.
Bond, M. and Holland, S. (1998) *Skills of Clinical Supervision for Nurses.* Buckingham: Open University Press.
Butterworth, T., Carson, J., White, E., Peacock, J., Clements, A. and Bishop, V. (1997) *Clinical Supervision and Mentorship. It's Good to Talk: An Evaluation Study in England and Scotland.* Manchester: University of Manchester.
Butterworth, T. and Faugier, J. (1992) *Clinical Supervision and Mentorship in Nursing.* London: Chapman & Hall.
Carroll, M. (1996) *Counselling Supervision.* London: Cassell.

Casement, P. (1985) *On Learning From the Patient*. London: Tavistock.

Clarkson, P. and Gilbert, M. (1991) 'Training counsellor trainers and supervisors', in W. Dryden and B. Thorne (eds), *Training and Supervision for Counselling in Action*. London: Sage.

Cutcliffe, J. R., Butterworth, T. and Proctor, B. (eds), (2001) *Fundamental Themes in Clinical Supervision*. London: Routledge.

Department of Health (DoH) (1984) *Psychiatric Services — Planning for the Future*. Dublin: Stationery Office.

Department of Health and Children (DoHC) (2006) *A Vision for Change: Report of the Expert Group on Mental Health Policy*. Dublin: Government Publication Office.

Department of Health (DoH) (UK) (1993) *Vision for the Future: The Nursing, Midwifery and Health Visiting Contribution to Health and Health Care*. London: HMSO.

Department of Health (DoH) (UK) (1995) *Clinical Supervision* (conference proceedings from a national workshop at the National Motorcycle Museum). London: NHS Executive.

Driscoll, J. (2000) *Practising Clinical Supervision. A Reflective Approach*. London: Bailliere Tindall.

Edwards, D., Cooper, L., Burnard, P., Hanningan, D., Adams, J., Fothergill, A. and Coyle, D. (2005) 'Factors influencing the effectiveness of clinical supervision'. *Journal of Psychiatric and Mental Health Nursing*, 12, 404–14.

Faugier, J. (1994) 'Thin on the ground', *Nursing Times*, 18 May 18, 90, 64–5.

Fowler, J. (1995) 'Nurses' perceptions of the elements of good supervision'. *Nursing Times*, 91(22), 33–7.

Green, A. (1999) 'A utilization focused evaluation of a clinical supervision programme for nurses and health visitors in one National Health Service trust'. *Journal of Vocational Education and Training*, 51, 493–504.

Hawkins, P. and Shohet, R. (2005) *Supervision in the Helping Professions* (2nd edn). Berkshire: Open University Press.

Jubb Shanley, M. and Stevenson, C. (2006) 'Clinical supervision revisited', *Journal of Nursing Management*, 14, 586–92.

Kelly, B., Long, A. and McKenna, H. (2001) 'A survey of community mental health nurses' perceptions of clinical supervision in Northern Ireland'. *Journal of Psychiatric and Mental Health Nursing*, 8, 33–44.

Lyth, G. (2000) 'Clinical supervision, a concept analysis'. *Journal of Advanced Nursing*, 31, 3, 722–9.

National Council for the Professional Development of Nursing and Midwifery (NCNM) (2003) *Agenda for the Future Professional Development of Nursing and Midwifery*. Dublin: NCNM.

Nursing Midwifery Council (NMC) (2001) *Clinical Supervision*, www.nmc-uk.org. London: NMC.

Page, S. and Wosket, V. (2001) *Supervising the Counsellor: A Cyclical Model*. London: Routledge.

Proctor, B. (1986) 'Supervision: a co-operative exercise in accountability', in M. Marten and M. Payne (eds), *Enabling and Ensuring Supervision in Practice*. Leicester: National Youth Bureau and Council.

Rolfe, G., Freshwater, D. and Jasper, M. (2001) *Critical Reflection for Nursing and the Helping Professions: A Users' Guide*. London: Palgrave Publishers.

Scaife, J. (2001) *Supervision in the Mental Health Professions: A Practitioner's Guide*. Hove: Brunner-Routledge.

Scanlon, C. (1998) 'Towards effective training of clinical supervision', in V. Bishop (ed.) *Clinical Supervision in Practice*. London: Macmillan.

Scanlon, C. and Weir, W. S. (1997) 'Learning from practice? Mental health nurses' perceptions and experiences of clinical supervision'. *Journal of Advanced Nursing*, 26 (2), 295–303.

Stoltenberg, C. D. and Delworth, U. (1987) *Supervision Counsellors and Therapists: A Developmental Approach*. San Francisco: Jossey-Bass.

United Kingdom Central Council for Nursing, Midwifery and Health Visiting (UKCC) (1996) *Position Statement on Clinical Supervision for Nursing and Health Visiting*. London: UKCC.

Winstanley, J. (2000) 'Manchester Clinical Supervision Scale', *Nursing Standard*, 14, 19: 31–2.

Winstanley, J. (2001) 'Developing methods for evaluating clinical supervision', in J. R. Cutcliffe, T. Butterworth and B. Proctor (eds.) (2001) *Fundamental Themes in Clinical Supervision*. London: Routledge.

Winstanley, J. and White, E. (2003) 'Clinical supervision: models, measures and best practice'. *Nurse Researcher*, 10(4):7–38.

Yegdich, T. (1999) 'Lost in the crucible of supportive clinical supervision: supervision is not therapy'. *Journal of Advanced Nursing*, 29(5), 1265–75.

26
Mental Health Nursing in an Ethnically Diverse Society

Padraig Byrne

> Of all the forms of inequality, injustice in health is the most shocking and inhumane.
>
> (Martin Luther King Jr 1966)

Ireland has been transformed by the growing presence of non-Irish-born, ethnically diverse minority groups, most of whom have come to Ireland as economic migrants or political asylum seekers. Currently Ireland is host to about 160 different ethnic minorities, with UK nationals, Poles and Lithuanians being the largest groups (CSO 2006). The differences and similarities that distinguish and unite people, though generally seen in a positive light, also serve to challenge our intellect, emotions and skills as we strive to provide equitable health care in a diverse society. The principle of equity in health care, which underpins the policies of the World Health Organisation (WHO 1981), the Irish national health strategy *Quality and Fairness* (DoHC 2001) and the national policy framework for Irish mental health services *A Vision for Change* (O'Connor 2006), is of particular significance when considering the mental health nursing care of ethnic minority groups.

Irish health services policies and Irish law provide for equity and diversity in mental health care. Irish equality legislation, comprising the Equal Status Acts of 2000 and 2004 and the Employment Equality Act 2004, prohibits discrimination on the basis of race, and provides for the accommodation of diversity and the assurance of equality in health service provision. However, despite the provisions for equitable health services in Ireland and elsewhere, widespread inequalities exist in the mental health care of ethnic minorities (Alegria *et al.* 2003). The aim of this chapter is to introduce mental health nurses to cross-cultural nursing in a rapidly diversifying Irish society in order to provide equitable and effective nursing care to diverse service users.

CONCEPTS IN CROSS-CULTURAL MENTAL HEALTH NURSING

Culture
The influence of culture on health status and behaviour is widely accepted. Culture can be defined as 'a learned world view or paradigm, shared by a population or group and transmitted socially, that influences values, beliefs, customs and behaviors, and is reflected in the language, dress, food, materials and social institutions of a group' (Rosenjack-Burchum 2002:7). We are all products of our culture and our cultural background influences many important aspects of our lives, including our beliefs and behaviours in relation to health and illness. Culture can both directly and indirectly influence a person's perceptions of health and illness, his/her help-seeking behaviour and treatment outcomes.

Ethnicity
The terms 'culture' and 'ethnicity' are often used interchangeably and although they may overlap, the concepts are not synonymous. Ethnicity is socially constructed and generally refers to people with a common ancestry, often linked to a specific geographical territory, and who perhaps share a language, religion or social customs (Culley and Dyson 2001). Ethnicity describes an active process of social construction of difference, by self-identification and categorisation by others, which takes place between and within groups and is characterised by a sense of belonging experienced by members of a group. Sometimes the term 'ethnic' is taken to refer to ethnic minority groups, but everybody is ethnic and belongs to an ethnic group.

Cultures of Nursing and Psychiatry
Nurses, in addition to their individual ethnic and cultural heritages, also construct identifiable nursing cultures through social processes such as professional socialisation. The values of the dominant societal culture permeate the practice of nurses as a result of the internalisation of that dominant position during nurse training (Narayanasamy 1999a). Similarly, as nursing practice reflects society, the theory and practice of Western psychiatry is also largely culturally determined (O'Brien and Morrrison-Ngatai 2003). Western mental health care, which is dominated by the 'biomedical model', conceptualises mental illness as an objective, physical state and postulates a biological basis for the cause and treatment of mental distress. This reductionistic approach and the use of a Eurocentric system of classification in the diagnosis of mental illness, based on the DSM-IV-TR (APA 2000) and the ICD-10 (WHO 1992), are often incongruent with the healthcare perspectives of ethnic minority groups (Huggins 2003).

ETHNIC INEQUALITIES IN MENTAL HEALTH

The mental health status and care of ethnic minorities are influenced by cultural factors originating from the ethnic minority group itself, mental health professionals, the mental health care system and society as a whole. Cultural factors have also been postulated in the creation of the widespread inequalities or disparities that have been observed in the mental health status and care of ethnic minorities (Iley and Nazroo 2001). Though Irish data is limited (Byrne 2006), the aetiology, presentation and manifestation of mental health problems among different ethnic minority groups, and the interaction of these groups with mental health services, are marked with inequalities internationally. Examples of unequal treatment of ethnic minorities abound in the literature and ethnic minorities complain of more coercive treatments and adverse experiences. Black people are over-represented among in-patients, have more complex pathways to specialist mental health care and are more likely to experience compulsory and emergency admission to psychiatric services with police involvement, compared to white people (Bhui *et al.* 2003). Generally, the main areas of disparities between minority and majority ethnic groups in mental health care relate to the mode of entry into psychiatric institutions, disease profile and treatment regimes.

Determinants of Inequalities

Although research supports a strong association between ethnicity and mental health disparities, ethnicity in and of itself is not seen as a sole determinant of the health status of ethnic minority groups (Iley and Nazroo 2001). Other mediating causal mechanisms of ethnic health disparities have been proposed, including racism, socio-economic status, access to services and migration. The roles played by racism and socio-economic factors are thought to be particularly significant.

Racism

Though the concept of 'race' is now rejected as having no scientific or rational basis, it still exerts an influence as a social construct (Mulholland and Dyson 2001) through the reality of racism and racial prejudice (LaVeist 2002). Racism refers to ideas (attitudes, beliefs and ideologies), actions and structures which serve to promote the exclusion of people by virtue of their being considered members of different 'racial' groups (Culley and Dyson 2001). Ethnic differences in mental health due to racism can result from: direct experience of discrimination and harassment; the social and material disadvantages that racism leads to; and experience of institutionalised racism in health service provision and delivery (Cortis 2003).

Socio-economic Factors

Economic and environmental circumstances which make up socio-economic status are widely seen to play a major role in the ethnic patterning of health. The influence of variables such as social class, income and standard of living is central in the determination of ethnic inequalities in health (Nazroo 1998). Nevertheless, social disadvantage alone does not offer a sufficient explanation for ethnic health disparities; the operation of cultural and societal influences must also be taken into account.

APPROACHES TO ETHNIC MINORITY HEALTHCARE AND HEALTH DISPARITIES

Nursing is well positioned to have a great impact upon the mental health care of ethnic minorities. Despite criticisms of poor preparation for cross-cultural practice (Cusack 2005) and racist practice (Baxter 2001), nursing has played a leading role in the development of cross-cultural health care. Generally, two main theoretical positions have been adopted in relation to ethnic minority health care and ethnic inequalities in health, multiculturalism and anti-racism.

Multiculturalism
Multiculturalism emphasises the existence and validity of different cultural traditions, recognises the positive value of ethnic differences and argues for the promotion of tolerance, understanding and harmony between different ethnic groups (Papadopoulous 2001). Health inequalities between ethnic groups are understood to be the result of a lack of knowledge and understanding of the cultural traditions of different groups.

Within nursing, Leninger (1995) adopted a multiculturalist approach in the development of the Sunrise Model of cross-cultural nursing care. This approach is founded on the basic principle that an understanding of cultural differences is essential to the provision of safe and effective nursing care. In the field of mental health nursing, Campinha-Bacote (1999) and Narayanasamy (1999b) have developed models of culturally responsive mental health nursing care, in the USA and the UK respectively. A fundamental concept of transcultural nursing is cultural competence, which has been defined as 'the process in which a healthcare provider continuously strives to achieve the ability to effectively work within the cultural context of a client' (Campinha-Bacote 1999:203).

Despite its growing influence, a number of important failings of multiculturalism have been noted. The lack of attention to the role played by the health practitioner's own ethnicity in interventions, the static and deterministic notion of culture, and the failure to recognise the nature of differences within ethnic groups, have been criticised as potentially leading to ethnocentricity, victim-blaming and stereotyping respectively (Mulholland and Dyson 2001). Furthermore, because the cultural attributes of ethnic minorities are focused on and pathologised, the roles played by racism or socio-economic factors are not dealt with (Culley 2001). Finally, claims by advocates of transcultural nursing that cultural competence is a means of reducing ethnic health disparities have not, as yet, been substantiated.

Anti-racism
Anti-racism developed primarily as a critique of the theoretical assumptions and political implications of multiculturalism. Multiculturalism is criticised as serving as a diversion from racism (Papadopoulous 2001), facilitating ethnic reductionism (i.e. the view that all ethnic minorities are similar), facilitating the unjust control

of ethnic minority groups, and promoting the practice of the resocialisation of culturally different ethnic minorities (Mulholland and Dyson 2001). Central to the anti-racism approach is the emphasis on ideology, power and racism within society and the role of racism in health and social inequality.

Anti-racist writers such as Ahmad (1996) criticise multiculturalism as aligning itself with racist ideologies and ignoring materialist and political causes of ethnic health disparities. In New Zealand, an anti-racist stance has emerged in the development of the concept 'cultural safety' as an alternative to 'cultural competence' (Richardson 2004). Cultural safety has been defined as 'the effective nursing of a person/family from another culture by a nurse who has undertaken a process of reflection on his/her own cultural identity and recognises the impact of the nurse's culture on his/her own nursing practice' (Nursing Council of New Zealand 1996). The significance of the nurse's power and cultural identity in any nursing intervention, and the local historical, social, economic and political context of the nursing care of ethnic minority groups are emphasised (O'Brien and Morrison-Ngatai 2003).

Anti-racism is criticised for over-emphasising the role of 'race' in the determination of people's identities and interests, for portraying ethnic groups as distinct and unchanging, and for limiting itself to a critique of racism and multiculturalism. Anti-racism fails to propose a positive agenda for dealing with ethnic inequalities (Mulholland and Dyson 2001) and to recognise the limited improvements in healthcare provision and people's attitudes that have actually taken place. Similarly, although the concept of cultural safety was developed within nursing as a means of addressing ethnic health differences, evidence is still needed to support the efficacy of cultural safety in healthcare practice.

MANAGING DIVERSITY AND ETHNIC MINORITY MENTAL HEALTH NURSING CARE

In psychiatry and mental healthcare, the multiculturalist approach to cross-cultural care has dominated, despite the influence of the anti-racist stance (Papadopoulous 2001). The development of this multiculturalist persepective, which recognises the interplay between cultural and social factors and mental health, has taken place over time. Historically, because traditional psychiatry has failed adequately to account for its own ethnocentric misconceptions, the service-user's model of illness or institutional racism, service users from ethnic minority groups have come to experience mental health services as culturally insensitive and racist (Gray 2005). The challenge for mental health nursing is to develop improved models of practice which provide appropriate and effective care for ethnic minority service users and contribute to the reduction of ethnic mental health disparities.

Generally, there is a need to avoid an essentialist and stereotypical approach to ethnically diverse groups, to challenge racism in mental heath care, to develop partnerships with ethnic minority service users (Richardson 2004), to support individual and group empowerment (Anderson *et al.* 2003), and to celebrate, rather than tolerate, cultural diversity (Parish 2000).

Consistent with current Irish health policy, dimensions of human diversity and inequality other than ethnicity (such as class, age and gender) must also be addressed (Mulholland and Dyson 2001). A focus on cultural competence in the nursing care of ethnic minorities seems to be giving way to a greater appreciation of the wide spectrum of human diversity and the need to develop diversity-competent nursing practitioners.

Campinha-Bacote Model of Cultural/Diversity Competence

Campinha-Bacote's (1999) model, which was developed from the background of transcultural nursing in the area of mental health, is widely used in nurse education (Huggins 2003). This model was primarily intended to underpin the mental health nursing care of ethnic minorities but may also be used in the nursing care of diverse groups generally. Rosenjack-Burchum defines cultural competence as:

> ... a process of development that is ... related to the attributes of cultural awareness, knowledge, understanding, sensitivity, interaction and skill ... it requires a caring and respectful provider–client relationship ... assures care that is culturally relevant and accommodating to the beliefs, values and practices of client ... equips clients with strategies for meeting their unique cultural needs and thus provide for self-empowerment.
>
> (Rosenjack-Burchum 2002:8)

Campinha-Bacote contends that the development of the components of the model (cultural desire, awareness, knowledge, skill and encounter), leads the nurse to become culturally competent.

Cultural Desire

Cultural desire stimulates the process of becoming culturally competent and refers to:
- the nurse's motivation and commitment to engage in culturally competent care
- a genuine wish to care for diverse service users, to accept difference and build on similarities
- the desire to be open and willing to learn from others.

Campinha-Bacote suggests that the mnemonic LEARN can be used as an aid in this process.
- Listen — the nurse listens non-judgementally to the client's perception of the problem.
- Explaining — the nurse explains his/her perception of the problem.
- Acknowledging — the nurse acknowledges the differences and similarities between his/her perceptions and the client's perceptions of the problem.
- Recommending — the nurse and the client make recommendations on how to deal with the problem.

- Negotiating — cognisant of the client's views, the nurse negotiates an intervention plan.

Cultural Awareness

This is a deliberate, cognitive, reflexive process by which the nurse becomes aware of the dynamics of culture and of how culture shapes values and beliefs. First, the nurse strives to become aware of his/her own values, beliefs, prejudices and practices in relation to diverse and minority groups. He/she also reflects upon the cultural values of the service user's culture, of the nursing profession and of the healthcare organisation. The nurse examines his/her own cultural background in an effort to avoid tendencies to ethnocentrism and cultural imposition. That is, to avoid being bound by his/her own culture and to assume that it is the norm from which others deviate and to avoid imposing his/her own values, beliefs and behaviour patterns upon others (Leninger 1995).

Coming to terms with one's own cultural heritage is necessary in order to eliminate one's biases, stereotypes and prejudices. For this purpose, the nurse may ask him/herself questions such as:

- What ethnic group, socioeconomic class and community do I belong to or feel a part of?
- To what extent do I recognise and understand my own ethnic or cultural background?
- What are the values of my ethnic group? What do we believe about mental health and illness?
- What are my earliest images of people who are different from me in appearance and behaviour? What are my attitudes towards them?
- What have been my personal experiences of other ethnic groups? What do I know about them?
- What are the values and beliefs of my nursing heritage and nursing colleagues? How deeply do I adhere to them?
- What are the values and beliefs of the organisation I work for? How deeply do I adhere to them?

Cultural awareness is seen by many to be the first essential step towards cultural competence (Craig 1999). It enables the nurse to undertake the journey from ethnocentricity to ethno-relativity; the appreciation of the equal value of all cultures.

Cultural Knowledge

Cultural knowledge is the process of continually acquiring information about diverse cultures. Through instruction and interaction with people of other cultures, an understanding and knowledge is developed of their health-related values, meanings, beliefs, behaviour patterns and, principally, their world views (Cortis 2003). World view refers to the way individuals or groups of people view reality to form values about their lives and the world about them; it explains how people interpret health and illness and guides their thinking, doing and being (Campinha-Bacote 2003). Cultural knowledge also involves learning about physical, psychological, psychiatric and social variations among peoples.

One area of specific relevance to mental health nursing care is ethno-pharmacology; the study of ethnic variations in drug pharmacokinetics. It is increasingly apparent that the findings of drug studies performed on subjects of European origin cannot be readily applied to other ethnic groups. Research has shown that, because of ethnic differences in drug metabolism, the efficacy of psychotrophic medications and the incidence of adverse effects vary between ethnic groups (Shives 2002). Ethnic differences in responses to drugs include the following:

- Compared to the white population, extrapyramidal side effects occur at lower doses in Asian groups.
- Lower effective dosage levels and lower thresholds for side effects for anti-depressants are seen among Hispanic peoples.
- A higher red-blood cell plasma-lithium ratio, and a lower therapeutic range, is observed in Black and Asian clients.
- Agranulocytosis, while associated with clozapine in one per cent of the general population, is seen in up to twenty per cent of Jewish people on treatment.

Other non-biological cultural variables such as diet, traditional herbal medicines and belief systems, which may influence drug absorption, drug interaction and treatment compliance respectively, must also be taken into account.

Generally, the bio-transformation and efficacy of psychotrophic medications depends on biological, cultural and environmental factors and the mental health nurse must be alert to the impact of these factors on the client's well-being and recovery. The nurse plays a key role in observing and reporting the therapeutic and adverse effects of prescribed medications upon diverse clients. Information is also sought by the nurse, in the initial assessment and in ongoing communication with the client and his/her family, as to the client's attitude to psychotrophic medication and on the use of any special foods or alternative treatments.

Culturally founded health-related beliefs are also of particular interest to the mental health nurse. The client's view of how mental illness is defined, caused, manifested and treated is derived from his/her cultural world view and may not be consistent with the Western model (Burr and Chapman 1998). To facilitate culturally safe and effective mental healthcare, the nurse must ascertain what constitutes normal or abnormal behaviours, feelings or states in a specific ethnic group. Mental health or normality can be seen as the degree to which an individual conforms to the cultural expectations of his/her ethnic group. For example, whereas 'speaking in tongues' is seen as a gift from God and mentally healthy in some cultures, it may be perceived as a sign of perceptual disorder and mental illness in others.

When treatment is required, what kind of treatment is expected and from whom is treatment acceptable for the client? Chinese people, for example, may see Western treatments as a last resort to be utilised only after first trying traditional methods within the family and community circle. Similarly, religion and spirituality play a central role in many ethnic groups' understanding of, and ways of coping with, mental illness.

Culturally specific manifestations of mental illness, referred to as culture-bound syndromes, are also relevant to client assessment. These refer to culture-specific patterns of abnormal behaviour which do not feature among conventional psychiatric diagnostic categories. The DSM-IV-TR (APA 2000) recognises the culture-bound nature of Western psychiatric diagnostic categories and includes a glossary of syndromes of abnormal behaviour limited to specific ethnicities and localities. 'Neurasthenia', for example, which is described by Chinese people, is characterised by somatic features of depression, such as anorexia, fatigue and insomnia, although feelings of depression are denied.

Generally, in drawing up an individual's nursing care plan, problems, needs and outcomes identified should be meaningful within the client's cultural context, and interventions planned must take account of the coping resources used within his/her ethnic group. Finally, it is important to remember that each individual is unique and it is not appropriate to apply cultural knowledge in a stereotypical fashion.

Cultural Skills
Cultural skills include the ability to draw up an individual plan of care which takes account of the diverse client's perspective. In using the nursing process, the nurse's ability to integrate cultural factors into client assessment is fundamental. This involves the gathering, in a culturally sensitive manner, of relevant cultural data regarding the client's presenting problems in order to determine the client's nursing care needs within his/her cultural context. Many cultural assessment tools are available (Campinha-Bacote 2003), though their applicability to the Irish context may be limited. The diagnosis of the client's nursing needs and the planning and implementation of nursing interventions are based upon information derived from the client's cultural assessment. A brief cultural assessment guide follows (Shives 2002):
- To what culture or ethnic groups do you belong?
- Who are your family and those important to you? How can they be contacted?
- Why do you think you became ill?
- Do you have any beliefs or practices that should be considered in planning your treatment?
- Would you like to involve anybody else in your treatment?
- What is your normal diet? Are there any specific foods you need?
- Have you any religious or spiritual needs that should be catered for?

Communication and the development of the therapeutic nurse–client relationship are skills central to cross-cultural mental health nursing. Language and cultural differences make it very difficult for the nurse to establish effective communication and develop rapport with the client. Research has shown that communication difficulties can adversely impact upon client assessment, treatment and outcomes in mental healthcare (Craig 1999). When the nurse and client experience language difficulties, knowledge of non-verbal communication can facilitate understanding. Non-verbal cues such as tone of voice, eye contact, facial expression, posture, gestures, silence, touch, and personal space can be effectively interpreted and used by the nurse to communicate and develop rapport. For example, it is important for the nurse to know that, although direct eye contact is considered professionally therapeutic in Western cultures, it is perceived to be disrespectful and insulting in many other cultures (Frisch and Frisch 2006). Information on verbal and non-verbal communication styles of the client can be gained from the cultural assessment, the client's family and friends and others familiar with the client's cultural background.

Basic communication guidelines (Arnold and Underman Boggs 2003) may also be of help where language is problematic. For example:
- Speak slowly and clearly.
- Do not raise your voice or exaggerate the mouthing of words.
- Use simple sentences and language the client will understand.
- Ask the same basic questions in the same sequence.
- Repeat the same phrases.
- Avoid slang and technical jargon.
- Use open- and closed-ended question as appropriate.
- Allow plenty of time for answers.
- Engage in active listening.
- Use picture cards if available.
- Learn and use a few words or phrases in the client's language.

When it is necessary to use interpreters, local policy is followed. In Ireland, though not ideal in the area of mental health, a telephone interpretation service is available to Health Service Executive staff. Whenever possible, trained interpreters who are familiar with mental health concepts should be used. Family members, especially children, may not be suitable interpreters as the accuracy of their account may be compromised by their lack of objectivity, lack of understanding, embarrassment or verbal ability. See Tribe and Morrissey (2004) for further suggestions when working with interpreters.
- Use qualified interpreters whenever possible.
- Use same-age, same-sex and same-ethnic group interpreters if possible.
- The client must approve of the interpreter.
- Speak directly to the client and not to the interpreter.
- Request general information before proceeding to sensitive areas.
- To assist the interpreter, be prepared and able to rephrase statements.
- Try to ensure that the interpreter is simply translating and not providing opinions or insights.
- Allow adequate time for interpretation and feedback.

Cultural Encounters

Cross-cultural nursing will commonly involve encounters with the service user's family. Because of the close bond between the individual and the family characteristic of many ethnic minority groups, a working relationship with the family is essential. Family members can provide invaluable information on issues such as personal history, health-related beliefs, communication styles, alternative remedies and dietary patterns. The family's co-operation and support are a vital aid to nursing interventions (Shives 2002).

In general, cultural competence implies an acceptance of human difference as normal and a respect for the diverse client's right to be different (Burford 2001). In cross-cultural mental health nursing care, the golden rule is: 'Never assume, ask'. The lesson is not to operate on the basis of prejudice or stereotypes but to respect the client's own definition of his own reality. Cultural competence is achieved when care is congruent with the individual service-user's own concerns (Nailon 2004). Campinha-Bacote (2003) offers a useful mnemonic device for clinical practice: 'Have I ASKED myself the right questions?'

- Awareness — Am I aware of my personal biases and prejudices towards other cultural groups?
- Skill — Do I have the skills necessary to communicate with, develop rapport with, and draw up a care plan of, a client of a diverse background?
- Knowledge — Do I know the world view and health-related attitudes and practices of a diverse client I am caring for?
- Encounters — Have I had sufficient direct personal experience of clients/people from diverse backgrounds?
- Desire — Have I a genuine desire to be culturally competent?

CONCLUSION

Though models of cultural competence are of educational and clinical utility, the need to further develop the concept of cultural competence is apparent. Aspects of anti-racism, cultural safety and the managing diversity approach could be incorporated into a more comprehensive and powerful model of diversity competence. Cultural safety offers some guidance with its emphasis on the patient as partner and on the role of the nurse in either reinforcing or challenging disadvantage. Seeing the client as a partner in the care process demands that power relationships are challenged and real choices are offered to the client by means of advocacy and empowerment. In the managing diversity approach, the valuing of diverse clients' differences paves the way towards a genuine nurse–client partnership, thus making appropriate and effective mental health more possible. While the scope for eliminating ethnic health disparities, which are determined to a large extent by socio-economic disadvantage and racism, lies largely outside the mental health service, the diversity-competent mental health nurse has, nevertheless, a valuable role to play in the provision of equitable nursing care to the diverse client.

Reflective Questions

1. A colleague remarks that there are too many immigrants in the country and that the immigrants already here should follow the maxim: 'When in Rome, do as the Romans do'. What do you think?
2. What cultural/ethnic biases might you bring into your nursing practice?
3. Can you describe a situation in which you might have provided better nursing care to a service user from an ethnic minority background?
4. How could you go about becoming familiar with the ethnic minority groups most common in your area?

Useful Websites

Websites that provide information on culture, health and associated issues:
www.jiscmail.ac.uk
www.mdx.ac.uk/www/retsh
www.kingsfund.org.uk/Library/Links/cfm
www.ethnicityonline.net/resources.htm
www.omhrc.gov
www.diversityrx.org
www.georgetown.edu/research/gucdc/nccc/
www.web.nmsu.edu/~ebosman/trannurs/index.shtml

References

Ahmad, W. I. U. (1996) 'The trouble with culture', in D. Kelleher and S. Hillier (eds), *Researching Cultural Differences in Health*. London: Routledge.

Alegria, M., Perez, D. J. and Williams, S. (2003) 'The role of public policies in reducing mental health status disparities for people of color'. *Health Affairs*, 22 (5), 51–9.

American Psychiatric Association (APA) (2000) *Diagnostic and Statistical Manual of Mental Disorders* (DSM-IV-TR) (4th edn). Washington DC: APA.

Anderson, J., Perry, J., Blue, C., Browne, A., Henderson, A., Khan, K. B., Kirkham, S. R., Lynam, J., Semeniuk, P. and Smye, V. (2003) '"Rewriting" cultural safety within the postcolonial and postnational feminist project: towards epistemologies of healing'. *Advances in Nursing Science*, 26 (3), 196–214.

Arnold, E. and Underman Boggs, K. (2003) *Interpersonal Relationships: Professional Communication Skills for Nurses* (4th edn). St Louis: Saunders.

Baxter, C. (2001) 'Diversity and inequality in health and health care', in C. Baxter (ed.), *Managing Diversity and Inequality in Health Care*. Edinburgh: Balliere Tindall.

Bhui, K., Stansfeld, S., Hull, S., Priebe, S. (2003) 'Ethnic variations in pathways to and use of specialist mental health services in the UK'. *British Journal of Psychiatry*, 182, 105–16.

Burford, B. (2001) 'The cultural competence model', in C. Baxter (ed.), *Managing Diversity and Inequality in Health Care*. Edinburgh: Balliere Tindall.

Burr, J. and Chapman, T. (1998) 'Some reflections on cultural and social considerations in mental health nursing'. *Journal of Psychiatric and Mental Health Nursing*, vol. 5(6), 431–7.

Byrne, P. (2006) *The Experiences of Migrant Ethnic Minority Users of Irish Mental Health Services: An Exploratory Study* (unpublished master's dissertation), University of Dublin, Trinity College.

Campinha-Bacote, J. (1999) 'A model and instrument for addressing culturally competent care'. *Journal of Nursing Education Thorofare*, 38 (5), 203–7.

Campinha-Bacote, J. (2003) 'Many faces: addressing diversity in health care'. Online *Journal of Issues in Nursing*, 8 (1), 1–8.

Central Statistics Office (CSO) *Census* (2006), www.cso.ie/census/ (accessed 3 April 2007).

Cortis, J. D. (2003) 'Culture, values and racism: application to nursing'. *International Nursing Review*, 50, 55–64.

Cortis, J. D. and Price, K. M. (2000) 'The way forward for transcultural nursing'. *Nurse Education Today*, 20, 233–43.

Craig, A. B. (1999) 'Mental health nursing and cultural diversity'. *Australian and New Zealand Journal of Mental Health Nursing*, 8, 93–9.

Culley, L. (2001) 'Nursing, culture and competence' in L. Culley and S. Dyson (eds), *Ethnicity and Nursing Practice*. Basingstroke: Palgrave.

Culley, L. and Dyson, S. (2001) 'Introduction: sociology, ethnicity and nursing practice' in L. Culley and S. Dyson (eds), *Ethnicity and Nursing Practice*. Palgrave: Basingstoke.

Cusack, R. (2005) 'A qualitative study of staff nurses' experiences in caring for patients from ethnic minority groups in psychiatric nursing'. *Psychiatric Nursing*, 3 (1), 22–7.

Department of Health and Children (DoHC) (2001) *Quality and Fairness: A Health System for You*. Dublin: DoHC.

Department of Justice, Equity and Law Reform (2005), www.orac.ie/pages/Stats/statistics.htm, accessed 7 May 2006.

Employment Equality Acts 1998 and 2004, www.irishstatutebook.ie/, accessed 18 April 2007.

Equal Status Acts 2000 to 2004, www.irishstatutebook.ie/, accessed 18 April 2007.

Frisch, N. C. and Frisch, L. E. (2006) *Psychiatric Mental Health Nursing* (3rd edn). New York: Delmar/Thompson Learning.

Gray, J. (2005) 'A blueprint for equality'. *Nursing Standard*, 19 (19), 3.

Huggins, M. (2003) 'Culture'. in: Mohr, W. K. (ed.) *Johnson's Psychiatric-Mental Health Nursing* (5th edn). Philadelphia: Lippincott.

Iley, K. and Nazroo, J. (2001) 'Ethnic inequalities in mental health' in L. Culley and S. Dyson (eds), *Ethnicity and Nursing Practice*. Basingstoke: Palgrave.

LaVeist, T. A. (2002) *Race, Ethnicity and Health*. San Francisco: Jossey Bass.

Leninger, M. (1995) *Transcultural Nursing: Concepts, Theories and Practices* (2nd edn). New York: Wiley and Sons.

Luther King, Martin, Jr (1966) (online), www.en.wikiquote.org/wiki/ Martin_Luther_King.jr, accessed 3 April 2007.

Mulholland, J. and Dyson, S. (2001) 'Sociological theories of "race" and "ethnicity"' in L. Culley and S. Dyson (eds), *Ethnicity and Nursing Practice*. Basingstoke: Palgrave.

Nailon, R. (2004) 'Expertise in the care of Latinos: an interpretive study of culturally congruent nursing practices in the emergency department'. *Journal of Emergency Nursing*, 30(5), 403–7.

Narayanasamy, A. (1999a) 'Transcultural mental health nursing 1: benefits and limitations'. *British Journal of Nursing*, 8 (10), 664–9.

Narayanasamy, A. (1999b) 'Transcultural mental health nursing 2: race, ethnicity and culture'. *British Journal of Nursing*, 8 (11), 741–5.

Nazroo, J. Y. (1998) 'Genetic, cultural or socio-economic vulnerability? Explaining ethnic inequalities in health' in M. Bartley, D. Blane and G. Davey Smith (eds), *The Sociology of Health Inequalities*. Oxford: Blackwell Publishers.

Nursing Council of New Zealand (1996) *Guidelines for Cultural Safety in Nursing and Midwifery Education*. Wellington: Nursing Council of New Zealand.

O'Brien, A. J. and Morrison-Ngatai, E. (2003) 'Providing culturally safe care' in P. Barker (ed.) *Psychiatric and Mental Health Nursing: The Art of Caring*. London: Arnold.

O'Connor, J. (2006) *A Vision for Change: Report of The Expert Group on Mental Health Policy*. Dublin: Stationery Office.

Papadopolous, I. (2001) 'Antiracism, multi-culturalism and the third way' in C. Baxter (ed.) *Managing Diversity and Inequality in Health Care*. Edinburgh: Balliere.

Parish, C. (2000) 'Celebrating diversity'. *Nursing Standard*, 15 (1), 15–16.

Richardson, S. (2004) 'Aoteaoroa/New Zealand nursing: from eugenics to cultural safety'. *Nursing Inquiry*, 11 (1), 35–42.

Rosenjack-Burchum, J. L. (2002) 'Cultural competence: an evolutionary perspective'. *Nursing Forum*, 37 (4), 5–15.

Shives, L. R. (2002) *Basic Concepts of Psychiatric-Mental Health Nursing* (6th edn). Philadelphia: Lippincott, Williams and Wilkins.

Tribe, R. and Morrissey, J. (2004) 'Good practice issues in working with interpreters in mental health', *Intervention*, 2, 2, 129–42.

World Health Organisation (WHO) (1981) *Global Strategy for Health for All by the Year 2000*. Geneva: WHO.

World Health Organisation (WHO) (1992) *The ICD-10 Classification of Mental and Behavioural Disorders. Clinical Descriptions and Diagnostic Guidelines*. Geneva: WHO.

27
Psychiatric Consultation Liaison Nursing
Mark Tyrrell

Psychiatric consultation liaison nursing (PCLN) is a sub-speciality of psychiatric nursing that has been developing over the past twenty to thirty years, mainly in the United States of America, the United Kingdom and, latterly, in Australia and New Zealand. In the closing years of the last millennium, PCLN also began to emerge as a sub-speciality of psychiatric nursing in Ireland, with developments particularly in the areas of suicide prevention, the emergency department and to a lesser extent in the areas of peri-natal mental health and substance misuse. PCLNs are clinical specialists who provide consultations to general hospital nurses and physicians on mental health matters, education about the care of general patients experiencing mental health problems, and specialist psychological care to patients and their families. They also liaise with other disciplines regarding the management of these patients (Nelson and Schilke 1976).

The aim of this chapter is to outline the context in which PCLN has evolved and to trace its development internationally up to and including recent developments in Ireland. The fundamental principles underpinning PCLN practice and a discussion of the areas of practice within which PCLN has been particularly well established will be presented.

HISTORICAL BACKGROUND

Psychiatric consultation liaison nursing originated from a number of forces that occurred in the latter half of the twentieth century. These were: the overall emergence of psychiatric nursing as a professional discipline, principally as a result of the work of Peplau; the establishment of departments of psychiatry in university hospitals; the emergence of crisis intervention techniques and brief therapies after the Second World War; and the community mental health movement and other socio-political trends in the 1950s (Robinson 1982).

The first references to liaison psychiatric nursing in the literature are those of the American nursing theorists Barbara Johnson in 1963 and Hildegarde Peplau in 1964 (Roberts 1997). Johnson described a specialist team of nurses that included a psychiatric nurse, who provided a liaison and consultation service to general hospital nurses to assist them in the management of patients with a dual diagnosis, or who were exhibiting some form of psychological distress. Over the next decade, psychiatric liaison nursing in the USA became established, with a firm educational base and a defined scope of practice and practitioners who expanded their range of operation into a number of diverse areas, especially in the area of emergency nursing (Sharrock 2006; Roberts 1997).

Some examples of PCLN areas of practice in the USA are:

- cardiac patients — Pranulis (1972)
- burns patients — Davidson and Noyes (1973)
- addictions — Leiker (1989)
- nursing home care — Smith *et al.* (1990)
- HIV/AIDS — Chisolm (1991)
- emergency department — McIndoe *et al.* (1994)
- general medical patients — Shahinpour *et al.* (1995)
- family therapy — Ragaisis (1996)
- obstetrics and gynaecology — D'Afflitti (2005).

In the UK, liaison psychiatric nursing has developed somewhat differently. Early references by Tunmore (1989) and Jones (1990) described the emergence of the role in oncology settings and the general hospital setting respectively, while Roberts (1997) has mapped the emergence of the psychiatric nurse consultant role in the accident and emergency (A&E) department in the UK. In the 1990s, UK government targets to reduce suicide (Department of Health (UK) 1992, 1994) heralded further development of liaison psychiatric nursing services focusing on the assessment of deliberate self-harm and suicide risk (Callaghan *et al.* 2003).

More recently, PCLN emerged in Ireland, initially as a specialist nursing service to assist in the reduction of suicide and self-harm, but it has begun to expand to include other areas of practice such as substance abuse, children and adolescents, and peri-natal mental health. In 2005, the National Strategy for Action on Suicide Prevention identified a need to establish a 'liaison psychiatric nursing service in all accident and emergency departments for responding to those who present following DSH [deliberate self harm] or who are acutely suicidal' (HSE and DoHC 2005:33). Current mental health policy in Ireland recommends that there should be 'a minimum of one liaison mental health team ... per 500 bed general hospital to provide a day time service', and an additional four teams nationally, one each for the regional hospitals (DoHC 2006:155). Currently, however, there are fewer than a dozen liaison mental health teams in the country, the majority of which are centred in the greater Dublin area, with some services available in other main cities such as Cork, Limerick and Waterford. A major limitation of these services, though, is that the majority are only available on a nine to five basis on weekdays. This is problematic, as staff (particularly those in emergency departments (EDs)) express concern that there is no service available when they most need it. The majority of liaison mental health services that are available in Ireland are delivered by a multidisciplinary team, typically comprising:

- one consultant liaison psychiatrist
- one doctor in training

- two clinical psychologists
- five clinical nurse specialists to include two specialist nurse behaviour therapists or psychotherapists
- two secretaries/administrators.

Other staff might include:
- one neuropsychologist
- one mental health social worker
- one occupational therapist with vocational rehabilitation skills
- one substance misuse counsellor
- one family therapist.

(Adapted from DoHC 2006)

The most common model of service delivery by these liaison teams is that of consultation and liaison, and most teams are led by a liaison psychiatrist. While literature is sparse on PCLN in the Irish context, there are some descriptions of PCLN models and evaluations of service provision such as that at Tullamore (Johnson and McDonald-Steenkist 2004), and the recently announced service at Mullingar (*Westmeath Examiner* 2006).

It is strongly recommended in the literature that PCLN is considered an area of advanced nursing practice and hence that practitioners are prepared to master's degree level. In addition, best practice advocates that practitioners should have an extensive knowledge and skills base in mental health and should be preceptored by an experienced PCLN during initial educational preparation for the role and for some time thereafter (Sharrock and Happell 2000). From the outset, consultation liaison nursing in the USA was established as an area of advanced nursing practice. Although advanced practitioners in the 1960s were not prepared to master's degree level, they did receive additional preparation, either by mentored clinical experience or by additional education (Robinson 1982). By the mid-1970s, however, master's degree programmes were established to prepare psychiatric liaison nurses (Robinson 1987).

In the UK, the role has developed differently and, in contrast to the USA, liaison psychiatric nursing is not as clearly defined and established at advanced practice level, although this is recognised as an ideal (Roberts 1997). As a result, the educational preparation for the role is less clear cut. Some argue that liaison mental health nursing is but an extended application of generic mental health nursing skills (Tunmore and Thomas 1992).

In Ireland the PCLN role has been developed at clinical nurse specialist (CNS) level (National Council 2001). According to the National Council (2002:1), a clinical nurse specialist is 'a specialist in clinical practice who has undertaken formal recognised post-registration education relevant to his/her area of specialist practice at higher diploma level'. This formal education must also be underpinned by extensive experience and clinical expertise in the area of specialist practice.

The core elements of the CNS role are:
- clinical focus
- patient advocate
- education and training
- audit and research
- consultant.

(Source: National Council 2002)

LIAISON AND CONSULTATION

Liaison is defined as 'communication and cooperative contact between groups' (*Collins Dictionary* 1998:546). In the PCLN context, liaison focuses on the collaboration between the PCLN and non-mental healthcare professionals, the aim of which is to assist the latter group in identifying actual or potential patient mental health problems, to instigate suitable interventions and to minimise the effects of the mental health problem for the client and for the staff involved in his or her care. This involves regular and sustained contact between the PCLN and the non-mental health staff. Much of the work is done through educational programmes provided by the PCLN and through formal meetings and informal discussions. Regular contact is also more likely to influence the culture of care on the unit, making it a more 'mentally aware and healthy unit for both patients and staff' (Sharrock and Happell 2000:24).

Consultation refers to the *act* of consultation, which involves the 'giving of advice on professional matters' (*Collins Dictionary* 1998:189). Caplan (1970) describes consultation as the process whereby a person, who is regarded as an authority or expert on a subject area (the consultant), assists another professional (the consultee) in solving some difficulty they are encountering in practice. The consultee initiates the request and the consultant, by virtue of their expertise, assists either directly or indirectly in solving the professional problem the consultee has encountered. In addition to being an expert in a given field of practice, however, the consultant must also possess expertise in helping others solve problems, the emphasis being on facilitating problem-solving rather than directly solving the problem for the consultee (Tunmore and Thomas 1992). Four types of consultation are outlined in Caplan's model, two case-centred and two organisation-centred:

1. *Client-centred case consultation* focuses on an individual client or patient. The consultee seeks the expert opinion of the consultant as to how to address a particular client problem. The consultant assesses the client and situation and makes recommendations to the consultee with the secondary aim of improving the consultee's skills in managing similar situations in the future. For example, a general ward nurse seeks the advice of the psychiatric liaison nurse on how to deal with the distress of a young woman who is recovering from an intentional but unsuccessful drug overdose.

2. *Consultee-centred case consultation.* The focus is on the *nature* of the difficulty the consultee is having with the client rather than the actual clinical problem

with which the client presents. Typically, the difficulty is due to deficiencies in the consultee's knowledge, skills or confidence in dealing with the situation, or occasionally to the consultee's inability to remain objective in the situation. The consultant focuses therefore on assisting the consultee to resolve these difficulties in order to enhance the quality of client care. For example, a ward nurse finds that they are getting emotionally involved and hence unable to remain objective in nursing a client who is a victim of abuse. The PCLN helps the nurse understand the dynamics at play. In this instance, the PCLN may not need to meet with the client or patient as the problem is located with the consultee.

3. *Programme-centred administrative consultation.* In this instance, the consultee is an organisation rather than an individual: a general hospital administrator requests the expertise of the consultant in setting up a patient care management programme. For example, a hospital administrator consults the PCLN on the establishment of a programme of mental health triage in the emergency department, the focus being on the processes involved. The PCLN may or may not remain involved with the programme after it has been established.

4. *Consultee-centred administrative consultation.* This is similar to number two above, except the consultee is the organisation and the focus of the consultant is on the nature of the difficulty the organisation is having in running or managing a particular programme. For example, the mental health triage programme is not working effectively because of lack of support from one of the clinical nurse managers (CNMs). This CNM rarely allocates a suitably qualified nurse to mental health triage. The focus of the consultation process would therefore be on the reasons behind this CNM's decisions. The aim would be to 'facilitate a change in the manager's knowledge, skill, confidence or professional objectivity that, in turn, increases the support given to and effectiveness of the programme' (Sharrock and Happell 2000:22).

THE ROLE OF THE PCLN

The role of the PCLN varies from country to country principally due to the different ways in which the service has developed internationally. Nelson and Schilke's (1976) typology captures the main focus of the PCLN role as it is practised in most countries:

- Expertise in mental illness and people's reactions to physical ill health, including an in-depth understanding of the relationship between physical illness and psychological states.
- Staff and client education.
- Interdisciplinary collaboration.
- Delivery of direct nursing care to clients and families.
- Advising and consulting with nursing staff on mental health care planning and assisting them in developing skills for practice.

(Adapted from Nelson and Schilke 1976)

A more contemporary view of the role in the UK is provided by Roberts (2002), who outlines four dimensions to the role:

1. *Consultation.* This concerns the working relationship between a consultant (in this case, a PCLN) and a consultee (e.g. a general nurse). While the consultant is not necessarily in a position of authority regarding the consultee, their authority is vested in their specialist knowledge, hence it is more a relationship between peers.
2. *Education.* The provision of education to non-mental health professionals on issues such as dealing with anxiety, depression, substance misuse and self harm.
3. *Research.* The identification of areas for research within PCLN practice, in particular engaging in collaborative interdisciplinary research.
4. *Supervision and Support.* In the context of PCLN practice, this is more a process of professional development than a process of management or appraisal. It is similar to the supervision processes used in psychotherapy.

AREAS OF PCLN PRACTICE

There is a growing body of literature internationally depicting a wide variety of areas in which consultation-liaison psychiatric nursing is practised (see above). Two of these areas (obstetrics and gynaecology, and the emergency department) will now be examined.

Obstetrics and Gynaecology

D'Afflitti (2005) presents a PCLN model within an obstetrics and gynaecology department in the United States that was established to support staff in the recognition and treatment of mental health problems in women. In this model, the PCLN has an office located in the obstetrics and gynaecology department and spends five hours per week receiving referrals from clinical nursing and medical staff from the obstetrics/gynaecology unit. The main reason for situating the PCLN's office within the department was to avoid the possible stigma for patients coming to a psychiatric department and also to enable staff to become familiar with the PCLN's work and thus accept her as part of the team. D'Afflitti describes her role as both an expert resource and educator to clinical staff and also a direct provider of mental health nursing care to patients.

Common reasons for referral to this liaison service include post-natal depression, pregnancy loss, infertility, puerperal psychosis, unwanted pregnancy, adoption, abortion, reproductive system cancer, sexually transmitted diseases and sexual dysfunction. There is also a strong emphasis on prevention. For example, the PCLN screens all post-partum women for post-natal depression and offers a pre-birth visit to women who have a history of depression or other mental illness. She also reviews psychotropic medication regimens for women who plan to breast feed and runs group counselling sessions for couples with primary infertility.

Emergency Department

The emergency department (ED) has been the setting for many PCLN services in the USA (Roberts 1997), Australia (Wand and Fisher 2006), the UK (Callaghan *et al.* 2001) and Ireland (Johnson and McDonald-Steenkist 2004). The main reason for their development in the ED was the recognition that many people with mental health problems were accessing mental health services through the ED, primarily because the large psychiatric hospitals were being closed and because the ED provided a 24-hour service. While many of these ED-based services have a broad focus addressing such diverse issues as aggression and violence, drug overdose, self harm, depression and psychotic illnesses, increasingly PCLN services situated in the ED have a focus on deliberate self-harm and suicide prevention (Barr *et al.* 2005). This focus on suicide prevention in both the UK and Ireland has come about as a result of government initiatives to reduce the incidence of deliberate self-harm (DSH) and completed suicide (HSE and DoHC 2005; DoH 1998).

Callaghan *et al.* (2001) outline a liaison mental health service provided by a multi-disciplinary team of nurses, social workers and psychiatrists in an East London ED. While a majority of referrals (66 per cent) come from within the ED, other referrals come from police, GPs and community mental health nurses, and there are also self referrals from people experiencing mental health difficulties.

Reasons for referral to this service include: self-harm; depression; alcohol and/or drug dependency; schizophrenia; anxiety; and overdose. Other activities undertaken by the liaison team include teaching, patient escorts, research, and liaison with other disciplines and community groups. Examples of this liaison include advice, information and support on how to manage certain clinical situations, and advice on aspects of the Mental Health Act.

NURSING INTERVENTIONS AND SKILLS FOR PRACTICE

The work of the PCLN has been described in the literature as being both *direct* and *indirect* (Roberts 2002; Sharrock and Happell 2001). Direct work relates to the actual hands-on delivery of care by the PCLN; indirect work is where the PCLN assists staff in the management of patient care. While the processes of direct and indirect care are interwoven, some studies suggest that the provision of indirect care is more common. Sharrock and Happell (2001), for example, reported that direct contact with clients occurred in fewer than one third of referrals in their study. Indirect consultation such as giving advice to nursing, medical and allied health staff on patient care issues formed the greater part of the PCLN's work. Clearly, therefore, in addition to having advanced knowledge and skills in the area of mental health, the PCLN must also have the capacity to assist others in solving problems.

Two examples from PCLN practice are looked at below: one focusing on DSH; the other dealing with psycho-oncology.

Example 1: Deliberate Self-Harm in the Emergency Department

Ryrie *et al.* (1997), in their study of the role of two liaison psychiatric nurses working in a central London ED, identify *brief counselling interventions* and *psycho-social assessment* as key interventions of particular merit in this area of practice. While the reasons for referral to this service varied widely and included people with alcohol/substance misuse, depression, disturbed/ aggressive behaviour and psychosis, the deliberate self-harm categories of overdose, cutting, stabbing, drowning and gassing accounted for the majority of presentations.

Brief Counselling Interventions

Brief problem-orientated therapies such as those based on a crisis intervention model are useful interventions in the management of those who present to the ED with deliberate self-harm in that they are 'flexible and adaptable to individual circumstances' (Whitehead and Royles 2002:116). These therapies commonly include: an exploration of the meaning and consequences of the self-harm; the instillation of hope and self-esteem; the facilitation and support of emotional expression; the modification of inflexible thinking; the promotion of new and adaptive coping strategies aimed at preventing further self-harm; and the formulation of a suicide prevention plan (Whitehead and Royles 2002).

Psycho-social Assessment

A 1994 UK consensus statement from the UK Health Advisory Service and the Royal College of Psychiatrists advocated that 'all patients attending hospital accident and emergency departments with a self-harm diagnosis should be offered adequate psycho-social assessment ... by members of staff with mental health training' (Barr *et al.* 2005:131). This involves an assessment with a specific focus on the person's mental state, their interpersonal relationships and their social situation at the time of presentation, the aim of which is to identify those at risk of completed suicide and those who are at risk of committing further acts of self-harm in the future.

Example 2: Psycho-oncology

Roberts (2002:132) defines psycho-oncology as 'the branch of psychiatry and mental health services dealing with cancer patients', pointing out that its focus is on both the psychosocial consequences of contracting cancer, and on the role that psychosocial factors play in the aetiology of cancer. Roberts (2002) cites Fawzy *et al.'s* (1995) categories of PCLN intervention in cancer care as including behavioural training, individual psychotherapy, group interventions and patient education. These are now briefly described:

Behavioural Training

This includes a number of strategies, such as guided imagery, hypnosis, biofeedback, meditation and systematic relaxation techniques, the aim of which is to assist the client to change their response to illness or the side effects of their cancer chemotherapy.

Individual Psychotherapy

This is a form of CBT called adjuvant psychological therapy, which is designed for cancer patients and focuses on the meaning of the experience of having cancer for the individual, and the harnessing of coping strategies to assist the client in dealing with their psychosocial distress.

Group Interventions

A group therapy approach that draws on support from other group members who themselves have or have had cancer. The aim is symptom reduction (anxiety, depression) and enhanced coping.

Education

The focus here is on empowering the individual by demystifying their illness and involving them in the management of their treatment. This is seen as affording the client a greater sense of control through the provision of accurate and timely information about all aspects of their illness.

In addition to the skills cited in the above clinical examples, the PCLN also draws on a wide repertoire of other skills such as routine mental health assessment, problem-solving skills, troubleshooting, advice on medication management and the skills associated with verbal de-escalation of pre-violent crises.

BENEFITS OF PCLN SERVICE

The majority of PCLN evaluation studies reported in the literature focus on outcomes relating to the patient and family (e.g. a reduction in distress, better adherence to treatment regimens, improved patient safety and better caregiver interaction); the staff (increased job satisfaction for the PCLN and other involved staff, increased mental health knowledge and skills, better nurse–patient interaction); and the institution (reduced length of stay, prevention of patient complications, fewer readmissions, and increased patient referral to a more appropriate service) (Yakimo *et al.* 2004). Some specific benefits are stakeholder satisfaction, cost-effectiveness and change in clinical status.

Stakeholder Satisfaction

Callaghan *et al.* (2003) conducted a systematic review of research (n=17 studies) on the structure, process and outcome of liaison mental health services and found that on the whole, both patient and staff respondents in these studies had a positive experience of the service. The main areas of satisfaction for staff that were identified included:

- the quality of the assessments and care provided
- ease of referral and promptness of the service
- speed of response from the PCLN once the referral was made
- availability and objectivity of the service
- the support they received from the PCLN.

Studies on physicians' views suggest that they are particularly satisfied with the advice they receive from the PCLN on patient management and the fact that follow-up visits are conducted. Interestingly, senior physicians were more likely to value the service than were junior physicians.

Studies on service users show that they value the information they received from the PCLN about their treatment and the quality of the care they received, expressing extreme satisfaction overall with the service. An evaluation of the service at Tullamore suggests that all key stakeholders 'place a high value on the efficient, effective and timely service provided by the PCLNs' (Johnson and McDonald-Steenkist 2004:13). This evaluation involved an audit of the patients referred to the service, an analysis of the perspectives of the staff referring patients to the service and semi-structured interviews with the two PCLNs running the service. The main benefits of the PCLN service that were identified included: faster assessment time; improvement in patient follow-up; and the perception that the PCLNs were professional, approachable, experienced and empathetic. In addition, benefits to the profession of nursing were also identified: in particular, the establishment of the post of PCLN at clinical nurse specialist level was seen as a significant advancement in autonomy and status for psychiatric nursing.

Cost Effectiveness
Lyons et al. (1989) studied general medical patients over a four-month period. Thirty patients received PCLN contact and sixty did not. They found that those receiving psychiatric consultation required significantly less nursing time than those who did not; the greater the amount of psychiatric consultation, the greater the decrease in nursing time required. In an earlier study of over 400 patients receiving PCLN services, Lyons et al. (1986) reported that patients who were referred early to the PCLN service had a significantly shorter length of stay in hospital, a clear result of which was again a decrease in healthcare cost. Other studies have attempted to quantify the actual cost savings of the PCLN service. Ragaisis (1996), for example, reported that over an eight-month period, a PCLN using a family therapy approach with ten families saved one hospital in excess of $65,000.

Change in Clinical Status
Morgan and Coleman (2000) evaluated the implementation of a nurse liaison service for people who presented with deliberate self harm (DSH) to an emergency department (ED) in the UK. Data were collected from the records of 142 individuals prior to implementation of the DSH liaison nursing service and from 198 after its implementation. There was a statistically significant reduction in re-presentations to the ED following the introduction of the nurse-led DSH service, including for those who had a known psychiatric diagnosis. For example, prior to the introduction of the service, all individuals with a known diagnosis of schizophrenia re presented to the ED with DSH over the following twelve months. After the implementation of the service, however, only two of the six people with schizophrenia re-presented to the ED.

CONCLUSION

The medical discipline of consultation liaison psychiatry has been established for over a century now, but psychiatric consultation liaison nursing is a relatively recent innovation, and here in Ireland it is still in the early stages of its development. The main impetus for the development of the role came from the recognition that many general hospital in-patients had concurrent psychiatric illness and that many general nurses and physicians lacked the knowledge and skills to deal with these patients' specific mental health needs. While the core elements of the role are similar in the various countries where PCLN practice is established, some differences exist, particularly in regard to: the degree of autonomy that PCLNs have; the educational preparation for the role; the level at which the role is established; and the relationships with other disciplines, especially with medicine.

While the majority of evaluations of PCLN practice have been favourable, most have been narrow in scope and some are methodologically weak. Hence, as Ireland progresses to establish PCLN practice further, it is imperative that rigorous audits of the service are conducted and that these address issues of structure, process and outcome from the perspective of all of the key stakeholders, not least the service users.

Reflective Questions

1. Reflecting on the types of intervention used by PCLNs in practice, what particular challenges might non-mental health professionals encounter in caring for individuals in a general hospital setting, who present with concurrent physical and psychiatric problems?
2. Reflect back on a general hospital placement you have undertaken in the past and some of the patients you met there. What particular contribution might a PCLN have made to the well-being of these patients if one were available?
3. How do you think the skills of a psychiatric liaison nurse might be best utilised when caring for patients who present to the emergency department with suicidal behaviour?
4. If you were in hospital recovering from disfiguring surgery and began to feel depressed about your situation, what professional help do you feel you would need and who do you feel would be best placed to give you this help?

References

Barr, W., Leitner, M. and Thomas, J. (2005) 'Psychosocial assessment of patients who attend an accident and emergency department with self-harm'. *Journal of Psychiatric and Mental Health Nursing*, 12,130–8.

Callaghan, P., Eales, S., Coates, T. and Bowers, L. (2003) 'A review of research on the structure, process and outcome of liaison mental health services'. *Journal of Psychiatric and Mental Health Nursing*, 10, 155–65.

Callaghan, P., Eales, S., Leigh, L., Smith, A. and Nichols, J. (2001) 'Characteristics of an accident and emergency liaison mental health service in East London'. *Journal of Advanced Nursing*, 35 (6), 812–18.

Caplan, G. (1970) *The Theory and Practice of Mental Health Liaison*. London: Tavistock.

Chisolm, M. (1991) 'The consultation-liaison nurse and the challenge of AIDS: caring for nurses'. *Clinical Nurse Specialist*, 5,123–9.

Collins Dictionary (1998) (*Collins Concise Dictionary and Thesaurus*). London: Harper Collins.

D'Afflitti, J. (2005) 'A psychiatric clinical nurse specialist as liaison to OB/GYN practice'. *JOGNN*, 34 (2), 280–5.

Davidson, S. and Noyes, R. (1973) 'Psychiatric nursing consultation in a burn unit'. *American Journal of Nursing*, 73, 1715–18.

Department of Health (DoH) (1998) *The Report of the National Taskforce on Suicide*. Dublin: Government Publications.

Department of Health and Children (DoHC) (2006) *A Vision for Change: Report of the Expert Group on Mental Health Policy*. Dublin: Government Publications.

Department of Health (UK) (1992) *The Health of the Nation: A Strategy for Health in England*. London: HMSO.

Department of Health (UK) (1994) *Working in Partnership: Report of the Mental Health Nursing Review Team*. London: HMSO.

Fawzy, F. I., Fawzy, N. W., Arndt, L. A. and Pasnau, R. O. (1995) 'Critical review of psychosocial interventions in cancer care'. *Archives of General Psychiatry*. 52, 100–13.

Health Service Executive (HSE) and Department of Health and Children (DoHC) (2005) *Reach Out – National Strategy for Action on Suicide Prevention 2005–2014*. Dublin: HSE.

Johnson, L. and McDonald-Steenkist, J. (2004) *Psychiatric Consultation Liaison Nursing: Midlands Regional Hospital at Tullamore* (unpublished one-year service evaluation (2001–2002)). Midland Health Board.

Jones, A. (1990) 'The nurse as therapist'. *Nursing*, 4, 40–2.

Leiker, T. (1989) 'The role of the addictions nurse specialist in a general hospital setting'. *Nursing Clinics of North America*, 24, 137–49.

Lyons, J., Hammer, J., Strain, J. and Fulop, G. (1986) 'The timing of psychiatric consultation in the general hospital and length of hospital stay'. *General Hospital Psychiatry*, 8, 159–62.

Lyons, J., Scherubel, J., Anderson, R. and Swartz, J. (1989) 'Isolating the impact of psychiatric consultation in the general hospital: psychiatric co-morbidities and nursing intensity'. *International Journal of Psychiatry in Medicine*, 19, 173–80.

McIndoe, K., Harwood, G. and Olmstead, C. (1994) 'Psychiatric crisis in emergency'. *Canadian Nurse*. May, 26–9.

Morgan, V. and Coleman, M. (2000) 'An evaluation of the implementation of a liaison service in an A&E department'. *Journal of Psychiatric and Mental Health Nursing*, 7, 391–7.

National Council for the Professional Development of Nursing and Midwifery (2001), *Clinical Nurse/Midwife Specialists – Intermediate Pathway*. Dublin: National Council.

National Council for the Professional Development of Nursing and Midwifery (2002), *Submission to the Expert Group on Mental Health Policy*. Dublin: National Council.

Nelson, J. and Schilke, D. (1976) 'The evolution of psychiatric liaison nursing'. *Perspectives in Psychiatric Care*, 14, 60–5.

Pranulis, M. (1972) 'A factor affecting the welfare of the coronary patient'. *Nursing Clinics of North America*, 7, 445–55.

Ragaisis, K. (1996) 'The psychiatric consultation-liaison nurse and medical family therapy'. *Clinical Nurse Specialist*, 10 (1), 50–6.

Roberts, D. (1997) 'Liaison mental health nursing: origins, definition and prospects'. *Journal of Advanced Nursing*, 25, 101–8.

Roberts, D. (2002) 'Working models for practice' in S. Regel and D. Roberts (eds), *Mental Health Liaison: A Handbook for Nurses and Health Professionals*. Edinburgh: Balliere Tindall.

Robinson, L. (1982) 'Psychiatric liaison nursing in 1962–1982: a review and update of the literature'. *General Hospital Psychiatry*, 4, 139–45.

Robinson, L. (1987) 'Psychiatric consultation liaison nursing and psychiatric consultation liaison doctoring: similarities and differences'. *Archives of Psychiatric Nursing*, 1, (2), 73–80.

Ryrie, I., Roberts, M. and Taylor, R. (1997) 'Liaison psychiatric nursing in an inner city accident and emergency department'. *Journal of Psychiatric and Mental Health Nursing*, 4, 131–6.

Shahinpour, N., Hollinger-Smith, L. and Peira, M. (1995) 'The medical-psychiatric consultation liaison nurse: Meeting psychosocial needs of medical patients in the acute setting'. *Nursing Clinics of North America*, 30, 77–86.

Sharrock, J. (2006) 'Perspectives on psychiatric consultation-liaison nursing'. *Perspectives in Psychiatric Care*, 42, (2), 137–9.

Sharrock, J. and Happell, B. (2000) 'The psychiatric consultation-liaison nurse: towards articulating a model for practice'. *Australian and New Zealand Journal of Mental Health Nursing*, 9, 19–28.

Sharrock, J. and Happell, B. (2001) 'An overview of the role and functions of a psychiatric consultation-liaison nurse: an Australian perspective'. *Journal of Psychiatric and Mental Health Nursing*, 8, 411–417.

Smith, M., Buckwalter, K. and Albanese, M. (1990) 'Psychiatric nursing consultation: a different choice for nursing homes'. *Journal of Psychosocial Nursing*, 28, 23–8.

Tunmore, R. (1989) 'Liaison psychiatric nursing in oncology'. *Nursing Times*, 85, 54.

Tunmore, R. and Thomas, B. (1992) 'Models of psychiatric consultation liaison nursing'. *British Journal of Nursing*, 1, 447–51.

Wand, T. and Fisher, J. (2006) 'The mental health nurse practitioner in the emergency department: an Australian experience'. *International Journal of Mental Health Nursing*, 15, 201–8.

Westmeath Examiner (2006) 'HSE's new psychiatric service will be of benefit to Mullingar patients', *Westmeath Examiner*, 11 November 2006.

Whitehead, L. and Royles, M. (2002) 'Deliberate self-harm: assessment and treatment interventions' in S. Regel and D. Roberts (eds), *Mental Health Liaison: A Handbook for Nurses and Health Professionals*. Edinburgh: Balliere Tindall.

Yakimo, R., Kurlowicz, L and Murray, R. (2004) 'Evaluation of outcomes in psychiatric consultation-liaison nursing practice'. *Archives of Psychiatric Nursing*, 16, (6), 215–27.

Index

ulcers, 335
UN Convention on Human Rights, 362
unconditional acceptance, 130–1
unconditional love, 130
unconscious mind, 124–5
urban environment, and schizophrenia,
    194
urinalysis, 336
utilitarianism, 51–2

vagueness, 249
validation therapy, 280
Valium, 165, 218
value systems, 48–51
Van Meijel, B. *et al.*, 149–51
vascular dementia, 273 *see also* dementia
Venlafaxine, 163
verbal abuse, 309
violence and abuse, 255, 363–4
    effects on mental health, 194, 224, 227,
        240, 260, 363–4
violence and aggression, 307–18
    definitions of, 308
    dementia and, 273, 280
    extent of, 308, 313
    managing, 249, 315–17
    nurse training, 310
    'occupational hazard', 308, 313
    passive-aggressive behaviour, 249
    prosecution and zero tolerance, 312–13
    psychosis and schizophrenia, 201, 310
    risk assessment, 311–12
    young people, 260–2
*Vision for a Recovery Model in Irish
    Mental Health Services*, 352
Vision for Change, 81, 93, 96, 204, 254,
    322, 352, 375, 386
visual analogue scale, 214, 217
voice hearing, 139–40, 195, 198
    antipsychotic drugs, 159
    BAVQ questionnaire, 69
    strategies of working, 143–7, 200, 203

volition, 201
voluntary admission, 36–7
    children, 44
vulnerability, stress vulnerability model,
    25, 140, 143, 145, 194–5, 323

Walsh, E. *et al.*, 310
Watson clock drawing test, 278
Watzlawick, P. *et al.*, 109
well-being, 78, 80
Wells, J., 50
Westbrook, D. *et al.*, 214–15, 216
White, M., 119
Whitehead, D., 84
Whitehead, L. and Royles, M., 407
Whittington, R., 312
Winstanley, J., 378, 382
Wolford, G. *et al.*, 326
working conditions, historical, 10–11
World Health Organisation (WHO), 7
    health definition, 77–8
    health promotion definition, 80
    mental health definition, 16, 79
world view, 392–3
Wortman, C., 114
Wright, H. and Giddey, M., 96

Xanax, 165, 218

Yusupoff, L. and Tarrier, N., 147

Zaleplon, 165
Zauszniewsky, J., 84
Zimovane, 165
Zispin, 163
Zoleptil, 158
Zolpidem, 165
Zopiclone, 165
Zotepine, 158
Zubin, J. and Spring, B., 140
Zuclopenthixol, 158, 159
Zyprexa, 158